P9-EDX-952

NURSE'S LEGAL HANDBOOK

Third Edition

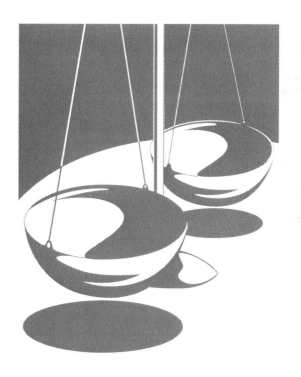

Springhouse Corporation
Springhouse, Pennsylvania

Staff

Executive Director
Matthew Cahill

Art Director
John Hubbard

Senior Editor
Michael Shaw

Clinical Manager
Judith Schilling McCann, RN, MSN

Clinical Editor
Cynthia Burlew, RN, MS, MBA

Editors
Marcia Andrews, Kathy Goldberg, Howard Kaplan

Copy Editors
Cynthia C. Breuninger (manager), Priscilla DeWitt, Christina P. Ponczek, Doris Weinstock

Designers
Stephanie Peters (associate art director), Elaine Ezrow, Anita Curry, Jacalyn Bove Facciolo, Susan Hopkins, Jeff Sklarow

Typography
Diane Paluba (manager), Joyce Rossi Biletz, Phyllis Marron, Valerie L. Rosenberger

Manufacturing
Deborah Meiris (director), Pat Dorshaw (manager), Andreas Hess, T.A. Landis

Production Coordination
Margaret A. Rastiello

Editorial Assistants
Beverly Lane, Mary Madden

The guidelines described and recommended in this publication are based on research and consultation with legal and nursing authorities. To the best of our knowledge, these guidelines reflect currently accepted practice; nevertheless, they can't be considered absolute and universal recommendations, nor can they be considered legal advice. For individual application, all recommendations must be considered in light of the unique circumstances of each legal or administrative situation. The authors and publisher disclaim responsibility for any adverse consequences from directly or indirectly following the suggested guidelines without first seeking legal advice, for any undetected errors, or for the reader's misunderstanding of the text.

© 1996 by Springhouse Corporation. All rights reserved. No part of this publication may be used or reproduced in any manner whatsoever without written permission except for brief quotations embodied in critical articles and reviews. For information, write Springhouse Corporation, 1111 Bethlehem Pike, P.O. Box 908, Springhouse, PA 19477-0908. Authorization to photocopy items for internal or personal use, or the internal or personal use of specific clients, is granted by Springhouse Corporation for users registered with the Copyright Clearance Center (CCC) Transactional Reporting Service, provided that the fee of $.75 per page is paid directly to CCC, 222 Rosewood Dr., Danvers, MA 01923. For those organizations that have been granted a license by CCC, a separate system of payment has been arranged. The fee code for users of the Transactional Reporting Service is 0874348498/96 $00.00 + $.75.
Printed in the United States of America.
NLH3-010396

Ⓡ A member of the Reed Elsevier plc group

Library of Congress Cataloging-in-Publication Data

Nurse's legal handbook, 3rd ed.
    p.   cm.
    Includes bibliographical references and indexes.
    1. Nursing ethics – Handbooks, manuals, etc.
[1. Ethics, Nursing – United States.   2. Legislation, Nursing – United States.]
    I. Springhouse Corporation.
ISBN 0-87434-849-8   96-67570

Contents

Contributors

Joseph T. Catalano, RN, CCRN, PhD, is a professor of nursing at East Central University in Ada, Oklahoma. He's a member of the American Nurses' Association, the Oklahoma Nurses Association, and the American Critical Care Nurses Association.

Ann Cotlar, RN, BSN, JD, is the director of risk management at St. Mary's Medical Center in Langhorne, Pennsylvania. She's a member of the Pennsylvania Bar Association, the American Society of Hospital Risk Managers, and the Pennsylvania Society of Healthcare Attorneys.

Janine Fiesta, BSN, JD, is vice president of legal services and risk management for Lehigh Valley Hospital in Pennsylvania. She's a member of the American Association of Nurse Attorneys; the American Society of Hospital Attorneys; the Hospital Attorneys of Southeastern Pennsylvania; the Lehigh Valley Risk Management Society; the American, Pennsylvania, and Lehigh County Bar Associations; the Professional Advisory Committee, Lehigh Valley Hospice; and the Risk Management Advisory Council of Voluntary Hospitals of America.

Irene Fleshner, RN, MHSA, is vice president of clinical program development at Genesis Health Ventures, Inc., in Kennett Square, Pennsylvania. She's a diplomate of the American College of Healthcare Executives and a member of Sigma Theta Tau.

Robert Fleshner, JD, is president of Incenter Strategies, a business development consulting firm that specializes in health care, located in Washington, D.C. He's a member of the District of Columbia Bar Association.

Ann Helm, RN, MS, JD, is an Associate Professor at the Oregon Health Sciences University in Portland. She's a member of the Oregon Women Lawyers, the Oregon Peace Institute, and the AON Direct Group Advisory Board.

Barbara E. Hirsch, RN, JD, is a senior associate with Freeman & Jenner, P.C., in Bethesda, Maryland. She's a member of the Association of Trial Lawyers of America, the Capitol-Area Network of Nurse Attorneys, and Sigma Theta Tau.

Carol Holmes, RN, BSN, JD, is a partner in the firm of Small, Toth, Baldridge & Van Belkum, P.C., in Bingham Farms, Michigan. She's an appointed mediator or arbitrator on medical malpractice and personal injury cases.

Linda Bangs Richey, RN, JD, is risk manager at St. Mary's Medical Center in Langhorne, Pennsylvania. She's a member of the American and Pennsylvania Bar Associations and the American and Philadelphia Area Societies for Health Care Risk Management.

Linda Rosen, RN, MA, JD, is an attorney with M. Mark Mendel Ltd. of Philadelphia. She's a member of the Nurses Association of the American College of Obstetrics and Gynecology; the American Association of Nurse Attorneys; the Pennsylvania and Philadelphia Bar Associations; and the American, Pennsylvania, and Philadelphia Trial Lawyers Associations.

Susan A. Salladay, RN, PhD, is director of the Center for Excellence in Bioethics at Bryan Memorial Hospital, Lincoln, Nebraska. She's a member of the Society for Health and Human Values and Sigma Theta Tau.

Linda Agustin Simunek, RN, ARNP, PhD, JD, is founding dean and professor at the School of Nursing of Florida International University. She's also a member of the Florida Board of Nursing and is a legal nurse consultant and associate attorney with the law firm of Rosen, Rosen & Kreiling, P.A., with offices in Hollywood, Fort Lauderdale, and Weston, Florida

Carole Taylor, RN, MSN, CSFN, is an assistant professor at Holy Family College in Philadelphia. She's a member of the American Nurses' Association and the National League for Nursing and is an associate member of the Kennedy Institute of Ethics. She's also a member of the Society for Law, Medicine, and Ethics and the Society for Health and Human Values and is a candidate for a PhD in philosophy from Georgetown University in Washington, D.C..

Phyllis B. Taylor, RN, ET, BA, is a nurse-educator and counselor at the Hospice of the Delaware Valley in Plymouth Meeting, Pennsylvania. She's a member of the Association of Nurses in AIDS Care, the Hospice Nurses Association, and Sigma Theta Tau.

Virgie M. Vakil, RN, BA, JD, is a partner in the firm of Kelly, Grimes, Pietrangelo & Vakil, P.C., in Media, Pennsylvania. She's a member of the American Inns of Court, the Pennsylvania Bar Association, the Delaware County Bar Association, and the board of the Delaware County Home Care Association.

Linda A. Webb, RN, BA, JD, is a partner in the law firm of Hagans, Ahearn & Webb in Anchorage, Alaska. She's a member of the American Association of Nurse Attorneys, the Health Lawyers Association, and the Alaska, Anchorage, and American Bar Associations.

Jerelyn Peixoto Weiss, RN, MA, FNP, JD, is director of advanced practice nursing at Memorial Sloan Kettering Cancer Center in New York City. She's a member of the American Nurses' Association, the New York Coalition of Nurse Practitioners, the American Bar Association, the American Association of Nurse Attorneys, and the American Society of Law, Medicine and Ethics.

Foreword

As the 21st century approaches, cost-cutting currents continue to stir waves of profound change in the American health care system. Managed care organizations, which operate by delivering health care services for a fixed fee, are now the most powerful force in health care delivery. The hospital environment is undergoing radical change. Patients are hospitalized only for the most acute phase of their illness and then are transferred to a less intensive level of care, including outpatient clinics and the patient's home.

Health care restructuring is having a tremendous effect on how nurses care for patients—and consequently causing profound changes in the legal and ethical dimensions of nursing practice. Providing high-quality care in a time of shrinking health care budgets and rapid industry-wide shifts poses enormous ethical and legal challenges. In fact, nurses' need for current, accurate information on nursing law and ethics has never been more pressing.

• Nurses must make do with less as declining operating budgets force hospitals to reduce nursing staffs. At the same time, nurses often are responsible for managing larger patient loads than before.

• Third-party payers have clamped down on long hospital stays, forcing nurses to provide more care for patients over a shorter duration.

• Nurses working in managed care arrangements are often being asked to manage their patients throughout the continuum of care, not merely through one episode of illness.

• Many health care facilities are replacing some RNs with lower-paid, unlicensed assistive personnel—and holding the remaining nurses responsible for the care provided by the unlicensed personnel. Without vigilant oversight, the use of such personnel could reduce the quality of patient care and lead to poor patient outcomes—posing a threat to a nurse's license and heightening nurses' legal liability.

These challenges further complicate the legal entanglements and moral dilemmas that already are an intrinsic part of contemporary nursing practice. The courts continue to expand the definition of liability, holding nurses to higher and higher standards. Even if you're meticulous in your practice and avoid unnecessary legal risks, there's no guarantee that you won't be named in a malpractice lawsuit.

What's more, patients are aggressive in asserting their rights and do not hesitate to pursue litigation if they feel their rights have been violated. Legal disputes about current health care practices have forced nurses to be especially conscientious when using restraints, witnessing informed consents, giving medications, obtaining personal information, providing discharge instructions, and performing other daily tasks.

In addition, delicate issues surrounding a patient's right to die continue to generate confusion and fear for nurses. Modern technology has created a moral and legal gray area between letting a patient die and killing him—a gray area where nurses are often caught.

Nurses also need ethical and legal guidance to meet their responsibility as advocates for the poor and uninsured, AIDS patients, children, abuse victims, and other disadvantaged patients, as well as to cope with the moral dilemmas created by medical research advances.

With little time to fully explore the legal and ethical implications of their actions, nurses must often make crucial choices during high-pressure patient care situations and then must act quickly. Thus, it's more important than ever for nurses to practice with an eye toward avoiding malpractice liability.

To be of use, information on law and ethics must be concise and readily accessible. Fortunately, you can now turn to a single source of practical information on legal risks and ethical dilemmas in nursing — the third edition of *Nurse's Legal Handbook*.

This handbook contains a wealth of up-to-date information presented in a straightforward, practical format. Becoming familiar with it will help you to recognize legal obligations and ethical choices, avoid potential conflicts, and choose an appropriate course of action. Numerous case studies, which describe how nurses act in real-life situations, provide vivid examples of your legal and ethical responsibilities. In addition, important legal and ethical terms are defined in the book's glossary. Throughout the text, glossary terms are highlighted in ***boldface italicized*** type.

The handbook is organized into 11 succinct and comprehensive chapters. The first 7 chapters focus on nursing and the law.

Chapter 1 provides fundamental information on the laws that directly govern nursing. It details state and provincial nurse practice acts and the role of the state board of nursing. It describes standards of care and how these standards may be used as evidence during malpractice litigation. This chapter also explains the legal significance of your nursing license and what to expect if you are disciplined for violating its provisions.

Chapter 2 discusses your legal obligation to uphold your patient's rights. It outlines your responsibilities in ensuring informed consent, protecting your patient's right to refuse treatment, and upholding his right to privacy. This chapter includes summaries of major U.S. Supreme Court rulings on the right to die and reproductive rights issues.

Chapter 3 describes the legal responsibilities and risks that nurses face on the job. You'll find information on the legal consequences of violating your hospital's policies and "legally safe" steps to take to help you cope with understaffing. You'll read about your responsibilities for maintaining patient safety, administering drugs, and upholding a patient's living will. You'll learn what to do when you encounter victims of child abuse, are forced to use restraints on a psychologically disturbed patient, or are asked by police to turn over a patient's belongings or blood samples for evidence.

Chapter 4 discusses your legal risks when providing off-duty nursing services. It includes a state-by-state chart describing Good Samaritan acts — the laws that protect you when you provide emergency care at an accident scene or in a disaster.

Chapter 5 presents straightforward facts about the greatest legal worry of the nursing profession — malpractice liability. It will help you understand malpractice law and recognize and avoid malpractice pitfalls. It includes advice on how to shop for professional liability insurance and how to identify patients who are likely to sue. If you're named in a lawsuit, this chapter provides guidelines on what steps to take to defend yourself.

Chapter 6 discusses your legal obligations regarding documentation. It includes guidelines for upholding standards and avoiding errors.

Chapter 7 will help you assert your employee rights. It focuses on two crucial issues: how to read and understand an employment contract and the pros and cons of joining a union.

In the next three chapters, the book's focus shifts from law to ethics. Chapter 8 outlines, in clear language, the principles of ethics that guide nursing practice. Chapter 9 covers six major areas of ethical conflict in clinical practice — the right to die, organ transplantation, critically ill neonates, AIDS, abortion and reproductive technology, and genetic engineering and screening.

Chapter 10 discusses three ethical obligations of professional practice: upholding your patient's rights, including the right to autonomy, the right to confidentiality, and the right to refuse treatment; blowing the whistle on misconduct by colleagues; and responding to the problem of widespread substance abuse among nurses.

Chapter 11 describes the rapid changes occurring in the health care marketplace and investigates their implications for the nursing profession. It compares types of managed care organizations, discusses how nursing practice is evolving, describes nurses' expanded roles in today's health care industry, and tells you how to cope with a radically different working environment.

But the *Handbook* doesn't stop there. Following Chapter 11, you'll find helpful appendices, the glossary, and an index of court case citations.

Both in format and content, the *Nurse's Legal Handbook,* Third Edition, is a clearly written, authoritative reference on nursing law and ethics. You'll find it will quickly become an indispensable aid that helps you to practice at your best while minimizing your legal risk and enhancing your ability to confront ethical dilemmas.

Linda Agustin Simunek, RN, ARNP, PhD, JD
Founding Dean and Professor
School of Nursing, Florida International University
Member, Florida Board of Nursing
Legal Nurse Consultant and Associate Attorney
Rosen, Rosen & Kreiling, P.A.
Hollywood, Fort Lauderdale, and Weston, Fla.

Nursing practice and the law

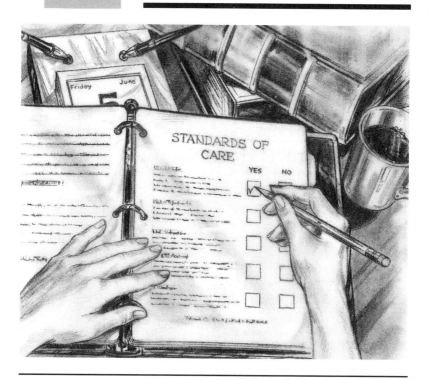

Like other professionals, nurses today want opportunities for personal advancement, increased economic benefits, and a sense that their profession will keep pace with the latest technologic advances. To realize these goals, each nurse must understand and accept the legal responsibilities of her practice. In doing so, she also can sidestep legal and professional pitfalls, such as malpractice. After all, ignorance of the law isn't a valid defense in any legal proceeding. The courts expect every nurse to know and obey the laws that directly and indirectly affect her practice.

This chapter will help you gain this necessary knowledge by providing fundamental information on the laws that directly govern nursing. It includes a detailed discussion of the nurse practice act—the state law that regulates nursing. You'll find coverage of how nursing law is applied in court and about the role of your state board of nursing. You'll learn about *standards of care* and how these standards may be used as evidence during *malpractice litigation.*

This chapter also explains the legal significance of your nursing license and what to expect if you are disciplined for violating its provisions. Finally, you'll find legal considerations for various nursing roles, such as a private-duty nurse and a *nurse practitioner.* Throughout the chapter, you'll find practical advice that reflects legal precedents or expected standards of care (see *Landmarks of nursing law*).

Levels of nursing practice

There are three levels of nursing practice—the *registered nurse* (RN), the *licensed practical* or *vocational nurse* (LPN or LVN), and a more specialized form of practice called the *advanced practice nurse*.

RNs complete a longer and more intensive educational program for entry into practice than LPNs and LVNs. Once licensed, the RN is responsible for developing and managing patient care. She also must make professional nursing judgments based on the nursing process—including patient assessment, planning, nursing diagnosis, implementation, and evaluation.

In 1987, the *American Nurses' Association* (ANA) published a statement on an RN's scope of clinical practice. According to the ANA, the *professional RN* is a graduate of a baccalaureate or higher degree program, and the *technical RN* is a graduate of an associate's degree program. The function of the professional RN is to develop *policies,* procedures, and *protocols* and to set standards for practice; the technical RN implements the policies, procedures, and protocols developed by the professional RN.

In state law, definitions of the RN's role vary, but basic responsibilities include observing patients' signs and symptoms, recording them, carrying out doctors' orders for patient treatments, and appropriately delegating patient care.

The LPN or LVN often is referred to as the "bedside nurse" because her role has traditionally centered on the patient's basic physical needs for hygiene and comfort. Many state *nurse practice acts* define LPN and LVN practice as the performance of duties that assist the professional nurse in a team relationship. In some states, the duties of LPNs and LVNs are more clearly defined in terms of *scope of practice*; for example, states may prohibit LPNs and LVNs from inserting I.V. lines.

Because of the current emphasis on cutting labor costs, the role of the LPN and LVN has expanded during the past decade. In the past 10 years, more than 30 states have authorized expanded roles for LPNs and LVNs. The Pennsylvania State Board of Nursing ruled, for example, that LPNs can "perform venipuncture and administer and withdraw I.V. fluids" and "administer immunizing agents and do skin testing."

Expansion of the LPN and LVN role is controversial. When Ohio and New York attempted to expand the role of the LPN, the professional nurses' association in each state sued to block such action. The associations argued that changes were taking place without public hearings and that proper *rule*-making procedures hadn't been followed.

Nursing practice in Canada

Canada permits *licensure* of registered nurses, *registered nursing assistants,* and—in some provinces—practical or vocational nurses. Some Canadian nursing associations recognize *clinical nurse specialists* (who usually have master's or doctoral degrees in specific specialties).

Landmarks of nursing law

Laws to establish minimum standards for entry into the nursing profession were introduced in the early 1900s. In the first part of the century, the standards and regulations that guided nursing practice were minimal at best. Beginning with World War II, rapid technological advances dramatically changed health care and nursing:

• To keep pace with advances in medical technology, nursing became more sophisticated and skill-oriented.

• Nurses took on greater responsibility for patient care and, consequently, became more accountable under the law.

• As health care became less personalized, patients became more inclined to use litigation as a means of retribution for harm resulting from treatments.

In today's litigious environment, every nurse needs to be aware of the professional goals and standards that define nursing practice. Like all other health care professionals, nurses cannot afford to be ignorant of their responsibility under the law.

The time line below lists some important dates in the evolution of nursing law.

1901: First state nurses' associations organize to work toward state laws to control nursing practice.

1903: North Carolina passes the first nurse registration act; New York, New Jersey, and Virginia soon follow. These acts were *permissive,* meaning that anyone could practice nursing but only those registered could use the initials "RN." By 1923, every state had some type of nurse registration law.

1938: New York passes the first mandatory nurse practice act. This law established two levels of nursing: licensed registered nurse and licensed practical nurse. It mandated that only professionals licensed under the act could practice nursing.

1952: By this time, all states, the District of Columbia, and all territories have enacted nurse practice acts.

1953: American Nurses' Association (ANA) adopts a statement on principles of legislation relating to nursing practice.

1955: ANA approves a definition of the practice of nursing to serve as a guide for nurses and for licensing legislation.

1970: ANA amends its definition of practice to eliminate the prohibition on nursing diagnosis.

1973: ANA publishes standards of nursing practice.

1977: By this time, 24 states have enacted new or additional amendments to their nurse practice acts, generally eliminating the prohibition on nursing diagnosis.

1979: ANA further amends its definition of practice to reflect nursing's broadening scope.

1988: By this time, all the states (except Arkansas, Georgia, Ohio, Oklahoma, Tennessee, West Virginia, and the District of Columbia) have revised their nurse practice acts to legalize expanded nursing practice. This revision allows nurses to perform nurse practitioner tasks.

1991: The Joint Commission on Accreditation of Healthcare Organizations (a voluntary organization that sets standards for the operation of health care institutions) establishes new standards for nursing care.

In most of Canada's 10 provinces, professional nurses' associations set requirements for graduation from an approved school of nursing, for licensing, for nurses' professional behavior, and for registration fees.

The Canadian registered nurse may receive her education in a diploma school (such as a hospital school of nursing), in a community college, or in a bachelor's degree program. The licensing examination she must take varies by province — some use the *National Council of Licensure Examination* (NCLEX) and some compile their own (thus complicating U.S.-Canadian nurse licensure reciprocity). Requirements for becoming a registered nursing assistant usually consist of a 10-month program and, in some provinces, a licensure examination.

Nurse practice acts

Each state has a nurse practice act, designed to protect the public by broadly defining the legal scope of nursing practice. Your state's nurse practice act is the most important law affecting your nursing practice. Every nurse is expected to care for patients within defined practice limits; if she gives care beyond those limits, she becomes vulnerable to charges of violating her state nurse practice act. Nurse practice acts also serve to exclude untrained or unlicensed people from practicing nursing. For a copy of your state's nurse practice act, contact your state nurses' association or the state board of nursing (see *State and provincial nurses' associations,* pages 5 to 9, and *State boards of nursing,* pages 10 to 12).

Contents of the nurse practice act

Most nurse practice acts begin by defining important terms, including "the practice of registered nursing" and "the practice of licensed practical and vocational nursing." These definitions differentiate between RNs and LPNs and LVNs according to their specific scopes of practice and their educational requirements. Some states have separate nurse practice acts for registered and practical or vocational nurses.

Scope of practice

Early nurse practice acts contained statements prohibiting nurses from performing tasks considered to be within the scope of medical practice. Nurses could not diagnose any patient problem or treat a patient without instructions from a doctor. More recently, interdisciplinary committees (consisting of nurses, doctors, pharmacists, dentists, and hospital representatives) have helped to ease this restriction on nursing practice. After reviewing some medical procedures that nurses commonly perform, these committees issued *joint statements* recommending that nurses be legally permitted to perform these procedures in specified circumstances. Some joint statements specifically recommend that nurses be allowed to perform venipunctures, cardiopulmonary resuscitation, and cardiac defibrillation. Still other joint statements (as well as interpretive statements issued by state boards of nursing and nursing organizations) specifically recommend that nurses be permitted to perform such functions as nursing assessment and nursing diagnosis. Such joint statements do not have the force of the law — unless state legislatures amend their nurse practice acts to include them. Many state legislatures have incorporated such state-

(Text continues on page 9.)

State and provincial nurses' associations

This chart lists the name, address, and telephone number of nurses' associations in the United States, its territories, and Canada.

Alabama State Nurses' Association
360 N. Hull St.
Montgomery, AL 36104-3658
(205) 262-8321

Alaska Nurses Association
237 E. Third Ave., Suite 3
Anchorage, AK 99501
(907) 274-0827

Arizona Nurses Association
1850 E. Southern Ave., Suite 1
Tempe, AZ 85282-5832
(602) 831-0404

Arkansas Nurses' Association
117 S. Cedar St.
Little Rock, AR 72205
(501) 664-5853

California Nurses Association
1145 Market St., Suite 1100
San Francisco, CA 94103
(415) 864-4141

Colorado Nurses' Association
5453 E. Evans Place
Denver, CO 80222
(303) 757-7483 Ext. 3

Connecticut Nurses' Association
Meritech Business Park
377 Research Parkway, Suite 2D
Meriden, CT 06450
(203) 238-1207

Delaware Nurses' Association
2634 Capitol Trail, Suite A
Newark, DE 19711
(302) 368-2333

Dist. of Columbia Nurses' Association
5100 Wisconsin Ave., N.W., Suite 306
Washington, DC 20016
(202) 244-2705

Florida Nurses Association
P.O. Box 536985
Orlando, FL 32853-6985
(407) 896-3261

Georgia Nurses Association
1362 W. Peachtree St., N.W.
Atlanta, GA 30309
(404) 876-4624

Guam Nurses' Association
P.O. Box 3134
Agana, Guam 96910
011 (671) 649-4930

Hawaii Nurses' Association
677 Ala Moana Blvd., #301
Honolulu, HI 96813
(808) 531-1628

Idaho Nurses Association
200 N. Fourth St., Suite 20
Boise, ID 83702-6001
(208) 345-0500

Illinois Nurses Association
200 S. Wacker, Suite 2200
Chicago, IL 60606
(312) 360-2300

Indiana State Nurses' Association
2915 N. High School Road
Indianapolis, IN 46224-2969
(317) 299-4575

(continued)

State and provincial nurses' associations continued

Iowa Nurses' Association
1501 42nd St., Suite 471
West Des Moines, IA 50266
(515) 225-0495

Kansas State Nurses Association
700 S.W. Jackson, Suite 601
Topeka, KS 66603-3731
(913) 233-8638

Kentucky Nurses Association
1400 South First St.
Louisville, KY 40201
(502) 637-2546

Louisiana State Nurses Association
712 Transcontinental Dr.
Metairie, LA 70001
(504) 889-1030

Maine State Nurses' Association
283 Water St.
P.O. Box 2240
Augusta, ME 04338-2240
(207) 622-1057

Maryland Nurses Association
849 International Dr.
Airport Square 21, Suite 255
Linthicum, MD 21090
(410) 859-3000

Massachusetts Nurses Association
340 Turnpike St.
Canton, MA 02021
(617) 821-4625

Michigan Nurses Association
2310 Jolly Oak Rd.
Okemos, MI 48864
(517) 349-5640

Minnesota Nurses Association
1295 Bandanna Blvd. N., Suite 140
St. Paul, MN 55108
(612) 646-4807

Mississippi Nurses' Association
135 Bounds St., Suite 100
Jackson, MS 39206
(601) 982-9182

Missouri Nurses Association
206 E. Dunklin St.
Jefferson City, MO 65102-0325
(314) 636-4623

Montana Nurses' Association
104 Broadway, Suite G-2
Helena, MT 59601
(406) 442-6710

Nebraska Nurses' Association
941 "O" St., Suite 707-711
Lincoln, NE 68508
(402) 475-3859

Nevada Nurses' Association
3660 Baker Lane, Suite 104
Reno, NV 89509
(702) 825-3555

New Hampshire Nurses' Association
48 West St.
Concord, NH 03301
(603) 225-3783

New Jersey State Nurses Association
320 W. State St.
Trenton, NJ 08618
(609) 392-4884

State and provincial nurses' associations continued

New Mexico Nurses Association
909 Virginia N.E., Suite 101
Albuquerque, NM 87108
(505) 268-7744

New York State Nurses Association
46 Cornell Rd.
Latham, NY 12110
(518) 782-9400

North Carolina Nurses Association
103 Enterprise St.
Raleigh, NC 27605-2025
(919) 821-4250

North Dakota Nurses' Association
212 N. Fourth St.
Bismarck, ND 58501
(701) 223-1385

Ohio Nurses Association
4000 E. Main St.
Columbus, OH 43213-2950
(614) 237-5414

Oklahoma Nurses Association
6414 N. Santa Fe, Suite A
Oklahoma City, OK 73116
(405) 840-3476

Oregon Nurses Association
9600 S.W. Oak, Suite 550
Portland, OR 97223
(503) 293-0011

Pennsylvania Nurses Association
2578 Interstate Dr.
Harrisburg, PA 17110
(717) 657-1222

Rhode Island State Nurses' Association
300 Ray Dr., Suite 5
Providence, RI 02906
(401) 421-9703

South Carolina Nurses' Association
1821 Gadsden St.
Columbia, SC 29201
(803) 252-4781

South Dakota Nurses' Association
1505 S. Minnesota, Suite 3
Sioux Falls, SD 57105
(605) 338-1401

Tennessee Nurses' Association
545 Mainstream Dr., Suite 405
Nashville, TN 37228-1207
(615) 254-0350

Texas Nurses Association
7600 Burnet Rd., Suite 440
Austin, TX 78757
(512) 452-0645

Utah Nurses' Association
455 East 400 South, Suite 402
Salt Lake City, UT 84111
(801) 322-3439

Vermont State Nurses' Association
Box 36 Champlain Mill, 1 Main St.
Winooski, VT 05404
(802) 655-7123

Virgin Islands Nurses' Association
P.O. Box 583
Christiansted, St. Croix 00821
(809) 773-2323 Ext. 119

(continued)

State and provincial nurses' associations continued

Virginia Nurses' Association
7113 Three Chopt Rd., Suite 204
Richmond, VA 23226
(804) 282-1808

Washington State Nurses Association
2505 Second Ave., Suite 500
Seattle, WA 98121
(206) 443-9762

West Virginia Nurses Association
P.O. Box 1946
Charleston, WV 25327
(304) 342-1169

Wisconsin Nurses Association
6117 Monona Dr.
Madison, WI 53716
(608) 221-0383

Wyoming Nurses Association
Majestic Building, Room 305
1603 Capitol Ave.
Cheyenne, WY 82001
(307) 635-3955

Canadian provincial and territorial nurses' associations

Registered Nurses Association of British Columbia
2855 Arbutus St.
Vancouver, British Columbia V6J 3Y8
(604) 736-7331

Alberta Association of Registered Nurses
11620 168 St.
Edmonton, Alberta T5M 4A6
(403) 426-0160

Saskatchewan Registered Nurses' Association
2066 Retallack St.
Regina, Saskatchewan S4T 2K2
(306) 527-4643

Manitoba Association of Registered Nurses
647 Broadway Ave.
Winnipeg, Manitoba R3C 0X2
(204) 774-3477

Registered Nurses' Association of Ontario
33 Price St.
Toronto, Ontario M4W 1Z2
(416) 923-3523

For information on registration and licensure in Ontario, contact:
College of Nurses of Ontario
101 Davenport Rd.
Toronto, Ontario M5R 3P1
(416) 486-4460

New Brunswick Association of Registered Nurses
231 Saunders St.
Fredericton, New Brunswick E3B 1N6
(506) 454-5591

Registered Nurses' Association of Nova Scotia
6035 Coburg Rd.
Halifax, Nova Scotia B3H 1Y8
(902) 423-6156

Association of Nurses of Prince Edward Island
P.O. Box 1838
Charlottetown, P.E.I. C1A 7N5
(902) 892-6322

State and provincial nurses' associations continued

Association of Registered Nurses of Newfoundland
55 Military Rd.
Box 6116
St. John's, Newfoundland A1C 5X8
(709) 753-6040

Northwest Territory Registered Nurses' Association
Box 2757
Yellowknife, Northwest Territory X0E 1H0
(403) 873-2745

Yukon Nurses Society
Box 5371
Whitehorse, Yukon Y1A 4Z2
(403) 667-4062

For information on registration and licensure in Quebec, contact:
L'Ordre des Infirmières et Infirmiers du Québec
4200 Dorchester Blvd. W.
Montréal, Québec H3Z 1V4
(514) 935-2501

---

ments into nurse practice acts. (See *Defining the boundaries of nursing practice,* page 13.)

Conditions for licensure

Your state's nurse practice act sets down the requirements for obtaining a license to practice nursing. To become licensed as an RN, LPN, or LVN, you must pass the NCLEX and meet certain other qualifications. All states require completion of a basic professional nursing education program. Your state may have additional requirements; examples include good moral character, good physical and mental health, a minimum age, fluency in English, and no drug or alcohol addiction.

In addition to specifying the conditions for RN and LPN or LVN licensure, your state's nurse practice act may specify the rules and regulations for licensure in special areas of nursing practice (usually termed *certification*).

State boards of nursing

In every state and Canadian province, the nurse practice act creates a state or provincial board of nursing. The nurse practice act authorizes this board to administer and enforce rules and regulations concerning the nursing profession and specifies the makeup of the board—the number of members as well as their educational and professional requirements. In some states, the nurse practice act requires two nursing boards—one for RNs and one for LPNs and LVNs.

The board of nursing is bound by the provisions of the nurse practice act that created it. The nurse practice act is the law; the board of nursing can't grant exemptions to it or waive any of its provisions. Only the state or provincial legislature can change the law. For example, if the nurse practice act specifies that, to be licensed, a nurse must have graduated from an approved school of nursing, then the board of nursing must deny a license to anyone who hasn't done so. This provision applies even to applicants who can provide evidence of equivalency and competence (*Richardson v. Brunelle,* 1979).

In many states and provinces, the board of nursing may grant exemptions and waivers to its own rules and regulations. For example, if a regulation states that all nursing faculty must have master's degrees, the board may

(Text continues on page 13.)

State boards of nursing

The list below includes boards of nursing for all 50 U.S. states and territories. For information on Canadian registered nurses jurisdictions (comparable to U.S. boards of nursing), contact the provincial nursing associations listed on pages 8 and 9.

Alabama
State Board of Nursing
RSA Plaza, Suite 250
770 Washington Ave.
Montgomery, AL 36130
(205) 242-4060

Alaska
Board of Nursing
Division of Occupational
Licensing
Dept. of Commerce and
Economic Development
3601 C Street, Suite 722
Anchorage, AK 99503
(907) 561-2878

Alaska Board of Nursing
P.O. Box 110806
Juneau, AK 99811-0800
(907) 465-2544

American Samoa
Health Service
Regulatory Board
LBJ Tropical Medical Center
Pago Pago, American Samoa
96799
(684) 633-1222 Ext. 206

Arizona
State Board of Nursing
1651 E. Morten Ave.
Suite 150
Phoenix, AZ 85020
(602) 255-5092

Arkansas
State Board of Nursing
University Tower Bldg.
Suite 800
1123 University Ave.
Little Rock, AR 72204
(501) 371-2751

California
Board of Registered Nursing
P.O. Box 944210
400 R Street, Suite 4030
Sacramento, CA 95814-6200
(916) 322-3350

Colorado
State Board of Nursing
1560 Broadway, Suite 670
Denver, CO 80202
(303) 894-2430

Connecticut
Board of Examiners for
Nursing
150 Washington St.
Hartford, CT 06106
(203) 566-1041

Delaware
Board of Nursing
Margaret O'Neill Bldg.
P.O. Box 1401
Dover, DE 19903
(302) 739-4522

District of Columbia
DC Board of Nursing
614 H St., N.W.
Washington, DC 20001
(202) 727-7468

Florida
Board of Nursing
111 Coastline Dr., East
Suite 516
Jacksonville, FL 32202
(904) 359-6331

Georgia
Board of Nursing
166 Pryor St., S.W.
Atlanta, GA 30303
(404) 656-3943 (RN)
(404) 656-3921 (PN)

Guam
Board of Nurse Examiners
P.O. Box 2816
Agana, Guam 96910
011-(671)-734-7295

Hawaii
Board of Nursing
P.O. Box 3469
Honolulu, HI 96801
(808) 586-2695

Idaho
Board of Nursing
P.O. Box 83720
Boise, ID 83720-0061
(208) 334-3110

Illinois
Department of Professional
Regulation
320 W. Washington St.
Springfield, IL 62786
(217) 785-0800

Indiana
State Board of Nursing
Health Professions Bureau
402 W. Washington St.
Room 041
Indianapolis, IN 46204
(317) 232-2960

State boards of nursing continued

Iowa
Board of Nursing
1223 E. Court Ave.
Des Moines, IA 50319
(515) 281-3255

Kansas
State Board of Nursing
Landon State Office Bldg.
900 S.W. Jackson
Suite 551
Topeka, KS 66612-1230
(913) 296-4929

Kentucky
Board of Nursing
312 Wittington Parkway
Suite 300
Louisville, KY 40222-5172
(502) 329-7000

Louisiana
State Board of Nursing
912 Pere Marquette Bldg.
150 Baronne St.
New Orleans, LA 70112
(504) 568-5464

Maine
State Board of Nursing
35 Anthony Ave.
State House Station 158
Augusta, ME 04333-0158
(207) 624-5275

Maryland
Board of Nursing
4140 Patterson Ave.
Baltimore, MD 21215-2299
(410) 764-5124

Massachusetts
Board of Registration in
Nursing
Leverett Saltonstall Bldg.
100 Cambridge St.
Room 1519
Boston, MA 02202
(617) 727-9962

Michigan
Bureau of Occupational
and Professional Regulation
Michigan Department of
Commerce
Ottawa Towers North
611 W. Ottawa
Lansing, MI 48933
(517) 373-1600

Minnesota
Board of Nursing
2700 University Ave. W.
#108
St. Paul, MN 55114
(612) 642-0567

Mississippi
Board of Nursing
239 N. Lamar St.
Suite 401
Jackson, MS 39201
(601) 359-6170

Missouri
Board of Nursing
3605 Missouri Blvd.
P.O. Box 656
Jefferson City, MO 65102
(314) 751-0681

Montana
State Board of Nursing
111 N. Jackson
P.O. Box 200513
Helena, MT 59620-0513
(406) 444-2071

Nebraska
State Board of Nursing
P.O. Box 950007
Lincoln, NE 68509
(402) 471-2115

Nevada
Board of Nursing
P.O. Box 46886
Las Vegas, NV 89114
(702) 739-1575

New Hampshire
Board of Nursing
Div. of Public Health Services
Health and Welfare Bldg.
6 Hazen Dr.
Concord, NH 03301-6527
(603) 271-2323

New Jersey
Board of Nursing
P.O. Box 45010
Newark, NJ 07101
(201) 504-6493

New Mexico
Board of Nursing
4206 Louisiana Blvd., N.E.
Suite A
Albuquerque, NM 87109
(505) 841-8340

New York
Board for Nursing
State Education Dept.
Cultural Education Center
Albany, NY 12230
(518) 474-3843

North Carolina
Board of Nursing
Box 2129
Raleigh, NC 27602
(919) 782-3211

North Dakota
Board of Nursing
919 S. 7th St., Suite 504
Bismarck, ND 58504-5881
(701) 328-2974

(continued)

State boards of nursing continued

Northern Mariana Islands
Commonwealth Board of
Nurse Examiners
Public Health Center
P.O. Box 1458
Saipan, MP 96950
011-670-234-8950 to 8954

Ohio
Board of Nursing
77 S. High St., 17th Floor
Columbus, OH 43266-0316
(614) 466-3947

Oklahoma
Board of Nurse Registration
and Nursing Education
2415 N. Classen Blvd.
Suite 524
Oklahoma City, OK 73106
(405) 525-2076

Oregon
State Board of Nursing
800 N.E. Oregon St., Box 25
Suite 465
Portland, OR 97232
(503) 731-4745

Pennsylvania
State Board of Nursing
Box 2649
Harrisburg, PA 17105-2649
(717) 783-7142

Puerto Rico
Commonwealth of Puerto Rico
Board of Nurse Examiners
Call Box 10200
Santurce, Puerto Rico 00908
(809) 725-8161 or 725-7904

Rhode Island
Board of Nurse Registration
and Nursing Education
Cannon Health Bldg. Three
Capitol Hill, Room 104
Providence, RI 02908
(401) 277-2827

South Carolina
Board of Nursing
220 Executive Center Dr.
Suite 220
Columbia, SC 29210
(803) 731-1648

South Dakota
Board of Nursing
3307 S. Lincoln Ave.
Sioux Falls, SD 57105-5224
(605) 367-5940

Tennessee
State Board of Nursing
283 Plus Park Blvd.
Nashville, TN 37217-1010
(615) 367-6232

Texas
Board of Nurse Examiners
9101 Burnet Rd.
Austin, TX 78758
(512) 835-4880

U.S. Virgin Islands
Virgin Islands Board of Nurse
Licensure
P.O. Box 4247
Veterans Drive Station
St. Thomas, U.S. Virgin
Islands 00803
(809) 776-7397

Utah
Division of Occupational and
Professional Licensing
Heber M. Wells Bldg.
P.O. Box 45805
Salt Lake City, UT 84145
(801) 530-6628

Vermont
Board of Nursing
109 State St.
Montpelier, VT 05609-1106
(802) 828-2396

Virginia
Board of Nursing
6606 W. Broad St.
4th Floor
Richmond, VA 23230-1717
(804) 662-9909

Washington
State Nursing Care Quality
Assurance Commission
Department of Health
P.O. Box 47864
Olympia, WA 98504-7864
(360) 753-2686

West Virginia
Board of Examiners
for Registered Professional
Nurses
101 Dee Drive
Charleston, WV 25311-1620
(304) 558-3596

State Board of Examiners
for Practical Nurses
101 Dee Drive
Charleston, WV 25311-1688
(304) 558-3572

Wisconsin
Department of Regulation and
Licensing
1400 E. Washington Ave.
P.O. Box 8935
Madison, WI 53708-8935
(608) 266-0257

Wyoming
Board of Nursing
Barrett Bldg., 2nd Floor
2301 Central Ave.
Cheyenne, WY 82002
(307) 777-7601

Defining the boundaries of nursing practice

You may characterize your state's nurse practice act as traditional, transitional, or modern, depending on how it defines the boundaries of nursing practice.

Traditional

These nurse practice acts allow only conventional nursing activities. They limit the nurse's responsibilities to traditional patient care, disease prevention, and health maintenance. Traditional nurse practice acts do not allow registered nurses (RNs) to participate in such expanded nursing activities as diagnosis, prescription, and treatment. Only a few states continue to have such limited nurse practice acts.

Transitional

These nurse practice acts have broader boundaries, and may include a "laundry list" of permitted nursing functions. For example, Maine's act lists six specific RN activities:
- traditional patient care
- collaboration with other health professionals in planning care
- diagnosis and prescription delegated by doctors

- delegation of tasks to licensed practical nurses, licensed vocational nurses, and nurses' aides
- supervision and teaching
- carrying out doctors' orders.

Because it allows expanded duties such as diagnosis and prescription, Maine is edging toward a modern type of nurse practice act.

Other states with transitional acts, such as Massachusetts, broaden the nurse's role by including a separate definition for nurse practitioners. This wording allows nurse practitioners to diagnose and treat patients.

Modern

States with modern nurse practice acts— New York, for example—allow RNs to diagnose and treat health problems as well as to provide traditional nursing care. New York's definition of registered nursing is so broad that it encompasses not only current nursing activities, but also much of what nurses are likely to do in the future.

waive this requirement temporarily for a faculty member who's in the process of obtaining one.

In most states, the board of nursing (sometimes called the state board of nurse examiners) consists of practicing RNs. Many boards also include LPNs or LVNs, hospital *administrators,* and *consumers*—usually financial or legal experts. The state legislature decides on the board's mix; in almost every state, the governor appoints members from a list of nominees submitted by the state nursing association. One state, North Carolina, replaced this appointment process with an elective one, allowing licensed nurses to elect their own board members.

Violations

The nurse practice act also lists violations that can result in disciplinary action against a nurse. Depending on the nature of the violation, a nurse may face not only state board disciplinary action, but also *liability* for her actions.

Interpreting your nurse practice act

Nurse practice acts tend to be broadly worded, and the wording varies from state to state. Understanding your nurse practice act's general provisions will help you stay within the legal limits of nursing practice.

Interpreting the nurse practice act is not always easy. One problem stems from the fact that nurse practice acts are *statutory laws*. Any amendment to a nurse practice act, then, must be accomplished by means of the inevitably slow legislative process. Because of the time involved in pondering, drafting, and enacting laws, amendments to nurse practice acts lag well behind the progress of changes in nursing.

Nursing diagnosis dilemma

You may be expected to perform tasks that seem to be within the accepted scope of nursing but in fact violate your nurse practice act. Consider this common example: Most nurses regularly make nursing diagnoses, although in many cases, their state nurse practice acts don't spell out whether they legally may do so.

Even some nurse practice acts that do permit nursing diagnosis fail to define what the term means. For instance, the Pennsylvania Nurse Practice Act defines the practice of professional nursing as *"diagnosing and treating* human responses to actual or potential health problems through such services as case finding, health teaching, health counseling, and provision of care supportive to or restorative of life and well-being, and executing medical regimens as prescribed by a licensed physician or dentist. The foregoing shall not be deemed to include acts of medical diagnosis or prescription of medical therapeutic or corrective measures." This definition and others like it don't distinguish clearly between medical and nursing diagnoses.

Your state nurse practice act isn't a word-for-word checklist on how you should do your work. You must rely on your own education and knowledge of your hospital's policies and procedures. For example, you know that a nursing diagnosis is part of your nursing assessment. It's your professional evaluation of the patient's progress, his responses to treatment, and his nursing care needs. You perform this evaluation so you can develop and carry out your *nursing care plan*. And you know that nursing diagnosis is not a judgment about a patient's medical disorder. So, if your state nurse practice act permits you to make nursing diagnoses, your sound judgment in applying its provisions should help you avoid legal consequences. If your state practice act doesn't permit nursing diagnoses, or its wording permitting nursing diagnoses is unclear, request an official interpretation from your state board of nursing.

Limits of practice

Be sure you're familiar with the legally permissible scope of your nursing practice, as it's defined in your state's nurse practice act, and never exceed its limits. Otherwise, you're inviting legal problems.

Here's an example. The Pennsylvania Nurse Practice Act forbids a nurse to give an anesthetic unless the patient's doctor is present. The case of *McCarl v. State Board of Nurse Examiners* (1979) involved a hospital nurse who violated this provision. The Pennsylvania Board of Nursing received a complaint about the incident and conducted a hearing. The nurse admitted to knowing about the law's requirement but argued that the requirement was satisfied by the presence of another doctor—although this doctor did not supervise her actions. The board ruled that the nurse had willfully violated a section of the Pennsylvania Nurse Practice Act and issued a reprimand. The nurse appealed the reprimand, but the court upheld it.

When to act independently

Most nurse practice acts pose another problem: They state that you have a legal duty to carry out a doctor's or a dentist's orders. Yet, as a licensed professional, you also have an ethical and legal duty to use your own judgment when providing patient care.

In an effort to deal with this issue, some nurse practice acts give guidance on how to obey orders and still act independently. For example, the Delaware Nurse Practice Act states that the RN practices the profession of nursing by performing certain activities; among these are "executing regimens, as prescribed by a licensed physician, dentist, podiatrist, or advanced practice nurse, including the dispensing or administration of medications and treatments." Having said this, the Delaware statute defines the practice of professional nursing as "the performance of professional services by a person who holds a valid license" and "who bears primary responsibility and accountability for nursing practices based on specialized knowledge, judgment, and skill derived from the principles of biological, physical, and behavioral sciences." This wording may be interpreted to mean that a nurse practicing in Delaware is required to follow a doctor's or a dentist's orders, unless those orders are clearly wrong or the doctor or dentist is unqualified to give them.

When you think an order is wrong, tell the doctor. If you're confused about an order, ask the doctor to clarify it. If he fails to correct the error or answer your questions, inform your head nurse or supervisor of your doubts.

A similar problem may arise when you deal with *physician's assistants*

(PAs) or advanced practice nurses. Nurse practice acts in some states specify that you may only follow orders given by doctors or dentists — but those states' medical practice acts may allow PAs or advanced practice nurses to give orders to nurses. Washington and Florida, for example, have decided that a PA is a doctor's *agent* and may legally transmit the supervising doctor's orders to nurses (*Washington State Nurses Ass'n. v. Board of Medical Examiners,* 1980, and *Fla. Op. Atty. Gen.* [077-96, September 1977]). The state of Delaware permits nurses with advanced credentials to prescribe regimens executed by RNs. Find out if your hospital's policy allows PAs to give you orders. If it doesn't, do not follow such orders. If hospital policy does permit PAs to give you orders, check if such orders must be verified or *countersigned* by the doctor. The same question of verification may arise over a nurse practitioner's orders written in a patient's chart. For further clarification, check with your state board of nursing.

Conflicts with hospital policy

Nurse practice acts and hospital policies don't always agree. Hospital licensing laws require each hospital to establish policies and procedures for its operation. The nursing service department develops detailed policies and procedures for staff nurses. These policies and procedures usually specify the allowable scope of nursing practice within the hospital. The scope may be narrower than the scope described in your nurse practice act, but it should not be broader.

Keep in mind that your employer can't legally expand the scope of your practice to include tasks prohibited by your nurse practice act. For example, in the case of *Sheffield v. State Education Department* (1991), nurses who measured, weighed, compounded, and mixed ingredients in preparing peripheral I.V. solutions for parenteral nutrition and other I.V. solutions (a longtime hospital practice and procedure) were censured and reprimanded by the board of nursing. They were charged with the unlicensed practice of pharmacy in violation of the state of New York's Nurse Practice Act and placed on 18 months' probation.

You have a legal obligation to practice within your nurse practice act's limits. Except in a life-threatening emergency, you can't exceed those limits without risking disciplinary action. To protect yourself, compare your hospital policies and your nurse practice act.

Reading between the lines

Most nurse practice acts don't specify a nurse's day-to-day legal responsibilities with respect to specific procedures and functions. For instance, along with omitting any reference to nursing diagnosis, many nurse practice acts don't address a nurse's responsibility for patient teaching or the legal limitations on nurse-patient discussions about treatment. Yet, in a case in Idaho (*Tuma v. Board of Nursing*, 1979), a state board of nursing took disciplinary action against a nurse who discussed, at a patient's request, the possibility of using Laetrile as alternative therapy. The board suspended her license on the grounds of unprofessional conduct. The Supreme Court of Idaho revoked the suspension and ordered the board to reinstate the nurse's license. Why? Because the Idaho Nurse Practice Act contained no provision stating that such a nurse-patient discussion constitutes a violation of the nurse practice act.

Keeping nurse practice acts up to date

To align nurse practice acts with current nursing practice, professional nursing organizations and state boards

of nursing have lobbied for two types of legislation: amendments and redefinitions.

An *amendment* may be used to add to or subtract from a nurse practice act or its regulations, thereby giving nurses legal permission to perform certain procedures or functions that have become part of accepted nursing practice. Amendments have the same legal force as the original act. They do, however, have a disadvantage: They represent a piecemeal approach that may allow an outdated nurse practice act to remain in effect.

Redefinition is a rewriting of the fundamental provision of a nurse practice act — the definition of nursing practice. This approach changes the basic premise of the entire act without amending or repealing it. Redefinition might be used, for example, to reverse a definition of nursing practice that prohibits diagnosis. How? By clarifying the term *diagnosis* to allow nurses to make nursing diagnoses. This type of change helps nurses understand exactly what is and isn't prohibited.

When a state legislature changes or expands the state's nurse practice act, it also must repeal sections that conflict with its changes. For example, if a state legislature decides to adopt the board of nursing's recommendation for a newly broadened definition of nursing, it must repeal the old definition in the state nurse practice act before it can enact the new definition into *law.*

Be aware of changes

Be aware that nurse practice acts are constantly being changed. For example, in 1989, Delaware amended its nurse practice act to allow an RN to make a pronouncement of *death* when "caring for terminally ill patients in the home or place of residence of the deceased as a part of a *hospice* program or a certified home health care agency devoted primarily to caring for the terminally ill, or in a hospice; and provided that the attending *physician of record* has agreed in writing to permit the attending registered nurse to make a pronouncement of death." The state further amended its nurse practice act in July 1994 to add the practice of the advanced practice nurse.

To help protect yourself legally, you need to thoroughly understand your nurse practice act and keep up with any changes in it.

Standards of nursing care

Standards of care set minimum criteria for your proficiency on the job, enabling you — and others — to judge the quality of care you and your nursing colleagues provide. States may or may not refer to standards in their nurse practice acts. Unless included in a nurse practice act, professional standards aren't laws — they're guidelines for sound nursing practice.

Some nurses regard standards of nursing care as pie-in-the-sky ideals that have little bearing on the reality of working life. This is a dangerous misconception. You're expected to meet standards of nursing care for every nursing task you perform.

For example, if you're a medical-surgical nurse, minimal standards require that you develop a nursing care plan for your patient based on the *nursing process,* including nursing diagnoses, goals, and interventions for implementing the care plan. Standards also call for documentation, in the patient's record, of your completion and evaluation of the plan. When you document your patient care, you're really writing a record of how well you've met these standards.

Evolution of nursing standards

Before 1950, nurses had only Florence Nightingale's early treatments, plus reports of court cases, to use as standards. As nursing gradually became recognized as an independent profession, nursing organizations stressed the importance of having recognized standards for all nurses. Then, in 1950, the ANA published the "Code of Ethics for Nursing," a general mandate stating that nurses should offer nursing care without prejudice and in a confidential and safe manner. Although not specific, this code marked the beginning of written nursing standards.

In 1973, the ANA Congress for Nursing Practice established standards that could be applied to all nurses in all settings. (See *The ANA's standards of clinical nursing practice,* pages 18 to 21.) The *Canadian Nurses Association* (CNA) has established similar nursing standards. Some states and provinces have incorporated ANA and CNA standards into their nurse practice acts.

By 1974, each of the ANA divisions of nursing practice (such as community health, geriatrics, maternal-child, mental health, and medical-surgical) had established distinct standards for its specialty. The ANA Congress called these *specialty standards.* State nursing associations also helped develop specialty nursing standards. (See *ANA standards for nursing administration,* pages 22 to 24.)

Other organizations have contributed to the development of nursing standards. The *Joint Commission on Accreditation of Healthcare Organizations* (JCAHO), a private, nongovernmental agency that establishes guidelines for the operation of hospitals and health care facilities, also has developed nursing standards to be used in hospital audit systems. In some states, JCAHO standards have been in-

(Text continues on page 21.)

The ANA's standards of clinical nursing practice

The American Nurses' Association (ANA) developed the following standards of clinical nursing practice to provide guidelines for determining quality nursing care. These standards may be used by the courts, hospitals, nurses, and patients.

The standards of clinical nursing practice are divided into "standards of care," which identify the care that is provided to recipients of nursing services, and "standards of professional performance," which explain the level of behavior expected in professional role activities. Each standard is followed by measurement criteria that give key indicators of competent practice for that standard.

Standards of care

Standard I: Assessment

The nurse collects patient health data.

Measurement criteria

1. The priority of data collection is determined by the patient's immediate condition or needs.
2. Pertinent data are collected using appropriate assessment techniques.
3. Data collection involves the patient, family members, and health care providers when appropriate.
4. The data collection process is systematic and ongoing.
5. Relevant data are documented in a retrievable form.

Standard II: Diagnosis

The nurse analyzes the assessment data in determining diagnoses.

Measurement criteria

1. Diagnoses are derived from the assessment data.
2. Diagnoses are validated with the patient, family members, and health care providers, when possible.
3. Diagnoses are documented in a manner that facilitates the determination of expected outcomes and plan of care.

Standard III: Outcome identification

The nurse identifies expected outcomes individualized to the patient.

Measurement criteria

1. Outcomes are derived from the diagnoses.
2. Outcomes are documented as measurable goals.
3. Outcomes are mutually formulated with the patient and health care providers, when possible.
4. Outcomes are realistic in relation to the patient's present and potential capabilities.
5. Outcomes are attainable in relation to resources available to the patient.
6. Outcomes include a time estimate for attainment.
7. Outcomes provide direction for continuity of care.

Standard IV: Planning

The nurse develops a plan of care that prescribes interventions to attain expected outcomes.

Measurement criteria

1. The plan is individualized to the patient's condition or needs.
2. The plan is developed with the patient, family members, and health care providers.
3. The plan reflects current practice.
4. The plan is documented.

The ANA's standards of clinical nursing practice continued

5. The plan provides for continuity of care.

Standard V: Implementation

The nurse implements the interventions identified in the plan of care.

Measurement criteria

1. Interventions are consistent with the established plan of care.
2. Interventions are implemented in a safe and appropriate manner.
3. Interventions are documented.

Standard VI: Evaluation

The nurse evaluates the patient's progress toward attainment of outcomes.

Measurement criteria

1. Evaluation is systematic and ongoing.
2. The patient's responses to interventions are documented.
3. The effectiveness of interventions is evaluated in relation to the outcomes.
4. Ongoing assessment data are used to revise diagnoses, outcomes, and the plan of care as needed.
5. Revisions in diagnoses, outcomes, and the plan of care are documented.
6. The patient, family members, and health care providers are involved in the evaluation process, when appropriate.

Standards of professional performance

Standard I: Quality of care

The nurse systematically evaluates the quality and effectiveness of nursing practice.

Measurement criteria

1. The nurse participates in quality of care activities as appropriate to the individual's position, education, and practice environment. Such activities may include:
● identifying aspects of care important for quality monitoring.
● identifying indicators used to monitor quality and effectiveness of nursing care.
● collecting data to monitor quality and effectiveness of nursing care.
● analyzing quality data to identify opportunities for improving care.
● formulating recommendations to improve nursing practice or patient outcomes.
● implementing activities to enhance the quality of nursing practice.
● participating on interdisciplinary teams that evaluate clinical practice or health services.
● developing policies and procedures to improve the quality of care.
2. The nurse uses the results of quality of care activities to initiate changes in practice.
3. The nurse uses the results of quality of care activities to initiate changes throughout the health care delivery system as appropriate.

Standard II: Performance appraisal

The nurse systematically evaluates her own nursing practice in relation to professional practice standards and relevant statutes and regulations.

Measurement criteria

1. The nurse engages in performance appraisal on a regular basis, identifying

(continued)

The ANA's standards of clinical nursing practice continued

areas of strength as well as areas for professional and practical development.
2. The nurse seeks constructive feedback regarding her own practice.
3. The nurse takes action to achieve goals identified during performance appraisal.
4. The nurse participates in peer review as appropriate.

Standard III: Education

The nurse acquires and maintains current knowledge in nursing practice.

Measurement criteria

1. The nurse participates in ongoing educational activities related to clinical knowledge and professional issues.
2. The nurse seeks experiences to maintain clinical skills.
3. The nurse seeks knowledge and skills appropriate to her practice environment.

Standard IV: Collegiality

The nurse contributes to the professional development of peers, colleagues, and others.

Measurement criteria

1. The nurse shares knowledge and skills with colleagues and others.
2. The nurse provides peers with constructive feedback regarding their practice.
3. The nurse contributes to an environment that is conducive to clinical education of nursing students as appropriate.

Standard V: Ethics

The nurse's decisions and actions on behalf of patients are determined in an ethical manner.

Measurement criteria

1. The nurse's practice is guided by the *Code for Nurses*.
2. The nurse maintains patient confidentiality.
3. The nurse acts as a patient advocate.
4. The nurse delivers care in a nonjudgmental and nondiscriminatory manner that is sensitive to patient diversity.
5. The nurse delivers care in a manner that preserves and protects patient autonomy, dignity, and rights.
6. The nurse seeks available resources to help formulate ethical decisions.

Standard VI: Collaboration

The nurse collaborates with the patient, family members, and health care providers regarding patient care and nursing's role in the provision of care.

Measurement criteria

1. The nurse communicates with the patient, family members, and health care providers regarding patient care and nursing's role in the provision of care.
2. The nurse consults with health care providers for patient care as needed.
3. The nurse makes referrals, including provisions for continuity of care as needed.

Standard VII: Research

The nurse uses research findings in practice.

Measurement criteria

1. The nurse uses interventions substantiated by research as appropriate to the individual's position, education, and practice environment.

The ANA's standards of clinical nursing practice continued

2. The nurse participates in research activities as appropriate to her position, education, and practice environment. Such activities may include:

- identifying clinical problems suitable for nursing research.
- participating in data collection.
- participating on a unit, organization, or community research committee or program.
- exchanging research findings with others.
- conducting research.
- critiquing research for application to practice.
- using research findings in the development of policies, procedures, and guidelines for patient care.

Standard VIII: Resource utilization

The nurse considers factors related to safety, effectiveness, and cost in planning and delivering patient care.

Measurement criteria

1. The nurse evaluates factors related to safety, effectiveness, and cost when two or more practice options would result in the same expected patient outcome.

2. The nurse assigns tasks or delegates care based on the needs of the patient and the knowledge and skills of the provider selected.

3. The nurse assists the patient and partner in identifying and securing appropriate services available to address health-related needs.

corporated into law, resulting in broadly applicable standards of patient care (see *JCAHO standards,* pages 25 to 28). In addition, state nursing associations and the specialty nursing organizations actively work with hospital *nursing administrators* for adoption of standards.

Federal regulations for staffing *Medicare* and *Medicaid* services have influenced the development of standards, especially *nursing home* standards. By suggesting ethical approaches to nursing practice, ethics codes written by the ANA, the CNA, and the *International Council of Nurses* also influence how nursing care standards are developed.

Local standards

The courts also may use local standards—reflecting a community's accepted, common nursing practices—to judge the quality of nursing care.

Local standards are established in two ways: by individual hospitals, through their policies and procedures, and by *expert witnesses* who testify in court cases that involve nurses. Every hospital establishes standards to fit its own community's needs. An expert witness interprets local standards by testifying about how nursing is commonly practiced in her community.

Legal significance

Even if they aren't law, nursing standards have important legal significance. The allegation that a nurse failed to meet appropriate standards of care is the basic premise of every nursing malpractice lawsuit.

During a malpractice trial, the court will measure the *defendant*-nurse's action against the answer it obtains to

(Text continues on page 28.)

ANA standards for nursing administration

The standards below are adapted from standards for nurse-administrators published by the American Nurses' Association (ANA). In the original document, the ANA refers to nursing administration as "organized nursing services."

Philosophy and structure

The nursing administration is guided by a philosophy and structure that ensure the delivery of effective nursing care.

Rationale for standard
The philosphy is a statement of beliefs and values that gives direction to the delivery of nursing services. A consistent philosophy and structure ensure a framework for providing nursing care and for resolving problems.

Criteria
1. The philosophy and structure are compatible with established professional, regulatory, and health care organization standards.
2. The philosophy ensures that individual nurses have accountability for and authority to manage nursing practice.
3. The administration's structure facilitates participative management.

Role of the nurse-administrator

The nursing administration is staffed by qualified and competent nurse-administrators.

Rationale for standard
The complex demands of the health care environment require the leadership and direction of qualified and competent nurse-administrators (nurse-executives and nurse-managers).

Criteria
1. The nurse-executive is an RN who holds a baccalaureate degree in nursing and a graduate degree in nursing or a related field from a program that includes organizational science and management concepts. Certification in nursing administration is recommended.
2. The nurse-executive is member of the policy-making body of the organization.
3. The nurse-manager is an RN prepared with a minimum of a baccalaureate degree in nursing. A graduate degree in nursing or a related field is recommended, as is certification in nursing administration.
4. Responsibilities of nurse-administrators include the following:
● maintaining knowledge of current technology and trends in health care.
● collaborating with the nursing staff at all levels to develop programs within the nursing administration.
● representing the nursing administration within decision-making bodies in the organization.
● advocating for the nurses they manage as well as for patients.

Use of the nursing process

Within the nursing administration, the nursing process is used as the framework for providing nursing care to patients.

ANA standards for nursing administration continued

Rationale for standard

The nursing process (assessment, diagnosis, care plan, intervention, and evaluation) enables the nurse to help patients reach established goals.

Criteria

1. A nursing information system is established and includes information on patient characteristics.
2. Documents used in recording data are accessible to nurses and are maintained in a confidential manner.
3. Record-keeping systems are based on the nursing process.
4. Resources are provided for staff to develop competence in and validate nursing diagnoses.
5. Independent nursing interventions within the scope of nursing practice are encouraged by the nursing administration.
6. Opportunities are provided for nurses to implement the plan of care in collaboration with the patient, the family, and the interdisciplinary team.
7. Resources are provided to allow the nurse to evaluate care and to develop alternative plans as necessary.

The working environment

An environment is created within the nursing administration that enhances nursing practice and facilitates the delivery of care by all nursing staff.

Rationale for standard

The nursing administration goal is to provide effective care to patients. To accomplish this, the practice climate must let nurses fully apply their education and expertise.

Criteria

1. A written organizational plan establishes lines of authority, accountability, and communication and is kept current.
2. Collaboration in the planning of care is encouraged by the nursing administration.
3. The nursing staff are oriented to the mission, objectives, and practices of the health care environment; the nurse's knowledge and skill are assessed and rewarded.
4. An environment is provided for staff to participate in decision making regarding clinical practice, procedures that affect nursing practice, and clinical issues such as requirements for care, including human and material resources.
5. Roles and responsibilities of practice are consistent with the nursing staff members' level of educational preparation or competence.
6. Nurse-administrators collaborate with the staff of human resources to develop and implement recruitment and retention programs for registered nurses, including continuing education.
7. There is an established system for identifying patient care requirements, allocating nursing resources, and evaluating the system's effectiveness.

Quality assurance and improvement

Rationale for standard

The nursing administration is obligated to provide effective nursing care to society. Standards provide the basis for evaluating care. A quality assurance and improvement program measures compliance with standards and provides opportunities to improve care and resolve problems.

(continued)

ANA standards for nursing administration continued

Criteria

1. Nurses are active in the ongoing monitoring and evaluation of nursing care.
2. Actions to resolve problems and improve care are documented and evaluated.
3. The quality assurance and improvement program is periodically evaluated and is an integral part of the facility's risk management and quality assurance effort.
4. Patients have the opportunity to express their satisfaction and perceptions of their care.

Ethics

The nursing administration has policies to guide ethical decision making based on the *ANA's Code of Ethics.*

Rationale for standard

Nurses providing care to patients are confronted with complex ethical dilemmas that require consideration of both the decision-making authority of patients and their requirements for care. The ANA's Code of Ethics provides the parameters within which the nurse makes ethical judgments.

Criteria

1. Nursing is represented in the formal mechanism for resolving ethical dilemmas.
2. Educational programs identify and support discussions of moral, ethical, and legal issues.
3. Mechanisms are in place for documentation of self-determination, informed consent, and treatment termination according to applicable laws and regulations.
4. Nurses are represented on the health care organization's decision-making bodies regarding ethical and legal issues.

Research

Within the nursing administration, research in nursing, health, and nursing systems is facilitated, and findings are integrated into the delivery of nursing care and nursing administration.

Rationale for standard

The continuing advancement of nursing practice and administration depends on the ongoing availability and application of a valid and current knowledge base.

Criteria

1. Nurses are encouraged by the nursing administration to conduct both nursing and interdisciplinary research.
2. A procedure is established to review proposed research studies, including protection of human subjects' rights.

Cultural, economic, and social differences

The nursing administration's policies and practices ensure equality and continuity of nursing services and recognizes patients' cultural, economic, and social differences.

Rationale for standard

The nursing administration must have policies that promote recognition of diversity among patients and their value systems.

Criteria

1. The policies and practices reflect the health-related values and traditions of various cultures.
2. Mechanisms are established for nurses and other personnel to identify and discuss their value conflicts.

JCAHO standards

The standards listed below are based upon the 1995 *Accreditation Manual for Hospitals* published by the Joint Commission on Accreditation of Healthcare Organizations (JCAHO). These standards are used by the JCAHO to evaluate and monitor the clinical and organizational performance of health care institutions.

Standards for patient assessment

Patients should receive nursing care based on a documented assessment of their needs.

Initial assessment

An initial screening or assessment of each patient's physical, psychological, and social status should be performed to determine the need for care, the type of care to be provided, and the need for any further assessment.
- The need for an assessment of the patient's nutritional status should be determined.
- The need for a discharge planning assessment of the patient should be determined.
- Initial assessment of each patient admitted should be conducted within a certain time frame preceding or following admission, as specified by policy.
- The patient's history and physical examination should be completed within 24 hours of admission as an inpatient.

Reassessment

- Each patient should be reassessed periodically.
- The patient should be reassessed when a significant change occurs in his condition.

Care decisions

- The information generated through the analysis of assessment data should be used to identify and prioritize the patient's needs for care.
- Care decisions should be based on the identified patient needs and on care priorities.

Structures supporting the assessment of patients

- Activities that comprise the patient assessment function should be defined in writing.
- An RN should assess the patient's needs in all settings in which nursing care is to be provided.

Standards for human resources planning

- The organization's leaders should define for their respective areas the qualifications and job expectations of the staff and a system to evaluate how well expectations are met.
- The organization should have an adequate number of staff members whose qualifications are commensurate with defined job responsibilities and applicable licensure, law, and regulation and certification.
- Processes should be designed to ensure that the competence of all staff members is assessed, maintained, demonstrated, and improved on an ongoing basis.
- The organization should assess each individual's ability to achieve job expectations as stated in her job description.

(continued)

JCAHO standards continued

Standards for planning and providing care
- The care, treatment, and rehabilitation planning process should ensure that care is appropriate for the patient's specific needs and the severity of his disease, condition, impairment, or disability.
- Qualified individuals must plan and provide care, treatment, and rehabilitation in a collaborative and disciplined manner, as appropriate for the patient.

Patient's rights
The organization should have a functioning process to address ethical issues.
- The process should be based on a framework that recognizes the interdependence of patient care and organizational ethical issues.
- The process should include mechanisms that address the patient's involvement in all aspects of care.

Standards for organizational planning
The leadership should provide for organizational planning.
- Planning should include setting a mission, a vision, and values for the organization and providing the strategic, operational, programmatic, and other plans and policies to achieve that mission and vision.
- When the organization is composed of many subunits, there should be a mechanism for the leaders of each individual organization to participate in policy decisions affecting the organization.

Patient care services
- The plan should include patient care services in response to identified patient needs and should be consistent with the organization's mission.

- The organization's leaders and, as appropriate, community leaders and organizations should collaborate to design services.
- The design of patient care services throughout the organization should be appropriate for the scope and level of care required by the patients served.
- The leaders should collaborate with representatives from the appropriate disciplines and services to develop an annual operating budget and, at least as required by applicable laws and regulations, a long-term capital expenditure plan, including a strategy to monitor the plan's implementation.
- The budget review process should consider the appropriateness of the organization's plan for providing care to meet patient needs.
- The leaders and other representatives of the organization should participate, as appropriate, in the organization's decision-making structure and processes.
- The organization's leaders should develop programs to promote the recruitment, retention, development, and continuing education of all staff members. These programs should include mechanisms for promoting at least the job-related educational and advancement goals of staff members.

Directing departments
Each department of the organization should have effective leadership. Department directors are responsible, either personally or through delegation, for:
- developing and implementing policies and procedures that guide and support the provision of services
- recommending a sufficient number of qualified and competent persons to provide care, including treatment

JCAHO standards continued

• continuously assessing and improving the performance of care and services provided
• maintaining quality-control programs, as appropriate
• orienting and providing in-service training and continuing education of all persons in the department.

Integrating services

Patient care services must be appropriately integrated throughout the organization. The leaders should individually and jointly develop and participate in systematic and effective mechanisms for:
• fostering communication among individuals and components of the organization and coordinating internal activities
• communicating with the leaders of any health care delivery organization that is corporately or functionally related to the organization seeking accreditation.

Improving performance

The organization's leaders should set expectations, develop plans, and manage processes to assess, improve, and maintain the quality of the organization's governance, management, clinical, and support activities.

Standards for information management planning

Information management processes should be planned and designed to meet the health care organization's internal and external information needs.
• The information management processes within and among departments, the medical staff, the administration and governing body, and with outside services and agencies should be appropriate for the organization's size and complexity.

• Based on the organization's information needs, appropriate staff members should participate in assessing, selecting, and integrating health care information technology and, as appropriate, using efficient interactive information management systems for clinical and organizational information.

Information management planning

• The information management function must provide for information confidentiality, security, and integrity.
• The organization should determine how data and information can be retrieved easily and quickly without compromising its security and confidentiality.

Patient information

The information management function should provide for the definition, retrieval, analysis, transformation, transmission, and reporting of individual patient information related to the process and outcome of the patient's care.

The medical record must contain sufficient information to identify the patient, support the diagnosis, justify treatment, document the course and results accurately, and ease continuity of care among health care providers. Each medical record should contain at least the following:
• the diagnosis or diagnostic impression
• diagnostic and therapeutic orders, if any
• all diagnostic and therapeutic procedures and tests performed and the results
• progress notes made by the medical staff and other authorized individuals
• all reassessments, when necessary
• the response to the care provided.

(continued)

JCAHO standards continued

At discharge, a clinical resume should concisely summarize the reason for hospitalization, the significant findings, the procedures performed and treatment rendered, the patient's condition, and any specific instructions given to the patient and family, as pertinent.

Standards for nursing

Nursing services should be directed by a nurse-executive who is an RN qualified by advanced education and management experience.

The nurse-executive

If the organization's structure is decentralized, an identified nurse leader at the executive level should provide authority and accountability for, and coordination of, nurse-executive functions.

● The nurse-executive has the authority and responsibility for establishing standards of nursing practice.

● The nurse-executive and other nursing leaders should participate with leaders from the governing body, management, medical staff, and clinical areas in planning and conducting organization-wide performance-improvement activities.

Policies and procedures

● Nursing policies and procedures, nursing standards of patient care, and standards of nursing practice must be created in a logical sequence.

● Policies, procedures, and standards should be developed by the nurse-executive, RNs, and other designated nursing staff members. These documents must be in writing.

● Policies, procedures, and standards should be approved by the nurse-executive or a designee.

---

the following question: *What would a reasonably prudent nurse, with like training and experience, do under similar conditions in the same community?*

To answer this question, the *plaintiff*-patient, through his attorney, must determine that certain standards of care exist and that the defendant-nurse should have applied those standards to him. He also must prove the appropriateness of those standards, show how the nurse failed to meet them, and show how this failure caused him injury.

When the standard of care is at issue, the plaintiff-patient must present expert witness testimony to support his claims. The defendant-nurse and her attorney also will produce expert witness testimony — in support of her claim that her actions did not fall below accepted standards and that she acted in a reasonable and prudent manner.

The court may consider written standards when considering the standards of care involved in a nursing malpractice lawsuit. The court may seek information about relevant national or state standards as well as information about the policies of the defendant-nurse's employer.

Because of two trends — uniform nursing educational requirements and standardized medical treatment regimens — national standards are gaining increasing favor with the courts. These trends have made the ANA's standards more influential than local standards or the standards of other organizations. For example, in the case of *Planned Parenthood of Northwest Indiana v. Vines* (1989), a nurse practitioner who inserted an intrauterine device was held to the minimum standard of care that was uniform throughout the country.

How nursing standards are applied in court

In *Story v. St. Mary Parish Service District* (1987), a 66-year-old man was admitted to the hospital complaining of abdominal distention and pain, nausea, and vomiting. Throughout the next 2 days, he complained several times to the nurses and attendants about shortness of breath and severe pain in his elbows and chest.

One evening, the staff nurse (a new graduate who had only recently taken her nursing boards) wrote in her *nurses' notes,* "Complains of both elbows hurting severely, denied pain anywhere else. Slightly irritable and confused. Assisted back to bed. Admits to arthritis. Slight shortness of breath noted. Abdominal distention in moderation noted; soft to touch. Blood pressure 150/98; pulse 88. Will have medicated." She did not indicate any consultation with the charge nurse. The patient died at 11:45 p.m.; *autopsy* revealed a myocardial infarction.

Pretrial testimony revealed that the patient had stated that the nurses did not listen to his reports of pain. In the pretrial memorandum, the plaintiff's attorney cited a variety of nursing practice standards, including the following:
• the Louisiana Nurse Practice Act, which describes the nurse's responsibility for performing patient assessment and intervening as appropriate
• a board of nursing rule stating that graduate nurses must have RN supervision when they provide care
• nursing care standards established by JCAHO.

Although this case was settled out of court, it provides a good example of the extensive use of nursing practice standards as evidence in a lawsuit.

In *Hodges v. Effingham County Hospital* (1987), a woman entered the emergency department and complained to the nurses of chest pains. No doctor was present. After conferring with the nurses by telephone, the doctor on call decided to discharge the patient. The nurses didn't tell the doctor that the patient had a history of heart disease and had recently taken a nitroglycerin tablet. The patient later died.

The plaintiff alleged that the nurses in the emergency department were *negligent* because they failed to obtain an accurate medical history and to "fully report known and observable symptoms to the doctor on call." The doctor was not sued: The plaintiff thought that the doctor had treated the patient appropriately based on the information given to him.

Although the nurses won the lower court decision, the higher court found the nurses liable. The court stated that because the nursing action in question involved nursing judgment rather than the adequacy of services or facility, the question was whether the nurses followed general standards of nursing care.

Drug administration

If you administer medication when the prescribing doctor isn't present, you're legally responsible for clarifying the doctor's instructions. The courts have strictly upheld this standard of nursing practice. In the Louisiana case *Norton v. Argonaut Insurance Co.* (1962), a doctor left an incomplete order for administration of 3 ml of digoxin to a young patient. A nurse supervisor helping out on the pediatric floor picked up the order. Unsure of the amount of digoxin the doctor had prescribed, she asked two doctors on the ward if 3 ml was an excessive dose. One of the doctors, believing that the nurse was describing an *oral* dose, told her that 3 ml was correct; the other doctor thought that she intended to administer only 1 ml. The nurse gave the patient 3 ml of digoxin *by injection,* and the young patient died.

In a subsequent malpractice lawsuit against the nurse, the court ruled that she violated a standard of practice that holds that each nurse has the *duty* to make certain that the dose and route of administration of every medication she administers are correct. The court made this decision based on the following evidence:

• The nurse attempted to administer a medication with which she wasn't familiar.

• The nurse failed to call the attending doctor for clarification of his orders.

Nonnursing professionals

During a malpractice trial, nonnursing professionals may provide expert witness testimony with regard to standards of nursing care. For example, in *Hiatt v. Groce* (1974), a patient sued an obstetric nurse for failing to notify a doctor when the patient was about to deliver a baby. The court permitted a doctor to testify about the adequacy of the nurse's care. In *Gugino v. Harvard Community Health Plan* (1980), the court allowed a doctor to testify about the standards for a nurse practitioner.

In *Jones v. Hawkes Hospital* (1964), the court instructed jurors to rely on their own common sense to judge whether a nurse met standards of practice instead of relying on expert testimony. In this case, a nurse left a sedated patient who was in labor to assist a doctor with another patient in labor. She did this because the hospital had a rule that no doctor could attend a woman in labor unless a nurse was present. Left alone, the plaintiff-patient got out of bed, fell, and suffered serious injuries. The nurse wanted the court to allow expert testimony to establish what standard of care should have been applied. But the court ruled that any reasonably prudent person could determine this case on the basis of ordinary experience and knowledge and that the jurors could decide on their own

whether the defendant-nurse's nontechnical nursing tasks met reasonable standards of care. The jury found the nurse negligent.

In a similar case, *Larrimore v. Homeopathic Hospital Association* (1962), a nurse was found liable for failing to read a new order or for reading it negligently. The court stated that the jury could apply ordinary common sense, without an expert witness, to establish the applicable standard of care.

Nursing licensure

Your nursing license entitles you to practice as a professionally qualified nurse. But like most privileges, your nursing license imposes certain responsibilities. As a licensed RN, LPN, or LVN, you're responsible for providing quality care to your patients. To meet this responsibility and to protect your right to practice, you need to understand the professional and legal significance of your nursing license.

Licensing laws

Each nurse practice act contains licensing laws. They establish qualifications for obtaining and maintaining a nursing license. They also broadly define the legally permissible scope of nursing practice.

Although they vary somewhat from state to state, most licensing laws specify the following:

• the qualifications a nurse needs to be granted a license

• license-application procedures for new licenses and reciprocal (state-to-state) licensing arrangements

• application fees

• authorization to grant use of the title *registered nurse* or *licensed practical or vocational nurse* to applicants who receive their licenses

• grounds for license denial, revocation, or suspension
• license-renewal procedures.

Most state licensing laws do not prohibit nursing students, a patient's friends, or members of his family from caring for him on a routine basis, provided no fee is involved. They also permit a newly graduated nurse to practice for a specified period while her license application is being processed, and they allow unlicensed people to give care (such as administering cardiopulmonary resuscitation) in an emergency. According to state and federal constitutional requirements, state laws must exempt the following types of nurses from state licensure requirements:
• nurses working in federal institutions
• nurses practicing in accordance with their religious beliefs
• nurses traveling with patients from one state to another.

Legal significance of the license

Licensing laws help you to avoid civil and criminal liabilities by defining the scope of your professional nursing practice. If you're named in a malpractice lawsuit, your state licensing laws will be used as partial evidence to determine whether you acted within the legal limits of your profession.

In *Barber v. Reinking* (1966), the court used the licensing laws in the Washington state nurse practice act to rule against the defendant-nurse. In this case, a boy age 2 was taken to a doctor's office for a polio booster shot. The doctor (who also was named in the suit) delegated this task to the LPN who worked in his office. While the nurse was administering the shot, the child moved suddenly and the needle broke off in his buttock. Despite attempts to remove it surgically and with a magnet, the needle remained lodged in the child's buttock for 9 months.

During the trial, the licensing law for practical nurses became the crucial factor in the court's decision. The court declared that the nurse had violated the nurse practice act by performing services beyond the legal limit of her practice. (Until the 1970s, the Washington state nurse practice act did not allow a practical nurse to legally give an injection.) The nurse's attorney attempted to introduce as evidence the fact that LPNs and LVNs in the local community commonly gave injections. This evidence was not allowed. Instead, the judge instructed the jury to consider the violation of the nurse practice act along with other evidence in the case, including the doctor's liability under the *respondeat superior* doctrine, to determine if the nurse was negligent.

Canadian licensing laws

Because each province in Canada has its own nurse practice act, the laws vary somewhat from province to province. Licensing laws in all provinces except Ontario require nurses to join provincial nursing associations to obtain their licenses.

In all provinces, Canadian licensing laws establish the following:
• qualifications for membership in the provincial nurses' association
• examination requirements
• applicable fees
• conditions for reciprocal licensure
• penalties for practicing without a license
• grounds for denial, suspension, or revocation of a nurse's license.

Within those provinces that license practical nurses, licensing laws for LPNs and LVNs are similar to those for RNs.

Keeping the license current

When you begin a new job, your employer is responsible for checking your credentials and confirming that you're properly licensed. Make sure your nursing license is current, and be prepared to furnish proof that you've renewed your license, if necessary.

If you fail to renew your license, you can no longer legally practice nursing. In the United States and Canada, you can be prosecuted and fined for practicing without a license; fines usually range from as little as $5 to as much as $2,000. Fines vary from state to state. For example, section 223 of the Professional Nursing Law of Pennsylvania states that practicing nursing without a license is a *misdemeanor*. For a first violation, the nurse must pay a fine of up to $1,000; if she doesn't pay the fine, she faces a 6-month prison term. For a second violation, the penalty may be a fine of up to $2,000, 6 months to 1 year in prison, or both. In addition to the criminal penalty, the nurse may be required to pay a *civil penalty* of up to $1,000.

License renewal and the law

The courts have addressed questions concerning license renewal, usually during an appeal of disciplinary action taken by a state board of nursing. The courts do not always agree with the boards' decisions. In *Kansas State Board of Nursing v. Burkman* (1975), an RN failed to renew her license and continued to practice nursing. No evidence existed to suggest that she had intentionally not renewed her license or knowingly practiced without it. The state board of nursing ruled that her actions constituted a violation of state licensing laws and suspended her license for 6 months. After several appeals, a high court ruled that the board of nursing had erred, and instructed the board to renew the license.

In *Oliff v. Florida State Board of Nursing* (1979), the court also ruled in the nurse's favor. In this case, the board of nursing refused to renew an LPN's certificate because her application had

not arrived on time. Evidence indicated that the nurse had mailed her application before the date specified by the board. The court ruled that the date adopted by the board was a deadline for applications to be mailed, not received.

Failure to renew

If you discover that you've forgotten to renew your license, several simple measures can help you avoid legal repercussions:
• Notify your employer.
• Find your original license application and immediately notify the state board of nursing of your oversight. Ask them for a temporary license or for authorization to continue nursing until you receive your license.
• If you can't find your license application, write to the state board of nursing for a renewal application and instructions on how to proceed. Then, follow the board's instructions exactly.

Working in a different state

Until the *National League for Nursing* established the first standardized examination for nursing licensure, each state had its own qualifications for entry into nursing practice. As a result, arranging to obtain a license in a different state often was difficult.

All candidates for licensure currently are required to pass the NCLEX, administered under the auspices of the National Council of State Boards of Nursing. Thanks to the establishment of national standards, nurses are able to move more freely to new jobs in different states.

When you move to another state to practice nursing, you must obtain a license or *temporary practice permit* from that state before you may legally practice. Most state boards of nursing will license you if you're currently licensed to practice nursing in another state or territory; if you're licensed to practice in Canada, most boards will license you if your education fulfills the issuing state's requirements. The policy of accepting out-of-state licensure is called *endorsement.* Many state boards waive reexamination if you're licensed in Canada and want to practice in the United States. The same usually applies if you hold a U.S. license and want to practice in Canada.

If you move to another state before its board of nursing has had time to approve your application, you may be granted a temporary license. Check both the time limit of the temporary license and the specific nursing functions it authorizes.

If you travel with a patient from one state to another, your license is valid for the duration of the trip in most states and Canadian provinces.

Failure to qualify

If the state board finds that you don't have the necessary qualifications to practice nursing in that state, it may reject your application or require that you complete a written examination — regardless of your education or the laws of the state in which you live.

In *Richardson v. Brunelle* (1979), an LPN who had practiced in Massachusetts for 15 years brought suit after being refused a license to practice in New Hampshire. In her New Hampshire application, she requested a *decree of educational equivalency.* Although she had originally taken and passed a Massachusetts state licensing examination, she had never graduated from an approved school of practical nursing. At that time, only nursing school graduates were permitted to practice in New Hampshire, so her request was denied. Her lawsuit was unsuccessful in reversing the New Hampshire decision, and subsequent appeals upheld the original ruling.

A similar case, *Snelson v. Culton* (1949), involved Maine's licensing requirements, which also require a successful applicant to be a graduate of a state-approved school of nursing.

Federal law and licensure

Even though no federal law has jurisdiction over state boards of nursing, federal laws may affect nursing licensure. For example, if you're a nurse in the armed forces who often is subject to transfer, you're required by federal law to hold a current state license — but not necessarily in the state to which you are assigned.

A federal public health code requires all state boards that license health care professionals to develop systems for verifying those professionals' continued competence.

Foreign licensure

If you move to a foreign country, your U.S. nursing license will be reviewed by the appropriate authority, which will either reject or accept it (possibly with conditions). If you're a nurse in the American armed forces working in an American installation, you're exempt from this review.

In a non-English-speaking country, the licensing authority may require you to complete a language-proficiency examination.

If you're an RN, an LPN, or an LVN licensed in a foreign country, you can't practice nursing in any state, territory, or province until the appropriate licensing authority has approved your application and issued your nursing license. When you're granted licensure in the United States or Canada, you function at the same legal status as a U.S.- or Canadian-educated RN, LPN, or LVN. You're also equally accountable for your professional actions.

Many states are beginning to require that foreign nurses pass the examination prepared by the *Commission on Graduates of Foreign Nursing Schools* (the CGFN examination). If a foreign nurse successfully completes this examination — which includes an English-proficiency segment — she may then take the NCLEX examination. If she passes, she qualifies for licensure and a work visa.

Disciplinary action

The state board of nursing can take disciplinary action against a nurse for any violation of the state's nurse practice act. In all states and provinces, the board of nursing has authority to discipline a nurse if she endangers a patient's health, safety, or welfare.

Depending on the severity of the violation, a state board may formally reprimand the nurse, place her on probation, refuse to renew her license, or suspend, or even revoke, her license. Other types of disciplinary action include imposing a probationary period or fine and restricting the nurse's scope of practice.

The list of punishable violations varies from state to state. The most common are:

• conviction of a crime involving *moral turpitude,* if the offense bears directly on whether the person is fit to be licensed

• use of fraud or deceit in obtaining or attempting to obtain a nursing license

• *incompetence* because of negligence or because of physical or psychological impairments

• habitual use of or addiction to drugs or alcohol

• unprofessional conduct, including (but not limited to) falsifying, inaccurately recording, or improperly altering patient records; negligently administering medications or treatments; performing tasks beyond the limits of the state's nurse practice act; failing to take appropriate action to safeguard the patient from incompetent health care; violating the patient's *confidentiality;* taking on nursing duties that require skills and education beyond one's competence; violating the patient's dignity and human rights by basing nursing care on prejudice; abandoning a patient; and abusing a patient verbally or physically.

Administrative review process

When a nurse is accused of professional misconduct, the state board of nursing usually investigates by conducting an *administrative review.*

As an administrative body, the state board of nursing wields broad *discretionary powers.* Court proceedings — and possibly legal penalties — may result from the board's administrative review findings. Because it lacks legal authority, the state board of nursing can't issue a final decision. You have the right to appeal, through the court system, for reversal of the nursing board's decision. (See *Disciplinary proceedings for nurse misconduct.*)

Steps in administrative review

In most states and provinces, the nurse practice act specifies the steps the board of nursing must follow during an administrative review. In some states, a general administrative procedure act (separate from the nurse practice act) specifies the steps; in still other states, the board of nursing determines protocol.

An administrative review begins when a person, a health care facility (the nurse's employer), or a professional organization files a signed *complaint* against a nurse with the state board of nursing — or when the board itself initiates such action.

The board then reviews the complaint to decide if the nurse's action

Disciplinary proceedings for nurse misconduct

The flow chart below shows what happens when the state board of nursing takes disciplinary action against a nurse for violation of the state's nurse practice act.

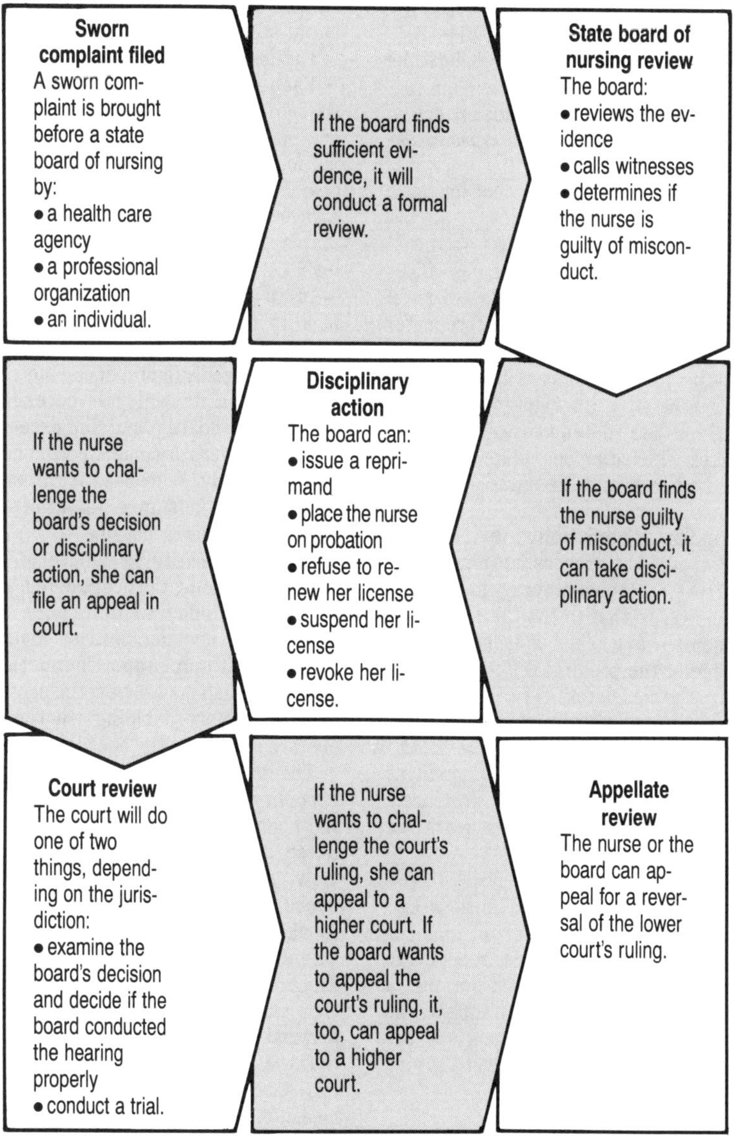

Sworn complaint filed
A sworn complaint is brought before a state board of nursing by:
- a health care agency
- a professional organization
- an individual.

If the board finds sufficient evidence, it will conduct a formal review.

State board of nursing review
The board:
- reviews the evidence
- calls witnesses
- determines if the nurse is guilty of misconduct.

If the nurse wants to challenge the board's decision or disciplinary action, she can file an appeal in court.

Disciplinary action
The board can:
- issue a reprimand
- place the nurse on probation
- refuse to renew her license
- suspend her license
- revoke her license.

If the board finds the nurse guilty of misconduct, it can take disciplinary action.

Court review
The court will do one of two things, depending on the jurisdiction:
- examine the board's decision and decide if the board conducted the hearing properly
- conduct a trial.

If the nurse wants to challenge the court's ruling, she can appeal to a higher court. If the board wants to appeal the court's ruling, it, too, can appeal to a higher court.

Appellate review
The nurse or the board can appeal for a reversal of the lower court's ruling.

appears to violate the state's nurse practice act. If it does, the board prepares for a formal hearing, including *subpoenaing witnesses.* When these preparations begin, the accused nurse's *due process rights* include the right to receive timely notice of both the charge against her and the hearing date.

At the hearing, the nurse has the following due process rights:
• to have an attorney represent her
• to present evidence and *cross-examine* witnesses
• to appeal the board's decision to a court.

At the formal hearing, an impartial attorney may act as a hearing officer (in lieu of a judge), or the board itself may hear the case. A court reporter documents the entire proceeding, or it may be taped. Members of the board act as the plaintiffs bringing the claim against the defendant-nurse. Witnesses — including co-workers — testify for the board and the nurse.

Canadian administrative review

In Canada, the process for administrative review of complaints against nurses is similar to that in the United States. In some provinces, a complaints committee of the provincial nursing board hears the complaint first and either dismisses or endorses it. If the complaints committee endorses it, the complaint is sent along to a discipline committee for a full hearing. In other provinces, only a discipline committee hears the complaint.

Note that in many provinces, an employer who terminates a nurse's employment for incompetence, misconduct, or incapacity must report the *termination* to the board of nursing in writing (this rule does not apply if the nurse's employer is a patient). If the employer fails to do this, the board may impose a fine.

Judicial review process

In every state, nurses have the right to challenge the board's disciplinary decisions by the process of appeal through the courts. This basic right cannot be revoked by any means; in many states, this right is spelled out in the nurse practice act.

Each state and court jurisdiction sets its own rules on how to file this type of appeal. In some jurisdictions, the nurse, through her attorney, must appeal to a special court that handles only cases from state agencies. In other states, she must appeal to the lowest level court.

In an appeal, the court reviews the legality of the state board's original decision against the nurse — not the nurse's allegedly improper conduct. The court attempts only to determine whether the board of nursing exceeded its legal powers or conducted the hearing improperly. It decides if the state board's decision is unlawful, arbitrary, or unreasonable according to law, or whether it constitutes "abuse of discretion" (meaning the board didn't have enough evidence to determine unprofessional conduct, and so made a decision without proper foundation). The court also may review the original evidence before deciding whether to sustain or reverse the board's decision.

The court also may allow a *trial de novo,* in which the *appellate court* hears the board's complete case against the nurse, as though the administrative review had never happened. New evidence, if it exists, may be introduced by the plaintiff (the board) or by the defendant-nurse, through her attorney. The court hears the case and then either sustains or reverses the board's original decision.

If the defendant-nurse loses this appeal, she may — depending on the jurisdiction — appeal to a higher court. (If the nurse wins, the board of nursing can appeal to a higher court.) To begin the new appeal, the nurse's attorney must file it with the lower court that ruled against the nurse; this court will send the trial transcript and the appeal to the higher court. All states have rules and regulations governing appeals, and abiding by them is an attorney's legal responsibility.

The higher court decides whether to hear the appeal, based on its merits. The appeal usually must establish that the lower court made an error of law in admitting — or not admitting — certain evidence; otherwise, the higher court may dismiss it. The higher court will not hear the case a second time, but the defendant-nurse and her attorney may continue to appeal through all higher courts up to the state's highest court. Exceptional cases may reach the U.S. Supreme Court.

Note that Canadian nurses may also challenge disciplinary action through the court system. An appeal involves a written application to a superior court. The application states that an error was made by the disciplinary tribunal and requests that the superior court correct the decision of the tribunal or modify it.

Court cases

Consider the following two cases, which describe the experience of two nurses during the administrative and judicial review.

In a Connecticut case, *Leib v. Board of Examiners for Nursing* (1979), a nurse was accused of improper conduct: charting the administration of meperidine hydrochloride to her patient, but using the drug herself. After voluntarily admitting to this action, she testified on her own behalf at the board hearing. The board issued an order revoking her nursing license. The nurse appealed the revocation order to the court of common pleas. When this court

dismissed her appeal, she appealed to the Supreme Court of Connecticut. This higher court also ruled that the evidence supported the board's findings of unprofessional conduct. The nurse's license was revoked. Other cases in which courts have upheld boards' decisions include *Tighe v. State Board of Nurse Examiners* (1979) and *Ullo v. State Board of Nurse Examiners* (1979).

In *Colorado State Board of Nurse Examiners v. Hohu* (1954), a doctor filed a complaint of incompetence against a nurse, claiming that her failure to admit a patient quickly and to contact the doctor caused the patient's injury. The board of nursing ordered the nurse's license revoked. But when the nurse appealed, the court reversed the board's revocation order. This court ruled that the board of nursing had abused its discretionary powers because the evidence did not support the doctor's charges.

License reinstatement

License revocation, if sustained despite all appeal efforts, usually is permanent. Check to see whether your state's nurse practice act provides for revoked-license reinstatement.

If your license is suspended, you may petition for reinstatement. Every nurse practice act contains a provision allowing reinstatement of a suspended license, and some license-suspension orders specify a date when the nurse may apply. In most states, after a suspension has been in effect for more than a year, the board of nursing will consider reinstatement.

Your first step would probably be to petition the board for reinstatement. Then the board would have to decide whether you're qualified to practice nursing again. In some states, you have the right to another hearing before the board makes this decision.

The board usually bases its decision on current evidence of the nurse's fitness to practice. For example, in a drug violation case, the board may consider whether a nurse has successfully completed a drug rehabilitation program.

Distinguishing between nursing and medical practice

Could you describe, in a simple sentence, how nursing practice and medical practice relate to each other? Don't try. Each state's and province's nurse practice act and medical practice act are intended to distinguish between the two professions. But social, professional, and judicial forces have blurred the distinction. More and more, the public expects you to perform many tasks formerly reserved for doctors. And the law allows you to perform them. Sometimes.

Knowing precisely where nursing and medical practice acts differ and where they overlap can be difficult; relevant statutes may lack specific detail. Be aware that not knowing exactly where your practice begins and ends can create some legal risks.

When state legislatures began writing medical and nursing practice acts, a doctor could legally perform any task a nurse performed. That remains true, although many doctors today are unfamiliar with certain nursing practices. Legislatures also reserved certain tasks exclusively for doctors. In theory, a nurse performs such actions at her own legal peril. The blurring of nursing and medical responsibilities has forced corresponding changes in the law.

Forces causing change

In part, the law is responding to patients' changing expectations of nurses. Increasingly, patients are filing (and winning) lawsuits that express their expectation that nurses provide expanded patient care, including some forms of medical diagnosis, treatment, and referral. In addition, hospitals and doctors have delegated more authority to nurses. For example, nursing responsibilities in *intensive care units* (ICUs) and *critical care units* (CCUs) include diagnosis (reading electrocardiograms) and treatment (performing cardiopulmonary resuscitation).

Reductions in health care funding also have led to increased responsibilities for nurses, whose lower salaries make them less expensive than doctors.

Defining medical practice

Medical practice acts may be divided into two types: those that define medical practice and those that don't. Both types forbid non-MDs from practicing medicine. (No Canadian law related to medical practice defines it.)

When a state's medical practice act includes a definition, it usually defines medicine as any act of diagnosis, prescription, surgery, or treatment. Not every definition includes all four elements, and some states' definitions add other elements.

Legislative response

Some states have solved the problem of overlap between the nursing and medical professions by passing laws making some functions common to both. New York's law, for example, allows both RNs and doctors to diagnose and treat patients—with the *proviso* that a nursing diagnosis should not alter a patient's medical regimen. Almost all states permit you to perform any patient care a doctor requests, as long as a written or oral order exists and the requested action is reasonable and safe.

Some state medical practice acts limit doctors' rights to delegate tasks. For example, Texas's medical practice act permits doctors to delegate tasks only to "any qualified and properly trained person or persons," and then only if doing so is "reasonable and prudent," and then only if the delegating doesn't violate any other state laws. Most state courts would probably interpret their state medical practice acts similarly, even if this restriction isn't written into the acts.

In most provinces, the boards of nursing and medicine jointly determine which medical tasks may be delegated to nurses and specify the requirements for appropriate delegation.

Court rulings

The courts are regularly called on to decide if a specific action constitutes medical practice. One area of considerable overlap between nursing and medicine is *midwifery;* in the past, the courts usually decided that delivering babies was a medical rather than a nursing function. In the early case of *Commonwealth v. Porn* (1907), a Massachusetts state court upheld the conviction of a *nurse-midwife* for *practicing medicine without a license.* In the more recent case of *Leigh v. Board of Registration in Nursing* (1985), however, the same court said that the basis for conviction in the *Porn* case was not the practice of midwifery per se, but the nurse's use of obstetric instruments and prescription formulas. The court went so far as to hold that the practice of midwifery, in ordinary circumstances, isn't to be considered the practice of medicine.

Some court decisions have concluded that a doctor need not be present during patient care once he's delegated a task

to a nurse. These decisions have been interpreted to mean that a nurse may perform some medical tasks on the basis of *standing orders* and nursing protocols, as well as on the basis of doctors' written and oral orders. Consequently, a nurse's scope of actions, when working under standing orders or nursing protocols, can be broad in certain practice settings, no matter how restrictive her state nurse practice act.

Standing orders and nursing protocols usually allow you to perform tasks that involve overlap of nursing and medical practices — such as ICU, CCU, and I.V. team practice — in states where the nurse practice acts don't grant nurses clear-cut independent authority to treat patients.

Argument over anesthesia

Many court cases that test principles involving the overlap of nursing and medical practice concern anesthesia treatment and emergency department diagnosis. Interestingly, courts seldom give more than a passing reference to their state practice acts when dealing with these problems.

In *Mohr v. Jenkins* (1980), the patient sued a *nurse anesthetist,* claiming that she incorrectly injected diazepam (Valium) into his arm and so caused phlebitis. The court dismissed the suit, saying that the nurse "performed the procedure correctly and conformed to accepted medical practice." The patient appealed, but the appellate court affirmed that the standard for "specialists in similar circumstances" is "accepted medical practice," and that the defendant-nurse had met the appropriate standards.

A similar result occurred in *Whitney v. Day* (1980). In this case, a Michigan court said — without reference to the practice acts — that nurse anesthetists are professionals with expertise in an area akin to medical practice. As such, the court said, they can be held to the

---

Supervising unlicensed assistive personnel

If you supervise unlicensed assistive personnel, they are essentially practicing on your license. Limit your liability by educating yourself and encouraging your employer to establish policies that clearly delineate the responsibilities of RNs, LPNs, and unlicensed assistive personnel.

● Attend all educational programs that your employer sponsors about supervising unlicensed assistive personnel.

● Encourage your supervisors to establish a written policy that defines the actions unlicensed assistive personnel may take.

● Work cooperatively with unlicensed assistive personnel in your clinical setting. If your employer decides to use unlicensed

assistive personnel, it is in your patients' best interest to establish a solid working relationship with them.

● Educate your patients about what unlicensed assistive personnel can and cannot do for them during your assigned work time. This will help patients ask the appropriate individuals to assist them with their needs.

● If there are problems or disagreements about the appropriate functions for unlicensed assistive personnel, report them to your nurse-manager for immediate resolution.

● Stay current with your state nursing board's recommendations on the use of unlicensed assistive personnel.

---

same practice standards—those of the "similar specialist."

Avoiding medical decisions may be illegal

In some situations, you have no alternative to practicing medicine without a license, and the courts expect you to do so when a patient requires treatment. In *Cooper v. National Motor Bearing Co.* (1955), a California nurse was accused of failing to make a medical diagnosis of cancer in one of her patients. The nurse defended herself by arguing that state law at that time prohibited her from making diagnoses of any sort. The court ruled against her, finding that nurses were supposed to have sufficient education to tell whether a patient had signs or symptoms of a disease that would require a doctor's attention. In *Stahlin v. Hilton Hotels Corp.* (1973), a federal court in Illinois reached a similar conclusion when a nurse failed to recognize that her patient's complaint resulted from a sub-

dural hematoma rather than from drunkenness.

Do not assume, however, that courts always ignore the difference between medical practice and expanded nursing roles. A case in point is *Hernicz v. Fla. Dept. of Professional Regulation* (1980), which involved an advanced practice nurse who examined and treated two patients without doctors' orders. The state board of nursing suspended his license, and the court decision upheld the suspension.

In general, the courts interpret the law in ways most likely to protect patients. If protecting patients means not strictly interpreting nursing and medical practice acts, the courts usually follow that course.

Nursing practice and unlicensed assistive personnel

In addition to defining the scope of nursing practice with respect to the medical profession, nurses must also now define their responsibilities with respect to supervising unlicensed assistive personnel.

Pressures to limit health care costs are causing employers to use more unlicensed assistive personnel to help in patient care. Unlicensed assistive personnel are not new to the health care system. For years, hospitals and extended care facilities have employed nurse's aides and assistants; both of these groups fall into the category of unlicensed assistive personnel. The problem is that educational requirements and on-the-job responsibilities for unlicensed assistive personnel are not uniformly defined by statute. RNs may not have a clear understanding of what unlicensed assistive personnel are capable of doing or how to use such personnel.

The ANA has defined unlicensed assistive personnel as "individuals who are trained to function in an assistant role to the registered professional nurse in the provision of patient care activities, as delegated by and under the supervision of that nurse." Therefore, nurses are responsible for the education, training, and supervision of unlicensed assistive personnel who participate in direct patient care. However, many questions remain unanswered, including what are the educational requirements for unlicensed assistive personnel and to what extent can unlicensed assistive personnel participate in direct patient care? (See *Supervising unlicensed assistive personnel*.)

Working as an advanced practice nurse

The title of advanced practice nurse encompasses many types of practitioners, including clinical nurse specialists, certified nurse midwives, certified nurse-anesthetists, and nurse practi-

tioners. Depending on the specialty area, advanced practice nurses regularly perform functions that formerly were doctors' exclusive responsibilities. They are specially trained to make independent judgments, under a doctor's direction or order, about a patient's condition.

State boards of nursing establish requirements for obtaining an advanced practice nurse license. The board may require an advanced practice nurse to have national certification or a master's degree in a clinical specialty. For example, the nurse practice act of the state of Delaware defines an advanced practice nurse as "an individual whose education and certification meet criteria established by the board of nursing, who is currently licensed as an RN, and who has a master's degree or a post-basic program certificate in a clinical nursing specialty with national certification."

This expanded role offers nurses exciting new challenges. In addition to the tasks regularly performed by hospital staff nurses, advanced practice nurses evaluate patients' therapeutic procedures, assess changes in their health status, and manage their medical care regimens. However, anyone contemplating becoming an advanced practice nurse should first consider the legal, financial, and professional implications.

Becoming an advanced practice nurse

Depending on the specialty (such as nurse-midwife, nurse practitioner, or clinical specialist), the requirements for certification vary. Generally, an advanced practice nurse will require:
• an RN license
• a college or university degree
• at least 2 years' experience working as a nurse

• a passing grade on the specialty licensing degree.

Sitting for the licensure exam usually requires the completion of a postbaccalaureate certificate or degree program. Many state certification programs also require that you obtain approval from a hospital's medical board if you want to work in that hospital.

In addition, many states require advanced practice nurses who work in an extended care facility or clinic to meet with the facility's administrator and doctors at least once a year to review procedures, standing orders, and documentation regulations.

Limits of advanced practice nursing

Significantly, the majority of advanced practice nurses are allowed to practice only under a doctor's direction or with his orders. Without a doctor's order, these nurses can perform only traditional nursing tasks.

Because expanded roles for nurses are fairly new, questions about scope of practice frequently lack clear-cut answers. Many questions about the scope of practice are being addressed by legislation. For example, many state legislatures are writing practice guidelines regarding the authority to diagnose and treat. One of the most significant issues has been the authority to prescribe drugs. Ten states and the District of Columbia now allow nurse practitioners to prescribe drugs (including controlled substances) independent of the doctor's involvement. Another 22 states allow nurse practitioners to prescribe drugs (including controlled substances) with some degree of doctor involvement. Other states delegate some prescription writing (excluding controlled substances) to nurse practitioners, while other jurisdictions have no statutes in place to allow any prescribing authority.

Where the state legislature does not meticulously define advanced practice nursing, the court has set its own limits on the scope of practice. For example, the New Jersey Board of Medical Examiners reviewed the complaints of two patients who charged two nurse practitioners in a *health maintenance organization* with prescribing drugs and making a medical diagnosis. The ANA supported the nurses, stating that they were acting well within the nurse practice act. Although the parties settled, those complaints were the basis for stricter definitions of doctors' and nurse practitioners' responsibilities.

In a Missouri case, *Sermchief v. Gonzalez* (1983), doctors on the Board of Registration of Healing Arts accused two nurse practitioners who provided family planning services of practicing medicine. Two consulting doctors were accused of contributing to the nurses' alleged illegal practice by delegating medical tasks to them. The tasks included performing pelvic examinations and Pap smears, treating vaginitis, counseling, providing contraceptives, and inserting intrauterine devices. The nurses claimed that their tasks were valid under protocols signed by the consulting doctors. The court ruled in favor of the defendants, stating that the acts were performed pursuant to standing orders and fell within legislative standards established by statute.

As the nurse's expanded role gains more acceptance, her legal risks probably will decline — although they'll always be higher than a staff nurse's.

Liability

In lawsuits, an advanced practice nurse's liability depends on whether she is:

• an employee of an institution, such as a hospital or public health agency

PRO AND CON

Should you practice as an independent contractor?

Thousands of nurses in the United States, including advanced practice nurses and private-duty nurses, have chosen to become independent contractors. They work directly for patients (or patients' families) and bill their patients (or third-party insurers) on a fee-for-service basis. If you're considering practicing on an independent contractor basis, first weigh the pros and cons.

Pro

• You can schedule your work hours to suit your life-style.
• You can put your nursing philosophy into practice by independently planning each patient's nursing care.
• You'll be relatively free from institutional politics and bureaucracy.
• You can negotiate your own contract with each patient and set your own fee.
• You'll assume a more prestigious role in the health care community, and your working relations with other professionals may improve.
• You'll keep more of your earnings because tax laws favor self-employment.
• You can tailor your benefits package to your own personal needs.
• You can become more involved in the total care of your patient.

Con

• You'll lose the security provided by continuous employment.
• You may experience strained working relations with professionals who feel threatened by your autonomy.
• You'll have to compete for work with other nurses who also are independent contractors.
• Your patients may be admitted to hospitals or other health care institutions at which you don't have privileges.
• You'll have to educate yourself about the financial and legal aspects of running a business.
• You'll have to deal with getting patients to pay their bills.
• You'll carry the full responsibility for your liability and, if named in a lawsuit, you'll be obligated to pay the entire cost of any damages awarded to the plaintiff.

• an employee of a doctor or part of a *joint practice*
• an *independent contractor.*

If you choose to work as an advanced practice nurse, the circumstances of your employment are important in determining the type and amount of *professional liability insurance* to buy.

If you work for an institution or a doctor and lose a malpractice suit, the court applies the traditional nurse-employer doctrine — called *respondeat superior* — to determine liability. The doctrine doesn't necessarily relieve you

of *professional liability.* But if you were working within the scope of your employment, application of the doctrine makes your employer responsible for all damages a court may award to the plaintiff.

If you're sued for malpractice while working as an independent contractor, you carry the full responsibility for your liability. That means you'll have to pay the entire cost of any cash damages awarded to the plaintiff. (See *Should you practice as an independent contractor?*)

Special protection for the advanced practice nurse

If you choose to work as an advanced practice nurse, be aware of special forms of protection. For example, a written contract can offer some protection. Have an attorney draw up a contract before you begin caring for patients. Be sure it defines such important conditions as what services you're expected to perform, your fees, how and when you'll be paid, the amount of professional liability insurance (if any) your employer will carry, and how disputes will be handled. To be valid, the contract must have a legal purpose and the willing consent of both parties.

The best protection comes with maintaining the highest competence in your practice. Consider taking advanced courses and classes to improve your professional credentials and to strengthen your defense in a lawsuit.

Financial concerns

Many insurance carriers won't provide reimbursement for an advanced practice nurse's services, even though state and professional nurses' organizations have lobbied to persuade carriers to provide coverage. If you're an advanced practice nurse, or if you become one, have your patient check whether his health insurance covers your services. If it doesn't, he may not want your services — or you may have difficulty collecting your fee.

As advanced practice nursing service gains wider acceptance, insurance reimbursement will become more common.

If you work as an independent contractor, no employer withholds federal, state, or local taxes; unemployment compensation; or social security payments. You're solely responsible for keeping track of these obligations and making payments on schedule.

If you have your own office, you'll also need property liability insurance. This will protect you if someone is injured on your property. Also, establish contact with an accountant who's familiar with business-finance regulations. And consider asking an attorney to help set up your business along sound legal lines.

Professional challenges

As an advanced practice nurse, you will encounter professional challenges that are foreign to the staff nurse. For example, to be effective as an advanced practice nurse, you'll need a certain degree of cooperation and acceptance from the community in which you practice. Some communities will oppose your practice because the people feel uncomfortable with your increased responsibilities.

If you work as an independent contractor, you'll have to request local hospitals and health care institutions to grant you patient care privileges. But what if one of your patients is admitted to a hospital that won't grant you privileges? You can appeal the hospital's decision through the hospital's nursing department committee, depending on your state laws. The hospital has a legal responsibility to tell you how its appeal process works. By appealing the hospital's decision, you can learn why your request for privileges was denied. If the denial is found to be baseless, designed to limit competition with medical staff, or obliged by an exclusive contract between the hospital and another practitioner, then you have grounds for charging the hospital with unfair competition or *restraint of trade.*

Remember, you may face opposition from staff nurses concerned that your expanded role could implicate them in a malpractice lawsuit. You'll have to work at winning their trust and confidence.

Outlook for advanced practice nurses

In the future, economics will largely determine the extent of the advanced practice nurse's influence on health care. If advanced practice nurses can provide efficient medical and nursing services at reduced cost to consumers, it's likely that this expanded role for nurses will find a secure place in our health care system.

Working as a private-duty nurse

A private-duty nurse is any RN, LPN, or LVN that a patient or his family hires for total nursing care. Working as a private-duty nurse allows you to devote all your nursing skills to the care of one patient. Other advantages of working as a private-duty nurse include choosing where you work, when you work, and the type of patient you care for and setting your own fee.

Employment status is the major factor that distinguishes a private-duty nurse from an *agency* nurse. A private-duty nurse is an independent contractor. She bills her patient or a third-party insurer directly. A hospital or other health care institution also may hire a private-duty nurse. (See the discussion of *Emory University v. Shadburn*, 1933, page 46.)

Patients are referred to a private-duty nurse through *nurse registries* and referrals from other nurses and doctors who are familiar with the nurse's practice. Many hospitals maintain referral lists of private-duty nurses. If you work as a private-duty nurse long enough, you will build up a clientele of hospitals, other health care institutions, nurses, doctors, and families.

A private-duty nurse performs most of the tasks a hospital staff nurse performs, and she's expected to have the same degree of skill. She plans a patient's care, observes and evaluates his condition, reports signs and symptoms, carries out treatments under a doctor's direction, and keeps accurate records so that the patient's doctor has the data he needs to diagnose and prescribe. It is a private-duty nurse's obligation to perform her job within the scope of her state nurse practice act — the same as a staff nurse. A private-duty nurse working in a hospital can expect the hospital to provide her with adequate equipment and support services for proper patient care.

Legal risks

A private-duty nurse faces legal risks not encountered by the hospital staff nurse. For example, a private-duty nurse doesn't retain professional liability insurance through an employer. As an independent contractor, she's solely liable for any damages assessed as the result of a lawsuit — although a court may decide a hospital shares liability for her actions. So, if you work as a private-duty nurse, you must purchase professional liability insurance.

Home care

As an independent contractor, your legal risks are highest when you care for a patient in his home. You're responsible not only for providing proper care, but also for obtaining and correctly using any equipment the patient care requires, and for recognizing and acting on the need for appropriate referral. These added responsibilities naturally increase your chances of making a mistake. And because you're self-employed, legally you're solely responsible for paying court-ordered damages if you're sued and found negligent.

Making written contracts with your patient can help to reduce your legal risks. A contract spells out the conditions of your employment — but remember, having a contract doesn't prevent a lawsuit, nor can it provide evidence that definitely will exonerate you if you're sued.

Hospital care

The case of *Emory University v. Shadburn* (1933) set the precedent for a hospital's liability for a private-duty nurse's wrongful conduct. A patient jumped out a window after the assigned private-duty nurse—who had reason to know that his condition warranted continuous watching—left him unattended. The court ruled that the hospital was liable for this nurse's negligence because the hospital had hired and paid the nurse on a private-duty basis.

A hospital usually insists on tight control of a private-duty nurse's practice, both to protect patients and to demonstrate "reasonable supervision" in case of a lawsuit. Because of the trend to make hospitals share liability, you'll probably face liability alone only if you commit a negligent act despite the hospital's reasonable supervision.

Hospital controls include checking every private-duty nurse's credentials and approving her nursing qualifications. The case of *Ashley v. Nyack Hospital* (1979) established that a hospital has the right to refuse practice privileges to a nurse if the hospital doesn't approve her qualifications. Most hospitals also establish policies to govern how private-duty nursing practice relates to hospital nursing practice. Hospitals are obligated to inform all health care team members about private-duty nurses' responsibilities and rights in the hospital.

Financial burdens

If you work as an independent contractor, you must manage certain financial burdens. For example, you'll be responsible for making social security payments and for paying federal, state, and local taxes on schedule. If you're injured on a job, you won't be eligible for *workers' compensation benefits.* The courts have repeatedly rejected private-duty nurses' claims for workers' compensation. For example, in a Maryland case, *Edith Anderson Nursing Homes, Inc. v. Bettie Walker* (1963), a private-duty nurse was hurt caring for a nursing home patient who was in a wheelchair. The nurse attempted to collect workers' compensation benefits from the nursing home because her injury occurred there. The nurse was an independent contractor who was paid by the patient's family, did no work for the nursing home, and took her orders only from the patient's doctor. As an independent contractor, the court ruled, she wasn't entitled to the benefits available to the nursing home's employees. A subsequent appellate court decision upheld the denial of the nurse's claim.

Working with a private-duty nurse

If you're working on a unit on which a private-duty nurse is working, you're responsible for seeing that the private-duty nurse receives any help she needs. But your responsibility doesn't end there—you're responsible for the patient as well.

Monitor the private-duty nurse's care. If you're a staff nurse and you see the private-duty nurse negligently performing care, inform your charge nurse. If you're the charge nurse, intervene immediately. Regardless of your staff position, if you see the private-duty nurse negligently performing emergency care when the patient's life is in danger, intervene immediately. If you ignore the private-duty nurse's negligence, you and the hospital could be liable if the patient or his family files a malpractice lawsuit.

If you're a charge nurse, remember that the private-duty nurse's contract outlines her responsibilities. Read over the contract and keep its provisions in mind when you make assignments. Never assign a private-duty nurse a job that involves responsibilities not included in her contract.

Working in geriatric facilities

U.S. census statistics show that by the year 2000, Americans over age 65 will make up about 13% of the population. This trend means that more and more patients will be cared for in geriatric facilities, including nursing homes and *extended care facilities.* In fact, more patients are in geriatric facilities than in hospitals.

The rapid growth in the number of nursing homes, and nursing home patients, began in 1965, when Congress passed the Medicare and Medicaid amendments to the Social Security Act. These amendments provided government reimbursement for geriatric care.

The Medicare and Medicaid amendments also provided reimbursement for skilled nursing care in extended care facilities. These facilities initially were planned to deliver short-term nursing care to elderly patients who no longer needed intensive medical and nursing care in a hospital. Today, most of the patients admitted to extended care facilities come directly from hospitals or other health care facilities. Because many patients remain in extended care facilities for long periods, the distinction between extended care and geriatric facilities has blurred.

Substandard care

Unfortunately, many geriatric facilities provide substandard care. (See *Helping your patient select an extended care facility.*) Many geriatric facilities fail to

Helping your patient select an extended care facility

Your elderly or disabled patient may need the care provided at an extended care facility. Help the patient and his family choose a facility by explaining the three types of extended care facilities available and what type of care each offers.

Residential care facility

Best for a patient who needs minimal medical attention, this type of facility provides meals, modest medical care, and assistance with housekeeping responsibilities. Some offer recreational and social programs as well.

Intermediate care facility

The best choice for a patient who can't manage independently, this type of facility provides room, board, and daily nursing care. The cost may be covered by government subsidy programs. Some offer rehabilitation programs as well as recreational programs.

Skilled nursing facility

Best for a patient who needs constant medical attention, this type of facility provides 24-hour nursing care, medical care when needed, and such rehabilitation services as physical and occupational therapies. Depending on the patient's eligibility, Medicare or Medicaid may subsidize the cost.

meet government standards for patients' safety, nutrition, medical care, and rehabilitation; all too often, patients' rights are violated. One major problem is that geriatric facilities employ only a small number of licensed nurses. An Institute of Medicine study states that sickness and disability have increased among nursing home patients, but employers' demands for nursing services haven't kept pace. Medicare and Medicaid payments aren't sufficient to pay for adequate nursing staff. Ironically, Medicare and Medicaid payments, intended by Congress to help elderly patients, have inadvertently resulted in substandard care.

Aware of these trying circumstances, many RNs, LPNs, and LVNs working in geriatric facilities are greatly concerned about their legal rights and responsibilities. Areas of concern include *staffing patterns,* quality of care, and patients' rights.

Staffing patterns

Health care professionals use the term *minimal licensed-personnel staffing* to describe the staffing situation in many geriatric facilities. Consider the following statistics:
• Only about 1 of every 20 nursing home employees is an RN.
• Only about 1 licensed *health care professional* is employed for every 100 nursing home patients.
• Doctors spend only about 2 hours a month with their nursing home patients.
• In some extended care facilities, about 6 of 10 charge nurses on the 3-to-11 p.m. shift and about 7 of 10 charge nurses on the 11 p.m.-to-7 a.m. shift are LPNs or LVNs.

Legal risks of inadequate staffing
In most geriatric facilities, RNs hold administrative positions, shouldering broad supervisory responsibility for the quality of care. LPNs or LVNs in many facilities work as charge nurses, performing most nursing procedures and supervising *nurses' aides.* Patients may depend on nurses' aides for a substantial amount of care. This arrangement creates potential legal problems concerning both supervision and the scope of nursing practice.

Legally, a supervisor is responsible for her supervisory acts and decisions. Suppose a supervisor knows — or should know — that a subordinate is inexperienced, untrained, or unable to perform a task safely. A court may find that supervisor liable in a malpractice lawsuit for delegating such a task to the subordinate. If the subordinate performs that task negligently, she'll be liable too. And if the court finds that the supervisor and the subordinate were working within the scope of their employment, the nursing home may share liability under the doctrine of *respondeat superior.*

In determining whether the defendant-nurse's actions met professional standards for her position, the courts may review details of the staffing situation. For example, a New York court found that nurses were negligent when an unsupervised patient jumped from a balcony (*Horton v. Niagara Falls Memorial Medical Center,* 1976). The court reached this conclusion after reviewing evidence detailing the number of patients on the unit, the number of staff members, and what each staff member was doing. During this review, the court discovered that a charge nurse had permitted the only available nurses' aide to go to supper when she had the authority to prevent it, leaving the disoriented patient unsupervised.

Guidelines for avoiding liability
As an RN, LPN, or LVN working in a geriatric facility, you must practice within the legal limits set by your state nurse practice act, meet professional standards for your position, and be familiar with state regulations for the type of facility in which you work. If you're an RN, be sure you possess the management and supervisory skills

required by your job. Keep in mind that if you're sued for malpractice, you'll be judged according to how a reasonably prudent nursing supervisor would act in similar circumstances. You can't defend yourself by claiming that you weren't trained to supervise.

If you're an LPN or LVN working in a geriatric facility, remember that no person or institution can force you to practice beyond the limits outlined in your state nurse practice act. If you exceed the legally permissible scope of nursing in your state, your state board of nursing can suspend or revoke your license. You won't be able to use your employer's expectations to excuse your actions.

Under the law, an LPN or an LVN who performs a nursing function legally restricted to RNs will be held to the RN standard if she's sued for malpractice. In *Barber v. Reinking* (1966), involving an LPN who had performed an RN function, the court stated, "In accordance with public policy of this state, one who undertakes to perform the services of a trained or graduate nurse must have the knowledge and skill possessed by the registered nurse."

Quality of care

Many nurses working in geriatric facilities are particularly concerned about fragmentation of the nursing process; although an RN remains responsible for overall patient assessment and evaluation, an LPN or an LVN decides on the daily assessments, planning, and evaluation and a nurses' aide implements the assessment plan.

Fragmenting the nursing process can greatly reduce the quality of patient care. It also can have legal consequences if nursing actions are performed improperly — or not performed at all. The following list describes poor nursing practices that plague geriatric facilities:
- failing to make a nursing diagnosis
- observing a patient's condition carelessly
- failing to document
- writing illegibly when documenting
- failing to keep up with geriatric nursing knowledge
- failing to use nursing consultants
- delegating improperly
- failing to insist on clear institutional policies
- failing to question a doctor's order
- taking a dangerous patient care shortcut
- excluding family from patient care
- failing to call the doctor whenever nursing judgment indicates that a patient needs medical attention.

Patients' rights

Many states have enacted patients' rights legislation patterned after the *Patient's Bill of Rights* published by the *American Hospital Association.* Most of these states have passed laws that make reporting maltreatment of patients a legal responsibility. Some states have even established an *ombudsman's* office that has the authority to investigate complaints of abuse and the obligation to post complaint procedures in all geriatric facilities.

On the federal level, the Omnibus Budget Reconciliation Act of 1987 dramatically strengthened the rights of nursing home residents. The law says that nursing home residents have the right to choose a personal attending physician, to participate in planning their own care and treatment, and to be free from physical or mental abuse, corporal punishment, and physical or chemical restraints imposed for purposes of discipline or convenience. The law also imposes new requirements for additional nursing staff. In 1989, the

Department of Health and Human Services, in an effort to carry out the 1987 law, issued new rules governing Medicare and Medicaid reimbursement for nursing homes.

Steps you can take

If you work in a geriatric facility, you should request that your institution:

• require a patient's signature for any release of information

• clearly specify who has access to medical records, and impose penalties for unauthorized disclosure of patient information

• foster a patient's right to know about his condition and provide for *informed consent* for his treatment

• help combat *drug abuse* and misuse by requiring that nurses administering drugs know the drugs' effects and know how to assess a patient's changing needs

• ensure prompt, effective communication between doctors and nurses

• acknowledge and respect a patient's right to refuse treatment

• encourage nurses to evaluate the quality of nursing services

• encourage nurses to work cooperatively with patient representatives and accreditation agencies

• restrict the use of chemical and physical restraints. Restraints should be used only when the patient's physical or mental status gives evidence that they're necessary (and even then only with a doctor's order).

Protecting your job

Most health care professionals are patient-rights advocates, but advocating your patient's rights may lead to conflicts with your co-workers and employers. This is one of the paradoxes of nursing practice: You have a professional obligation to protect your patient's constitutional rights — but doing so could cost you your job. Unfortunately, your legal protection in this situation is limited. If you're an employee working without a contract, you can be dismissed for any reason your employer wants to give. You do have legal grounds to protest your dismissal if:

• your contract clearly states that you can't be fired on these grounds

• your facility guarantees you the *right to notice* and a hearing before dismissal

• your state's laws prevent your employer from retaliating if you report violations to the appropriate agency

• you're a government employee and can claim the First Amendment right to free speech.

Opportunities and risks

In a geriatric facility, in which doctors' involvement with patients is limited, RNs, LPNs, and LVNs have a good opportunity to grow professionally and to affect the quality of patient care. If you're an RN, you'll learn not only geriatric nursing, but also good management. If you're an LPN or an LVN, you may have the chance to fill a charge nurse position and to expand your nursing skills. Depending on the limits of your nurse practice act, you also may learn how to perform nursing assessment and patient teaching. For all nurses, along with opportunity comes responsibility — for practicing within legal limits and for continuing your education to meet professional standards.

Working in an alternative practice setting

Practicing nursing outside of traditional settings — such as hospitals, clinics, and nursing homes — dates back to the 19th century; back then, most nurses worked outside hospitals: in doctors' offices, in patients' homes, and on battlefields. Today, many nurses choose to practice in alternative settings. Their employers include factories, schools, community *public health services,* insurance companies, and *claims review agencies* (see *Providing nursing care in alternative settings,* pages 52 and 53, and *Legal considerations in hospice care,* page 54).

When working in an alternative setting, you may not have anything like the legal services of a hospital's administration to help you out during a dispute. You must take on the special challenge of knowing your legal responsibilities.

Professional standards

Most state nurse practice acts don't discuss professional standards for nurses working in alternative settings. However, you still must meet the same practice standards as a hospital nurse. If you violate those standards, your state board of nursing may suspend or revoke your license, just as it would if you were a hospital nurse, and your patient may sue you for malpractice.

Courts have traditionally held nurses who work in alternative settings to state standards for nursing practice. A California malpractice case, *Cooper v. National Motor Bearing Co.* (1955), concerned an occupational health nurse who failed to diagnose suspected cancer and so didn't refer the patient for further evaluation and treatment. At the trial, the court ruled that the only point of law to be considered in deciding the case was whether the nurse met the standards of nursing practice in her area. When expert testimony showed that she had breached those standards, the court found her negligent. Her occupational setting was irrelevant to the court's decision. Similar court cases illustrating this principle include *Planned Parenthood of Northwest Ind. v. Vines* (1989), *Barber v. Reinking* (1966), and *Stahlin v. Hilton Hotels Corp.* (1973).

The Canadian approach to such cases is similar to the American approach.

In *Dowey v. Rothwell* (1974), a nurse who worked in a doctor's office knew that an epileptic patient was about to have a seizure, yet she failed to stay with the patient. This patient did have a seizure, fell, and fractured an arm. The court found that the nurse failed "to provide that minimum standard of care which a patient has a right to expect in an office setting." The court based its findings on testimony about the expected performance standards of experienced RNs in many settings.

Protection from liability

Nurses who work in alternative settings are sometimes protected against liability suits.

For example, if you work for a government agency, you may be immune from lawsuits because of the doctrine of *sovereign immunity.* Depending on the state in which you're working, this immunity may be complete or partial. Check with your personnel office or agency attorney. (See *Understanding sovereign immunity,* page 55.)

If you work for a privately owned business, such as an insurance company or small medical practice group, you are vulnerable to malpractice suits. In some states, however, you can't be sued by a fellow employee you've treated for a job-related injury. State workers' compensation laws, which protect the employer from excessive business costs, also protect you.

Purchasing professional liability insurance

Most private medical employers have coverage that includes the nurses they employ, but private industrial employers, especially small companies, may not. Check your employer's coverage thoroughly: If you have any doubt about whether you're fully protected, consider buying your own insurance.

(Text continues on page 54.)

Providing nursing care in alternative settings

Nurses choose to practice in alternative practice settings for many reasons: to take on greater challenges and achieve more responsibility, to increase their earning power, or to make an impact on public health policy.

The list below describes in detail some of the important options for nurses today: school nursing, occupational health nursing, community health nursing, and hospice nursing. You'll also find descriptions of nursing opportunities in the business world: working as a case coordinator for an insurance company, legal consultant, or making it on your own as an entrepreneur.

School nurse

When working in the schools, your responsibilities include providing nursing care for sick or injured students and giving first aid in emergencies. When authorized by the school doctor, you will administer medications to students. Other tasks include:
- helping the school doctor give routine examinations
- giving annual screening tests – for example, vision, audiometry, and scoliosis tests – and referring students for further testing or treatment when appropriate
- counseling parents and students
- meeting with teachers and other staff members about health problems and health education programs
- enforcing state immunization policies for school-age children
- visiting sick or injured students at home when necessary
- helping identify and meet special needs of handicapped students.

Occupational health nurse

Your primary responsibility as an occupational health nurse will be to provide nursing care for sick or injured employees. Other responsibilities include:
- giving first aid in emergencies
- performing medical screening tests or helping the doctor perform them
- referring sick or injured employees for appropriate treatment
- counseling employees on health matters
- meeting with management regarding health-related issues
- developing and maintaining employee medical records
- maintaining records for government agencies such as workers' compensation agencies, the Occupational Safety and Health Administration, and state or federal labor and health departments
- alerting management to potential health and safety hazards.

Community health nurse

Numerous opportunities exist for nurses willing to provide care for patients in the community. This frequently involves visiting the sick or injured in their homes. Other community health nursing responsibilities include:
- referring patients for treatment, when appropriate
- coordinating patient care services with patient, family, and health care staff
- communicating regularly with patients, families, and other health care staff
- supervising home health aides and other community health workers
- helping to plan community health care by helping your agency to define and set priorities

Providing nursing care in alternative settings   continued

• working with other professionals to identify and evaluate threats to community health, such as communicable diseases

• working with private-sector community health workers, such as visiting nurses

• working as a public school nurse, when needed.

Hospice nurse

Your most important responsibility will be to provide skilled nursing care to the terminally ill patient. Expect to focus on providing pain relief and symptom control. Your patient and his family will rely heavily on you for emotional and psychosocial support. Your professional satisfaction will come from knowing that you have helped the dying patient maintain dignity and make the most of the time he has left.

Nursing case coordinator for an insurance company

When working for an insurance company, your responsibilities may include reviewing records and assessing insurance claims by talking to the patient, his doctor, his family, and his employer. You may be asked to help design patient care plans. These care plans frequently include medical, nursing, social service, and payment goals. You also may monitor the patient's progress and prognosis by talking to the patient and his doctors. Other tasks may include:

• helping to coordinate medical, rehabilitation, and other services

• supervising other nursing case reviewers

• developing and maintaining insurance company records.

Nurse entrepreneur

To be an entrepreneur, you must organize and manage your own business undertaking. You take on the risk of failure for the sake of potential profit. Your opportunity to apply nursing skills as an entrepreneur is limited only by your own imagination. For example, nurses have established successful businesses providing such services as reviewing medical records and performing research for insurance companies and personal injury lawyers; finding medical experts for testimony in medical malpractice actions, personal injury litigation, and workers' compensation matters; and developing educational programs for use inside hospitals.

Nursing in the legal arena

Legal nurse consultants provide valuable support during the investigation and litigation of claims, serve as expert witnesses, and review medical records. Many nurses work as independent contractors to provide these services to law firms.

Nurse expert witnesses provide advice during litigation and testify in court about nursing issues. While there is no special training for the witness role, an attorney will consider nursing experience and credentials when choosing an expert witness.

Nurses who pursue additional education may become attorneys or paralegals. Nurse paralegals primarily research law and write reports as well as organize and examine medical records in medical negligence cases.

Legal considerations in hospice care

If you work in a hospice, be aware of these special legal responsibilities toward your patient:

Standing orders

A hospital staff nurse can follow standing orders for pain medication. When working in a hospice, however, never rely on standing orders as authorization to administer pain medication. Always obtain specific orders signed by the patient's doctor.

Advice on making a will

In a hospice, never give your patient advice concerning his will. If he asks for advice, tell him you can't help him. Suggest that he discuss the matter with his attorney or family members.

Living wills

Unlike the hospital nurse, whose duty with respect to living wills varies from state to state, the nurse who works in a hospice must respect the patient's living will. Don't violate it in any way, unless a court order instructs you to do so.

You also may need your own professional liability insurance if you work for a peer review organization or a state or federal government agency, unless the law grants you complete immunity from job-related lawsuits.

Your rights as an employee

If you choose to make your career in an alternative setting, take time to investigate your rights as an employee. Your legal position may be somewhat different than if you had chosen to work on a hospital staff.

Joining a union

You usually retain the right to join a union. In fact, if you work as an occupational health nurse in a factory with a *closed shop*, you may be required to join a union.

If you work for a state or local government, state laws may permit you to join a union but forbid your union to strike. Remember that the National Labor Relations Act exempts state and local government and so doesn't protect government nurses — such as community health nurses and public school nurses — in unionization disputes.

Termination of employment

Whether you work in an alternative setting or a hospital, nothing but a contract clause, a union agreement, or a civil service law can legally protect you from being fired. Even if you have such protection, you may be vulnerable to discretionary firing until after an initial probationary period. After this period, any of these forms of protection guarantees you the right to appeal your employer's decision.

Workers' compensation

If you work in an alternative setting, you should know what coverage your employer as well as your state, federal, or Canadian provincial government provide for on-the-job injuries. Workers' compensation will usually cover you. But not always.

Most states and provinces require that most privately owned businesses participate in workers' compensation plans. If you work for such a business, you'll probably receive workers' compensation for job-related injuries. But you should be aware that if the money you receive from this fund is inadequate, workers' compensation laws prevent you from suing your employer for additional *compensation.*

If you work for a small office
If you work for an employer with few employees or limited income (for instance, a doctor with a small practice), you may not be covered by workers' compensation. That's because some states don't require such employers to participate in the workers' compensation plan. If you're in this situation, you can sue your employer directly for any job-related injury.

Most of these employers buy their own insurance to cover workers' injuries. If your employer doesn't have such insurance, you can buy your own insurance.

If you work for the government
If you work for a state or federal government agency, you may receive compensation from the state workers' compensation plan or by making a claim under a state or federal *tort claims act,* depending on the applicable laws. However, if the sovereign immunity doctrine applies, you may not be eligible for any compensation.

If you are eligible for workers' compensation, it usually covers any on-the-job injury. For example, if you're a school nurse and a student kicks you, workers' compensation normally will cover you. You also usually have the legal right to sue the person who caused the injury.

Assuming that you win your lawsuit, the court will consider any money you've already received, either from workers' compensation or from other insurance, in deciding the amount of damages you should receive. Because lawsuits are costly and can take years to resolve, most nurses don't sue.

Understanding sovereign immunity

The doctrine of sovereign immunity goes back to the days when a person couldn't sue a sovereign or his agents unless the sovereign consented. In the United States, the courts transferred this privilege, applicable in most circumstances, to the elected government and its appointed agents—government employees. So government employees ordinarily can't be sued for their on-the-job mistakes.

Unfair results
In the past, this immunity has had some unfair results. A patient harmed in a private hospital could sue the hospital and its employees, but a patient harmed in a municipal or state hospital could not.

Perhaps because of this immunity, public hospitals gained a reputation for substandard practice; the public suspected that because public hospitals couldn't be sued for malpractice, their standards of care were lax.

Legislative action
In recent decades, most state legislatures have recognized the unfairness of this system. Many have passed laws that allow patients to sue public hospitals and other government agencies on a full or limited basis. In some states, legislatures have created special courts—usually called courts of claims—in which such lawsuits must be heard. Many state legislatures have set dollar limits on the amount a patient can recover from a government agency if he wins his suit.

Working as an agency nurse

Temporary-nursing service agencies represent an innovative approach to the delivery of nursing services — one response to the constant demand for practical, efficient, and cost-effective nursing care. Many nurses decide to work for a temporary-nursing service to achieve greater work schedule flexibility and the right to choose their own hours. In addition, most agencies pay higher salaries than hospitals.

When you work for an agency, you have an employee-employer relationship with that agency. The agency charges a fee for your services and pays your salary from that fee. It also may provide such benefits as social security and other tax deductions, workers' compensation, sick pay, and professional liability insurance. Traditional nursing registries don't enter into employee-employer relationships with private-duty nurses when they provide client referrals.

Few clear-cut policies
A nurse's professional responsibilities as an agency worker often are vague. No set of uniform policies and procedures has yet been formally identified or administratively defined. For example, if an RN and an LPN are assigned to care for the same patient in his home but on different shifts, what responsibility does the RN have for the LPN's work? Is the RN responsible for supervising home health aides? Also, should communication between the RN and the patient's doctor be direct or channeled through an agency supervisor?

Large agencies, especially those with nationwide placement, may have specific policies to deal with situations like these. But smaller regional agencies may not. Without clear-cut guidelines, you may have to rely heavily on your professional nursing judgment. But remember, the courts apply the same legal principles governing staff nurse malpractice cases to agency nurse malpractice cases.

Determining liability

A nurse is liable for her own wrongful conduct. She can't escape liability if a court makes that decision. But if an agency nurse is judged to have been working within the legally permissible scope of her employment, the agency is held vicariously liable and is required to pay any damages awarded to the plaintiff. The court may use the doctrine of *respondeat superior* to interpret the nurse's legal status. This doctrine makes an employer responsible for the negligent acts of his employees — so the agency is responsible for the actions of the nurses it employs. If the court finds that the nurse exceeded the scope of her employment, she is solely responsible for any damages.

As an agency employee, you may be assigned to work in a patient's home, to care for a single patient in a hospital or other health care institution, or to temporarily supplement an institution's staff. These different practice circumstances can influence how a court determines liability. Any malpractice lawsuit that involves an agency nurse will probably name as defendants the nurse, the temporary-nursing service agency and, if applicable, the hospital or other health care institution in which the alleged malpractice happened. When you work as an agency nurse in a patient's home, your agency-employee status usually is clear-cut. The same is true when you care for a single patient in a hospital or other health care institution.

The courts have more difficulty assigning legal liability in cases that involve agency nurses working as supplemental hospital or institutional staff. In this situation, you're still an agency employee, but you're also in the "special service" of another "employer"—the hospital or institution.

Courts may apply the "borrowed servant" (or *ostensible agent*) doctrine, holding that the regular employer (the agency) isn't liable for an injury negligently caused by the nurse-employee (the "servant") while in the special service of another employer (the hospital). When a court interprets a case this way, the legal liability shifts from the agency to the hospital or institution. However, under the doctrine of *dual agency*, the nurse may be held to be the agent of both the agency and the hospital.

Professional guidelines

To help protect yourself against a lawsuit, be sure you fully understand what's expected of you when you accept an agency job. Be prepared to adjust to different policies and procedures. When you work in a patient's home, for example, your agency's policies and procedures govern your actions. Be sure you understand them thoroughly and follow them carefully. How competently you follow procedures may affect such matters as whether a claim for workers' compensation is allowed or whether your agency will be included as a defendant with you in a malpractice suit. Don't perform any nonnursing functions when you work in a patient's home or arbitrarily change his nursing regimen from what your agency has specified. If you do and the patient or his family decides to sue, you may find yourself solely liable.

ANA guidelines

The ANA has issued guidelines outlining the responsibilities of temporary-nursing agencies and agency nurses. These guidelines say that an agency has a duty to select, orient, evaluate, and assign nurses and to provide them with professional development. According to these guidelines, agency nurses should:
• keep their licenses current
• select reputable employers
• maintain their nursing skills
• observe the standards of professional nursing practice
• document their nursing practice
• adhere to the policies and procedures of their agencies and clients.

The last point is particularly important if an agency assigns you to work in a hospital or other health care institution. As always, you must be sure you understand the hospital's or institution's policies and procedures for the nursing tasks you're expected to perform. Get to know the head nurse or unit supervisor, and seek clarification from her whenever you're in doubt.

The hospital or institution, in turn, is obligated to supply equipment you need for patient care and to keep its premises and equipment in safe condition.

Working with an agency nurse

If you're a hospital staff nurse and an agency nurse is assigned to your unit, your responsibilities as a co-worker are no different than when working with others on the health care team. If you see her performing a procedure in a way that may harm her patient, you have the same responsibility to stop the procedure that you'd have when working with your regular health team colleagues. If you see an agency nurse perform a procedure incorrectly but without potential harm to the patient, report your observation to your nursing supervisor.

Controversy over agency nursing

Because of the nursing shortage, health care institutions suffer frequent imbalances in the number of nurses available to work regularly scheduled shifts. Temporary-nursing service agencies provide a valuable service by supplying skilled nurses on short notice. However, use of agency-provided RNs, LPNs, and LVNs as supplemental staff in hospitals, nursing homes, and extended care facilities is a fairly new and controversial practice. Critics point out problems — for example, inequities in salaries between hospital and agency nurses performing the same functions may lead to morale problems. Proponents of agency-based supplemental staffing, on the other hand, stress the cost-effectiveness of the practice and believe that its flexibility helps to keep nurses working and prevents nurse burnout. Proponents and critics alike urge that nursing administrators plan supplemental staffing programs instead of bringing in agency nurses on a few hours' notice before a shift begins. Adequate planning helps to maintain quality and continuity of patient care.

Potential legal precedent

So far, no plaintiff in a lawsuit has ever charged a hospital with inadequate staffing caused by a failure to obtain available supplemental staff from an agency. But observers of the nursing profession believe that this may happen soon. Already, in the Louisiana case *McCutchon v. Mutual of Omaha Insurance Co.* (1978), a court has required an insurance company to pay the agency fees of two LPNs recruited to care for a critically ill patient whose doctor had ordered RNs (and whose insurance policy allowed payment only for RNs). The court reached its decision after reviewing evidence that neither the temporary-nursing service agency, the hospital, nor the insurance company could locate any available RNs at the time the LPNs were assigned. The court also considered the fact that the assigned LPNs were closely supervised by an RN at all times.

Working in home care

More and more patients are receiving nursing care in their homes. What's more, nursing care measures implemented in the patient's home are becoming increasingly sophisticated. While every hospital has similar characteristics, every home is unique. Each represents a different pattern of legal risks and an unknown constellation of personal relationships.

One factor that will clearly alter your potential liability as a home health nurse is your degree of control over the home environment. The home environment is much less controlled than the hospital environment. For example, situations that result in liability in the hospital, such as safety hazards, may have a different outcome in home care litigation because the health care provider has little control over the home setting.

If you work for a home health agency and your responsibilites include managing other home health workers, keep in mind that it is more difficult to evaluate personnel who work in the patient's home. Negligent training of a home health worker may form the basis for legal action. In *Loton v. Massachusetts Paramedical, Inc.* (1989), the patient was left unattended in a shower by a personal care worker employed by a home care company. The worker left the apartment to go to another part of the building to do laundry. While the patient was alone, the temperature of the water became very hot. As the patient tried to readjust the water, she fell from the shower seat and inadvertently moved the temperature control to the hot zone. Due to her underlying disability, she was unable to move away from the scalding water. When the worker returned, she was unable to reach her supervisor. She then applied ice to the burns and waited before calling an ambulance. The patient suffered third-degree burns over a large portion of her body, which necessitated many operations and skin grafts.

The plaintiff alleged that the home care agency was negligent in failing to educate personnel about managing patients with disabilities and also in not training staff for the appropriate response in emergency situations. The jury rejected the defense and awarded the plaintiff $1 million.

In addition to civil claims for malpractice and negligence, a home health provider or agency may be held for criminal actions in cases of serious neglect. In *Caretenders v. Commonwealth* (1991), the patient had been receiving home health service. She was admitted to the hospital with many pressure ulcers, some of which had extended to the bone. The woman looked unwashed and had an odor of necrotic material. An indictment was brought against the home care agency, the administrator of one of its offices, a visiting nurse employed by the company, and an LPN who worked in the agency's nursing and supportive care program. The charge involved knowingly and willfully neglecting the patient, causing serious mental and physical injury. Following a jury trial, the company was convicted of a class A misdemeanor and fined over $8,000.

Selected references

Auttonberry, D. "Risk Management and Non-employed Nurses," *Nursing Management* 26(9):70, 72, September 1995.

Brazen, L. "Continuing Professional Education: A State of Transition and Transformation," *Seminars in Perioperative Nursing* 4(1):31-37, January 1995.

Catalano, J.T. *Ethical and Legal Aspects of Nursing*, 2nd ed. Springhouse Notes Series. Springhouse, Pa.: Springhouse Corp., 1995.

Faherty, B. "Legal Nurse Consultants: Who Are They?" *Journal of Nursing Law* 2(1):37-50, 1995.

Iyer, P. "Mastering the Expert Witness Role," *Journal of Nursing Law* 1(2):35-45, Winter, 1994.

"Legislation Regarding Advanced Practice Nursing Abundant in Past Year," *AORN Journal* 59(3):707-08, 711, 713-14, March 1994.

Pearson, L.J. "Annual Update of How Each State Stands on Legislative Issues Affecting Advanced Nursing Practice," *Nurse Practitioner* 20(1):13-14, 16-18, 21-24, January 1995.

Pietro, J.B. "The Legal Side: Can a Lawsuit Cost You Your License?" *AJN* 95(2):70, February 1995.

Sellards, S., and Mills, M.E. "Administrative Issues for Use of Nurse Practitioners," *Journal of Nursing Administration* 25(5):64-70, May 1995.

Shaw, M.C. "The Discipline of Nursing: Historical Roots, Current Perspectives, Future Directions," *Journal of Advanced Nursing* 18(10):1651-56, October 1993.

Sullivan, G.H. "Home Care: More Autonomy, More Legal Risks," *RN* 57(5): 63-64, 67-69, May 1994.

2

Patient's rights

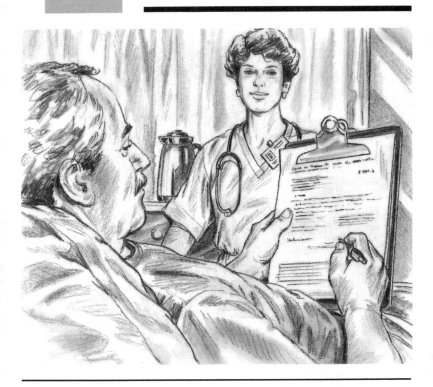

P atients are more knowledgeable, assertive, and involved in their health care than ever before. They question their diagnoses, seek assurances that their treatment is appropriate, and take action when care doesn't meet their expectations. When truly disgruntled with care, patients are more and more likely to initiate a *malpractice* suit. Sooner or later, health care providers must confront the reality that patients are prepared to assert their rights.

Your role in patient's rights

At one time, nurses were forbidden to give patients even the most basic information about their care or health. Doctors alone could answer questions about a patient's condition.

In the 1960s, large-scale questioning of authority caused a fundamental change in attitude. Patients began demanding more information about their care. Because nurses were the most approachable and most readily available health care providers, patients naturally turned to them as an information resource.

This chapter will help you apply sound legal principles when confronted with questions regarding your patient's rights in everyday nursing practice. It begins with a discussion of the evolution of patient's rights and goes on to outline your responsibilities in assuring *informed consent,* protecting your patient's right to refuse treatment, and upholding his right to *privacy.* You'll find summaries of major Supreme Court rulings on the right to die and reproductive rights issues. You'll learn when you *can* disclose confidential information, what steps to take when the patient leaves the hospital against medical advice, and how to avoid *false imprisonment* charges. Finally, you'll learn how to take responsibility for upholding the patient's dignity after his death.

Documents upholding patient's rights

Bills of rights for patients, endorsed by major health care providers and consumer groups, have helped to reinforce the public's assertive attitude. These documents define a person's rights while receiving health care. They help to protect his basic human rights at a time when he is most vulnerable.

Some consumers, civil rights activists, and attorneys believe that a patient's bill of rights is unnecessary. They claim that it simply reiterates the rights that already exist under the law. Proponents argue that these bills help to make patients aware that they have recourse to the health care institution's *grievance procedures.*

Bills of rights for patients are designed to protect such basic rights as human dignity, privacy, *confidentiality,* informed consent, and refusal of treat-

ment. They also assert the patient's right to receive a full explanation of the cost of medical care and to be fully informed before participating in experimental treatments.

Bills promoted by consumer groups focus on the patient's right to control his own health care. These bills emphasize the patient's right to information about all aspects of his care.

Strengthening patient's rights

The concept of a patient's rights is a relatively recent development in the health care field. (See *Landmarks in the evolution of patient's rights,* page 62.) The first professional group to publish a statement on patient's rights, in 1959, was the *National League for Nursing (NLN).* In its position statement, "What People Can Expect of Modern Nursing Practice," the NLN called the patient a partner in health care whose ultimate goal is self-care. Patient's rights received increasing public support during the 1960s as more people became aware of their rights as consumers. In a 1962 message to Congress, President John F. Kennedy further heightened this awareness when he outlined four basic consumer rights: the right to safety, the right to be informed, the right to choose, and the right to be heard.

The American Hospital Association *(AHA),* in 1973, issued its "Statement on a Patient's Bill of Rights." The statement — the result of a study the AHA had conducted with consumer groups — listed 12 patient rights. (See *AHA patient's bill of rights,* pages 63 and 64.) That same year, the Pennsylvania Insurance Department (PID) developed the "Citizens Bill of Hospital Rights," the first patient's bill of rights formulated by a government agency. This bill outlined the kinds of treatment a patient should expect in a hospital. It pointed out omissions in the AHA doc-

(Text continues on page 64.)

Landmarks in the evolution of patient's rights

A spirit of paternalism dominated health care until the 1970s and severely limited the rights of patients. Thanks in part to the growth in consumer activism, more attention is being paid to the rights of consumers of health care. It is interesting to note that despite the progress that has been made to date, nowhere is a person guaranteed an absolute right to health care.

1959: The National League for Nursing issues first patient's bill of rights, outlining seven points to help patients understand nursing care.

1973: The American Hospital Association (AHA) draws up patient's bill of rights, listing 12 patient rights.

The same year, Pennsylvania Insurance Department issues the "Citizens Bill of Hospital Rights," the first bill developed by a government agency that told patients what they had a right to expect from hospitals.

Also in 1973, Minnesota passes a patient's bill of rights, modeled after the AHA bill, becoming the first state to establish a bill of rights as law.

1973–1978: Congress enacts a series of laws designed to protect the rights of handicapped people. These laws include the Rehabilitation Act of 1973, the Community Mental Health Amendment of 1975, Education for Handicapped Children Act of 1975, the Developmentally Disabled Assistance and Bill of Rights Act, and the Rehabilitation Comprehensive Services and Development Disability Amendment of 1978.

1976: The New Jersey Supreme Court rules in the *Quinlan* case, granting the parents of Karen Ann Quinlan, who was in a persistent vegetative state, permission to remove her ventilator. This is the first court case to use the constitutional right to privacy as a basis for withdrawing life support.

1980: The U.S. government passes the Mental Health Systems Act (MHSA), which includes a bill of rights for patients receiving mental health services. Although much of this statute is later repealed, several states adopt recommendations found in the MHSA bill of rights.

1987: President Ronald Reagan signs the the Omnibus Budget Reconciliation Act, which includes provisions to protect the rights of patients receiving long-term care. Under the law, nursing homes can be fined up to $10,000 a day for violating a patient's rights.

1990: The U.S. Supreme Court rules in the *Cruzan* case. The parents of Nancy Cruzan requested that their daughter's feeding tube be removed after she had spent several years in a persistent vegetative state. The Supreme Court refused their request, saying that under the Constitution, a state had the right to require clear and convincing evidence that the patient wanted life-sustaining treatment withheld. This ruling implies that when there is such evidence, the patient's desires will be respected.

1991: The Patient Self-Determination Act goes into effect. This federal law calls for hospitals, nursing homes, health maintenance organizations, hospices, and home health care agencies that participate in Medicare and Medicaid to inform patients of their right (under state law) to refuse treatment if they become incapacitated.

AHA patient's bill of rights

The document below outlines the rights of the hospitalized patient. Although the American Hospital Association (AHA) patient's bill of rights has no enforcement mechanism, many hospitals use it as a model when establishing guidelines for patient care.

A patient's bill of rights

1. The patient has the right to considerate and respectful care.

2. The patient has the right to obtain from his doctor complete current information about his diagnosis, treatment, and prognosis in terms the patient can be reasonably expected to understand. When it is not medically advisable to give such information to the patient, it should be made available to an appropriate person in his behalf. He has the right to know, by name, the doctor responsible for coordinating his care.

3. The patient has the right to receive from his doctor information necessary to give informed consent prior to the start of any procedure or treatment. Except in emergencies, such information for informed consent should include but not necessarily be limited to the specific procedure or treatment, the medically significant risks involved, and the probable duration of incapacitation. Where medically significant alternatives for care or treatment exist, or when the patient requests information concerning medical alternatives, the patient has the right to such information. The patient has the right to know the name of the person responsible for the procedures or treatment.

4. The patient has the right to refuse treatment to the extent permitted by law and to be informed of the medical consequences of his action.

5. The patient has the right to every consideration of his privacy concerning his own medical care program. Case discussion, consultation, examination, and treatment are confidential and should be conducted discreetly. Those not directly involved in his care must have the permission of the patient to be present.

6. The patient has the right to expect that all communications and records pertaining to his care should be treated as confidential.

7. The patient has the right to expect that within its capacity a hospital must make reasonable response to the request of a patient for services. The hospital must provide evaluation, service, or referral as indicated by the urgency of the case. When medically permissible, a patient may be transferred to another facility only after he has received complete information and explanation concerning the needs for and alternatives to such a transfer. The institution to which the patient is to be transferred must first have accepted the patient for transfer.

8. The patient has the right to obtain information as to any relationship of his hospital to other health care and educational institutions insofar as his care is concerned. The patient has the right to obtain information as to the existence of any professional relationships among individuals, by name, who are treating him.

9. The patient has the right to be advised if the hospital proposes to engage in or perform human experimentation affecting his care or treatment. The patient has the right to refuse to participate in such research projects.

10. The patient has the right to expect reasonable continuity of care. He has the right to know in advance what appointment times and doctors are available and where. The patient has the right to

(continued)

AHA patient's bill of rights continued

expect that the hospital will provide a mechanism whereby he is informed by his doctor or a delegate of the doctor of the patient's continuing health care requirements following discharge.
11. The patient has the right to examine

and receive an explanation of his bill, regardless of source of payment.
12. The patient has the right to know what hospital rules and regulations apply to his conduct as a patient.

Reprinted with permission from the American Hospital Association,© 1992.

---

ument. The PID also warned that it would enforce the bill by stopping Blue Cross and Blue Shield payments to hospitals and other health care institutions that failed to protect the rights described in the bill. Also in 1973, Minnesota became the first state to make patient's rights a law. That law requires all state health care facilities to post Minnesota's patient's bill of rights conspicuously and to distribute it to their patients.

Since these early milestones, many states, advocacy groups, and health care organizations have developed their own patient's bills of rights. In 1990, the Advisory Board of Directors of the Hospice Association of America approved a bill of rights for *hospice* patients. (See *ACLU patient's bill of rights*, pages 65 and 66, and *Hospice patient's bill of rights*, pages 67 and 68.)

Congressional action

In 1973, Congress passed the Rehabilitation Act, which guarantees the physically or mentally handicapped person the right to any service available to a nonhandicapped person. In 1990, an expanded version of this act, called the Americans with Disabilities Act, was passed. This act prohibits discrimination on the basis of disability by employers with 15 or more employees and restricts medical testing of employees and job applicants by employers.

Other laws passed by Congress to protect the rights of handicapped people include the Community Mental Health Amendment of 1975, the Education for Handicapped Children Act of 1975, the Developmentally Disabled Assistance and Bill of Rights Act, and the Rehabilitation Comprehensive Services and Development Disability Amendment of 1978.

In 1980, Congress enacted the Mental Health Systems Act (MHSA), a comprehensive federal law on mental health services. Although much of this statute was later repealed, the MHSA Patient's Bill of Rights, which recommended that states review their mental health laws in light of patient's rights, survived. Since then, the bill has been used as a model by several states when revising their laws concerning the rights of patients suffering from mental illness.

In 1987, Congress enacted the Omnibus Budget Reconciliation Act, which included provisions that imposed dozens of new requirements on *nursing homes* and home health agencies to protect the rights of residents receiving long-term care. This law established standards for minimum RN staffing and the training of nurses' aides. Congress also mandated that patients be granted the right to immediate access to relatives and to federal and state officials who investigate *complaints.*

ACLU patient's bill of rights

The American Civil Liberties Union (ACLU) developed this patient's bill of rights as a model for health care institutions.

Preamble

As you enter this health care facility, it is our duty to remind you that your health care is a cooperative effort between you as a patient and the doctors and hospital staff. During your stay a patient's rights advocate will be available to you. The duty of the advocate is to assist you in all the decisions you must make and in all situations in which your health and welfare are at stake. The advocate's first responsibility is to help you understand the role of all who will be working with you, and to help you understand what your rights as a patient are. Your advocate can be reached at any time of the day by dialing _____. The following is a list of your rights as a patient. Your advocate's duty is to see to it that you are afforded these rights. You should call your advocate whenever you have any questions or concerns about any of these rights.

Patient rights

● The patient has a legal right to informed participation in all decisions involving his health care program.
● We recognize the right of all potential patients to know what research and experimental protocols are being used in our facility and what alternatives are available in the community.
● The patient has a legal right to privacy regarding the source of payment for treatment and care. This right includes access to the highest degree of care without regard to the source of payment for that treatment and care.
● We recognize the right of a potential patient to complete and accurate information concerning medical care and procedures.
● The patient has a legal right to prompt attention, especially in an emergency situation.
● The patient has a legal right to a clear, concise explanation in layperson's terms of all proposed procedures, including the possibilities of any risk of mortality or serious side effects, problems related to recuperation, and probability of success, and will not be subjected to any procedure without his voluntary, competent, and understanding consent. The specifics of such consent shall be set out in a written consent form, signed by the patient.
● The patient has a legal right to a clear, complete, and accurate evaluation of his condition and prognosis without treatment before being asked to consent to any test or procedure.
● We recognize the right of the patient to know the identity and professional status of all those providing service. All personnel have been instructed to introduce themselves, state their status, and explain their role in the health care of the patient. Part of this right is the right of the patient to know the identity of the doctor responsible for his care.
● We recognize the right of any patient who does not speak English to have access to an interpreter.
● The patient has a right to all the information contained in his medical record while in the health care facility, and to examine the record on request.
● We recognize the right of a patient to discuss his condition with a consultant specialist, at the patient's request and expense.
● The patient has a legal right not to have

(continued)

ACLU patient's bill of rights continued

any test or procedure, designed for educational purposes rather than his direct personal benefit, performed on him.
• The patient has a legal right to refuse any particular drug, test, procedure, or treatment.
• The patient has a legal right to privacy of both person and information with respect to the hospital staff, other doctors, residents, interns and medical students, researchers, nurses, other hospital personnel, and other patients.
• We recognize the patient's right of access to people outside the health care facility by means of visitors and the telephone. Parents may stay with their children and relatives with terminally ill patients 24 hours a day.
• The patient has a legal right to leave the health care facility regardless of his physical condition or financial status, although the patient may be requested to sign a release stating that he is leaving against the medical judgment of his doctor or the hospital.
• The patient has a right not to be transferred to another facility unless he has received a complete explanation of the desirability of and need for the transfer. If the patient does not agree to transfer, the patient has the right to a consultant's opinion on the desirability of transfer.

• A patient has a right to be notified of his impending discharge at least 1 day before it is accomplished, to insist on a consultation by an expert on the desirability of discharge, and to have a person of the patient's choice notified in advance.
• The patient has a right, regardless of the source of payment, to examine and receive an itemized and detailed explanation of the total bill for services rendered in the facility.
• The patient has a right to competent counseling from the hospital staff to help in obtaining financial assistance from public or private sources to meet the expense of services received in the institution.
• The patient has a right to timely prior notice of the termination of his eligibility for reimbursement by any third-party payer for the expense of hospital care.
• At the termination of his stay at the health care facility we recognize the right of a patient to a complete copy of the information contained in his medical record.
• We recognize the right of all patients to have 24-hour-a-day access to a patient's rights advocate, who may act on behalf of the patient to assert or protect the rights set out in this document.

Reprinted with the permission of the American Civil Liberties Union.

Under the law, nursing homes can be fined up to $10,000 a day for violating a patient's rights.

Legal status

Bills of rights that have become *laws* or state regulations carry the most authority because they give the patient specific legal recourse. If a patient be-

lieves a hospital has violated his legal rights, the patient can report the violation to the appropriate legal authority, usually the state health department. If an investigation shows that the hospital violated the patient's rights, the state will demand that the institution modify its practices to conform to state law. (In Canada, the courts usually ac-

Hospice patient's bill of rights

In 1990, the Hospice Association of America issued a bill of rights for hospice patients.

Introduction

Patients have a right to be notified in writing of their rights and obligations before their hospice care begins. Consistent with state laws, the patient's family or guardian may exercise the patient's rights when the patient is unable to do so. Hospice organizations have an obligation to protect and promote the rights of their patients, including the following:

Dignity and respect

Patients and their hospice caregivers have a right to mutual respect and dignity. Caregivers are prohibited from accepting personal gifts and borrowing from patients, families, or primary caregivers.

Patients have the right:
- to have relationships with hospice organizations that are based on honesty and ethical standards of conduct
- to be informed of the procedure they can follow to lodge complaints with the hospice organization about the care that is, or fails to be, furnished, and regarding a lack of respect for property (to lodge complaints with us, call _____)
- to know about the disposition of such complaints
- to voice their grievances without fear of discrimination or reprisal for having done so.

Decision making

Patients have the right:
- to be notified in writing of the care that is to be furnished, the types (disciplines) of caregivers who will furnish the care, and the frequency of the services that are proposed to be furnished

- to be advised of any change in the plan of care before the change is made
- to participate in the planning of care and in planning the changes in the care, and to be advised that they have the right to do so
- to refuse services and to be advised of the consequences of refusing care
- to request a change in caregiver without fear of reprisal or discrimination.

Privacy

Patients have the right:
- to confidentiality with regard to information about their health, social, and financial circumstances and about what takes place in the home
- to expect the hospice organization to release information only as consistent with its internal policy, required by law or authorized by the patient.

Finances

Patients have the right:
- to be informed of the extent to which payment may be expected from Medicare, Medicaid, or any other payer known to the hospice organization
- to be informed of any charges that will not be covered by Medicare
- to be informed of the charges for which the patient may be liable
- to receive this information, orally and in writing, within 15 working days of the date the hospice organization becomes aware of any changes in charges
- to have access, upon request, to all bills for the service the patient has received regardless of whether they are paid out-of-pocket or by another party
- to be informed of the hospice's ownership status and its affiliation with any entities to whom the patient is referred.

(continued)

Hospice patient's bill of rights continued

Quality of care

Patients have the right:
- to receive care of the highest quality
- in general, to be admitted by a hospice organization only if it is assured that all necessary palliative and supportive services will be provided that are necessary to promote the physical, psychological, social, and spiritual well-being of the dying patient; however, an organization with less than optimal resources may nevertheless admit the patient if a more appropriate hospice organization is not available, but only after fully informing the patient of its limitations and the lack of suitable alternative arrangements

- to be told what to do in case of an emergency.

The hospice organization will assure that:
- all medically related hospice care is provided in accordance with physicians' orders and that a plan of care which is developed by the patient's physician and the hospice interdisciplinary group specifies the services to be provided and their frequency and duration
- all medically related personal care is provided by an appropriately trained homemaker-home health aide who is supervised by a nurse or other qualified hospice professional.

Reprinted with permission of the Hospice Association of America.

cept a professional tribunal's decisions about patient's rights violations.)

Bills of rights issued by health care institutions and professional associations aren't legally binding. But hospitals may jeopardize federal funding, such as *Medicare* and *Medicaid* reimbursement or research funding, if they violate federal regulations or the standards of the *Joint Commission on Accreditation of Healthcare Organizations.*

You should regard bills of rights for patients as professionally binding. If your hospital has a bill of rights, you're required to uphold those rights. You're also expected to uphold the bills of rights published by professional organizations.

Interpreting patient's rights

The theory of patient's rights is clear, but the practice is full of conflict. What happens if defending a patient's rights requires that you exceed the bounds of nursing practice?

Consider the case of *Tuma v. Board of Nursing* (1979). A patient with myelogenous leukemia was admitted to a hospital in Idaho for chemotherapy. Although she had agreed to this treatment, she was openly distressed about it. Instead of asking her doctor about alternative treatment, she asked Jolene Tuma, RN, MSN, a nursing instructor at the College of Southern Idaho who supervised nursing students at the hospital. Ms. Tuma had asked to be assigned to the patient because of her interest in the needs of dying patients.

Ms. Tuma told the patient, in detail, about alternative treatments. She discussed Laetrile therapy and various natural food and herbal remedies, comparing their side effects with those of chemotherapy. She also gave the patient the name of a therapist who practiced alternative treatments and offered to arrange an appointment.

Ms. Tuma did not encourage the patient to alter her treatment plan or indicate that alternative treatments were better than the prescribed therapy or would cure her.

At the patient's request, Ms. Tuma also discussed the alternative treatments with the patient's son and daughter-in-law. They told the patient's doctor, and, as a result, he interrupted the chemotherapy until he could discuss the situation with the patient. The next day the patient again agreed to undergo chemotherapy. Two weeks later, she went into a coma and died. The patient's doctor demanded that the hospital remove Ms. Tuma from her position as clinical instructor at the College of Southern Idaho.

At the hospital's request, the board of nursing conducted an investigation and hearing. The board interpreted Ms. Tuma's behavior as unprofessional. They agreed that she had interfered with the doctor-patient relationship, and suspended her nursing license for 6 months. Ms. Tuma appealed, lost, and appealed again. This time, 3 years after the incident, the Idaho State Supreme Court declared her not guilty of unprofessional conduct because the Idaho Nurse Practice Act neither clearly defines unprofessional conduct nor provides guidelines for avoiding it.

Unanswered questions

The decision failed to define the nurse's specific role in upholding a patient's right to information. This leaves several troubling questions unanswered. For example, Ms. Tuma's patient asked her, not the doctor, for information about alternative therapies. The doctor testified that he wasn't knowledgeable about these therapies, so what recourse did that give his patient? If a doctor won't answer such questions, does the patient have the right to get answers from a nurse? Until the courts or legislatures address such questions, you won't find any easy answers.

Guidelines for upholding patient's rights

The best guideline you can follow to protect your patient's interests is the NLN's position statement on nursing's role in patient's rights. (See *NLN patient's bill of rights,* page 70.)

The NLN recommends that you view your patient as a partner in the health care process. In planning your patient's care, recognize his right to participate in decisions. Help him set realistic goals for his health care, and teach him the various approaches he can use to achieve them.

Throughout the decision-making process, keep assessing the patient's understanding of his illness. When he needs and wants more information, first determine whether you or the doctor should provide it. Then, let the patient decide on his care plan. A care plan you formulate with your patient helps you to communicate and demonstrates your respect for his wishes and rights.

Added benefits

Upholding patient's rights provides additional benefits, such as opening health care to new ideas. For example, ***nurse-midwives*** and other maternity nurses have acted as advocates for patients who challenge traditional childbirth practices. As a result, many hospitals have introduced changes, such as:
- using birthing rooms as an alternative to traditional delivery rooms
- using less ***intervention*** and medication during delivery
- allowing patients to use a birthing chair or walk at will during labor
- encouraging the company and support of a "coach" — husband, other relative, or friend — during labor and delivery.

NLN patient's bill of rights

The National League for Nursing (NLN) believes that nurses are responsible for upholding these rights of patients:

• People have the right to health care that is accessible and that meets professional standards, regardless of the setting.

• Patients have the right to courteous and individualized health care that is equitable, humane, and given without discrimination as to race, color, creed, sex, national origin, source of payment, or ethical or political beliefs.

• Patients have the right to information about their diagnosis, prognosis, and treatment—including alternatives to care and risks involved—in terms they and their families can readily understand, so that they can give their informed consent.

• Patients have the legal right to informed participation in all decisions concerning their health care.

• Patients have the right to information about the qualifications, names, and titles of personnel responsible for providing their health care.

• Patients have the right to refuse observation by those not directly involved in their care.

• Patients have the right to privacy during interview, examination, and treatment.

• Patients have the right to privacy in communicating and visiting with persons of their choice.

• Patients have the right to refuse treatments, medications, or participation in research and experimentation, without punitive action being taken against them.

• Patients have the right to coordination and continuity of health care.

• Patients have the right to appropriate instruction or education from health care personnel so that they can achieve an optimal level of wellness and an understanding of their basic health needs.

• Patients have the right to confidentiality of all records (except as otherwise provided for by law or third-party payer contracts) and all communications, written or oral, between patients and health care providers.

• Patients have the right of access to all health records pertaining to them, the right to challenge and to have their records corrected for accuracy, and the right to transfer of all such records in the case of continuing care.

• Patients have the right to information on the charges for services, including the right to challenge these.

• Above all, patients have the right to be fully informed as to all their rights in all health care settings.

The National League for Nursing urges its membership, through action and example, to demonstrate that the profession of nursing is committed to the concepts of patient's rights.

Reprinted with permission of the National League for Nursing.

Increasing interest in patient's rights has led many hospitals to employ full-time patient advocates, or *ombudsmen.* They mediate between the patient and the hospital when a patient is dissatisfied with care. Patient advocates may help you uphold your responsibilities to your patient, but advocates don't diminish those responsibilities. Whether you're an *RN, LPN,* or *LVN,* you must respect and safeguard your patient's rights.

Informed consent and the law

Suppose you're caring for a patient scheduled for surgery. He's talked to his doctor and signed the *consent form.* But the night before surgery, he doesn't seem to understand the implications of the procedure. What should you do? To answer, consider first the question, What is informed consent?

Basics of informed consent

Informed consent has two elements: *informed* refers to information given to the patient about a proposed procedure or treatment; *consent* refers to the patient's agreement to the procedure or treatment. To be informed, a patient must receive, in terms he understands, all the information that would affect a reasonable person's decision to consent to or refuse a treatment or procedure. The information should include:
• a description of the treatment or procedure
• the name and qualifications of the person who'll perform the treatment or procedure
• an explanation of the potential for death or serious harm (such as brain damage, paralysis, or disfiguring scars) or for discomforting side effects during or after the treatment or procedure
• an explanation and description of alternative treatments or procedures
• a discussion of the possible effects of not having the treatment or procedure.

The patient also must be told that he has a right to refuse the treatment or procedure without having other care or support withdrawn, and that he can withdraw his consent after giving it. (See *Informed consent: A landmark ruling,* page 72.)

Standards for informed consent

The *duty* to provide informed consent raises a difficult question: How much information is enough? To help answer this question, the courts have developed two standards: the reasonable doctor standard and the reasonable patient standard.

Reasonable doctor standard

Also called the malpractice model, the reasonable doctor standard is the standard used by most courts today. This standard essentially is based on what another doctor would disclose to a similar patient under similar circumstances. A famous example is *Natanson v. Kline* (1960). In this case, the doctor failed to inform the patient of the side effects of cobalt radiation therapy. In a subsequent lawsuit, the court ruled that the doctor had a duty to disclose information "which a reasonable medical practitioner would disclose under the same or similar circumstances."

In *Kinikin v. Heupel* (1981), a Minnesota court provided a variation on the reasonable doctor standard. It ruled that a doctor must disclose as much information as any reasonable doctor would under similar circumstances, if he knew the particular patient's ability to understand.

Reasonable patient standard

The landmark decision using the reasonable patient standard occurred in *Canterbury v. Spence* (1972). In this case, a patient had a laminectomy and then fell and developed paralysis. The patient sued the doctor for failing to warn him of the inherent risks. The court ruled that the doctor had a duty to disclose as much information as he knew—or should have known—a reasonable patient would need to make an informed decision.

COURT CASE

Informed consent: A landmark ruling

The right of informed consent didn't exist at the beginning of this century. At that time, a patient had no established legal right to information about his medical treatment. If a doctor performed surgery without the patient's consent, the patient could sue for battery—legally defined as one person touching another without consent. A patient could claim battery only if he'd refused consent or hadn't been asked to give it, but not if he hadn't had enough information to make an appropriate decision.

Rare exceptions

Most battery lawsuits were unsuccessful; courts usually took the doctor's word over the patient's. Two cases that patients did win were *Mohr v. Williams* (1905), in which the patient consented to surgery on one ear, but the doctor performed it on both, and *Schloendorff v. Society of New York Hospitals* (1914), in which the patient consented to an abdominal examination, but the doctor performed abdominal surgery.

Establishing a patient right

The right to receive informed consent wasn't expressed until 1957, when the California Supreme Court introduced the theory in the case of *Salgo v. Leland Stanford, Jr. Univ. Board of Trustees*. This case involved a patient who had acute arterial insufficiency in his legs. The doctor recommended diagnostic tests but failed to describe the tests or their risks. The day after the patient underwent aortography, his legs became permanently paralyzed. The court found the doctor negligent for failing to explain the potential risks of aortography.

This decision established a basic rule: A doctor violates "his duty to his patient and subjects himself to liability if he withholds any facts that are necessary to form the basis of an intelligent consent by the patient to the proposed treatment."

Since this landmark ruling, a patient can sue for *negligent nondisclosure* if his doctor fails to provide enough information to enable him to make an informed decision.

Courts have continued to develop variations of the reasonable patient standard. The courts weigh such personal factors as a patient's intelligence, educational level, hopes, fears, and idiosyncrasies.

Informed consent under state law

Many state legislatures have passed laws supporting the standards of informed consent set by the courts. Several states have substantive laws—laws that define informed consent or specify the claims and defenses that can be made in informed consent cases.

(These include Alaska, Delaware, Hawaii, Kentucky, Nebraska, New Hampshire, Oregon, Pennsylvania, Tennessee, Texas, Utah, and Vermont.)

Many states have procedural laws on informed consent—laws that describe the *tort* of *negligent nondisclosure* and possible defenses to such a lawsuit. (These states include Florida, Maine, New York, North Carolina, and Rhode Island.) By comparison, Washington state has a law that is both substantive and procedural.

Other states, including Mississippi, Arkansas, Louisiana, Georgia, and Missouri, have laws that deal with consent but not informed consent. And still others, including Idaho, Iowa, Nevada, and Ohio, have laws limited to the legal effect of documents, such as consent forms.

Among state laws on informed consent, Georgia's is noteworthy. It states that a signed consent form disclosing the treatment in general terms is conclusive proof of a valid consent. Thus, in Georgia, a patient who signs a consent form has no legal right to claim that he didn't fully understand a medical treatment or that the doctor didn't explain the information in the consent form.

In many other states, a signed consent form is evidence of informed consent, but it's not conclusive proof. Even if a patient signs a form, he may still challenge his consent's validity in court, claiming, for example, that he didn't understand the information or that he wasn't given relevant information. Most state laws don't even require a signed consent form. Some states accept as evidence of informed consent a doctor's handwritten progress notes, stating that he discussed the proposed procedure and its risks, benefits, and alternatives with the patient, and that the patient understood and consented to the procedure.

When informed consent becomes controversial

Informed consent is required before any treatment or procedure is performed. As a nurse, you obtain consent by explaining the procedure before you perform it. At that point, any conscious, mentally competent *adult* has a right to refuse to let you perform the nursing treatment or procedure.

Controversy over informed consent centers on medical and surgical treatments and procedures that are invasive, risky, experimental, or unlikely to succeed. For these, the doctor must obtain express consent, unless delaying treatment to get consent will adversely affect the patient's health.

Therapeutic privilege

The doctrine of informed consent assumes that an informed patient can act in his own best interests. But what if information about his condition seems likely to jeopardize the patient's health? In these situations, the law may recognize a doctor's *therapeutic privilege.* This legal concept permits the doctor to withhold information he believes would jeopardize the patient's health.

Therapeutic privilege has been viewed narrowly by the courts. A doctor who exercises it is required to document why he's withholding information from the patient. He also may be required to provide the information to the patient's *next of kin.*

Responsibility for obtaining informed consent

The responsibility for obtaining a patient's informed consent rests with the person who will carry out the treatment or procedure. This usually is the *attending doctor.*

Ideally, each doctor should disclose the information necessary for informed consent and then have the patient sign a consent form. The doctor's signature on the form indicates that he appropriately obtained the patient's signature.

Your signature as a *witness* means that you saw the doctor obtain the patient's signature on the consent form. In most states, a witness is not legally required, but some hospitals have a *policy* that requires their nurses to witness patients' signatures.

Answering the patient's questions

If the patient doesn't understand the information or wants more information, you can answer any questions that are within the scope of your knowledge.

You aren't obligated, however, to answer any of the patient's questions. As a witness, you are not legally responsible for disclosing all relevant information to the patient. The doctor retains this responsibility, and he cannot delegate it to you.

If you see that a patient is confused, and you can't provide the information he needs, document your observation in the patient's chart and make sure the patient gets the information from his doctor or another appropriate source.

Your potential liability

If you know a patient has not been informed and you do nothing, you can be held legally responsible.

If the doctor performs a procedure without the patient's consent and the patient sues for *battery,* the courts might hold you responsible if:
• you took part in the battery by assisting with the treatment
• you knew that it was taking place and didn't try to stop it.

If the doctor fails to provide adequate information for consent and the patient sues the doctor for negligent nondisclosure, the courts might hold you responsible if, knowing the doctor hasn't provided adequate information to a patient, you fail to try to stop the procedure by informing your supervisor.

Treating a sedated patient

If the doctor plans to seek consent from a patient who is receiving a sedative, narcotic, or tranquilizer, make sure he is aware of the patient's medication schedule. Then the doctor can select an appropriate time to explain the procedure or treatment and thus ensure a valid consent.

If the patient receives a sedative, narcotic, or tranquilizer before the doctor explains the procedure or treatment, the doctor should evaluate the patient's mental status. If the patient's mental status is impaired, his consent will be invalid.

Treating an incompetent adult

A *mentally incompetent* patient cannot understand explanations or comprehend the results of his decisions. When a patient is incompetent, the doctor has two alternatives. He may seek consent from the patient's next of kin, usually the patient's spouse. (Legal designation of next of kin varies from state to state.) Alternatively, the doctor or hospital may petition the court to appoint a *legal guardian* for the patient. When to appoint a legal guardian remains controversial. Doctors usually go to court when they aren't comfortable with the next of kin's decision.

Mental illness and incompetence

Don't assume that mental illness is the same as *incompetence.* An increasing number of courts have upheld the constitutional right of the alert, involuntarily confined mental patient to refuse medication and treatment, even if the treatment might ameliorate his mental illness. A confined mental patient may be forcibly medicated only in an emergency when he may cause harm to himself or others. A patient who has been *adjudicated incompetent* — declared incompetent by judicial authority — may still retain the mental capacity to make an informed decision about his care.

Treating a minor

In most situations, a *minor's* consent to treatment is legally invalid, so the doctor must obtain substitute consent from the minor's parents or legal guardians. The doctor is legally obligated to disclose all relevant information to the parents or legal guardians to ensure that their consent is informed.

In some situations, a minor can give valid consent. For instance, some states allow a minor to consent to treatment of a sexually transmitted disease. Most states allow an *emancipated minor* to give consent.

To avoid deciding whether a minor is legally emancipated, a doctor usually tries to get informed consent from both the minor and his parents.

Two exceptions

There are two situations in which the legal requirement for obtaining informed consent is waived. The patient himself may waive the requirement or the urgent nature of a medical or surgical emergency may supersede the requirement.

Patient discretion

A patient has the right not to be informed. He may exercise that right by telling his doctor that he doesn't want to know the details regarding a treatment or procedure. The doctor then has two responsibilities: He must make sure that the patient understands that risks and alternatives do exist. He also should clearly document the patient's waiver of his right to receive information. In some cases, the patient may direct that information be provided to the next of kin.

Emergencies

A doctor can legally provide immediate treatment without consent to save a patient's life or to prevent loss of an organ, a limb, or a function, if the patient is unconscious or, in the case of a minor, if the family can't be reached. In such situations, the law assumes that if a patient could decide, he would choose to receive treatment.

This exception is limited. It doesn't apply if the doctor knows the patient has previously said he'd refuse such treatment if and when offered. Nor does it apply if the doctor can wait for a proper consent from the patient or his family without increasing the patient's risk. For example, a doctor may admit a minor patient with acute appendicitis, but he can't do emergency surgery without consent if he has time to obtain consent from the parents.

If you assist in emergency treatment without the patient having given consent, make sure the doctor documents his reasons for proceeding, including the specific risks the patient would face without treatment. If the doctor wants to provide emergency care without consent, but you believe that the patient could wait, tell the doctor why. If the doctor insists on treating the patient anyway, evaluate the situation. If your refusal to help would harm the patient or create an unsafe situation (a doctor caring for a patient without assistance), you should assist. In all other situations, you should refuse to participate and then notify your nursing supervisor. She, in turn, should report the *incident* to hospital administration.

When informed consent becomes invalid

Informed consent can become invalid if a change in a patient's medical status alters the risks and benefits of treatment. In such situations, the doctor must explain the new risks and benefits to make sure the patient still consents to the treatment. The doctor also must explain any new risks or benefits to a nonconsenting patient to be sure the patient still wants to refuse the treatment.

In summary

Remember that the patient has a legal right to determine the treatment he receives, and you have a professional responsibility to protect that right. (See

Right to consent: From birth to adulthood.)

Right to consent: From birth to adulthood

A person attains more medical rights as he reaches the age of majority, defined as the age when a person is considered legally responsible for all his activities and becomes entitled to the legal rights held by citizens generally.

Birth rights

From birth, everyone has the right to:
- confidentiality concerning medical records
- privacy during treatment
- legal protection from malpractice.

Minors

Anyone under age 18 or 21 (depending on the state in which he lives) has the right to consent to treatment for sexually transmitted diseases, serious communicable diseases, and drug or alcohol abuse (although the minor's parents may have to be notified).

Mature minors

In certain instances, a doctor or judge may decide that a minor is mature—has a sufficiently developed awareness and mental capacity. If so, the minor has the right to make decisions about medical care.

Adults

Anyone who's reached majority, or who's legally emancipated, has the right to:
- consent to, or refuse, medical treatment
- consent to, or refuse, medical treatment for his children in most circumstances.

The patient who refuses treatment

Any mentally competent adult may legally refuse treatment if he's fully informed about his medical condition and about the likely consequences of his refusal. As a nursing professional, you may have difficulty accepting a patient's decision to refuse treatment. For example, you may become disturbed when a patient refuses treatment he can't live without, just to avoid unpleasant side effects. But as a professional, you must respect that decision. Laws and court rulings give almost all patients the right to refuse treatment.

When your patient refuses treatment, you must understand his rights and your responsibilities. (See *When a patient says no.*)

Legal right to refuse treatment

Most court cases related to the right to refuse treatment have involved patients with a terminal illness or their families who want to discontinue life support. In one of the best-known cases, Karen Ann Quinlan's parents argued that unwanted treatment violated their comatose daughter's constitutional right to privacy. In 1976, the Quinlans successfully petitioned the New Jersey Supreme Court to discontinue her life support.

In another landmark case, *Cruzan v. Director, Mo. Dept. of Health* (1990), the parents of Nancy Cruzan petitioned to have their comatose daughter's tube feedings discontinued. In 1990, the U.S. Supreme Court held that the state of Missouri has the constitutional right to refuse to permit termination of life-sustaining treatment *unless "clear and con-*

When a patient says no

A patient must give his consent before you can perform any treatment. If the patient refuses, take the following steps:

1. Tell him the risks involved in not having the treatment performed.

2. If the patient understands the risks but still refuses, notify your supervisor and the doctor.

3. Record the patient's refusal in your nurses' notes.

4. Ask the patient to complete a refusal of treatment release form, like the one shown below. The signed form indicates that the appropriate treatment would have been given had the patient consented. This form protects you, the patient's doctors, and your institution from liability for not providing treatment.

5. If the patient refuses to sign the release form, document this in your nurses' notes.

6. For additional protection, your institution's policy may require you to get the patient's spouse or closest relative to sign another refusal of treatment release form. Document whether or not the spouse or relative does this.

Refusal of treatment release form

I, _____ , refuse to allow anyone to
                      (patient's name)

_____(insert treatment).

The risks attendant to my refusal have been fully explained to me, and I fully understand the results for this treatment and that if the same is not done, my chances for regaining normal health are seriously reduced and that, in all probability, my refusal for such treatment or procedure will seriously endanger my life.

I hereby release _____ ,
                              (name of hospital)

its nurses and employees, together with all doctors in any way connected with me as a patient, from liability for respecting and following my express wishes and direction.

_____   _____
Witness   Patient or Legal Guardian

_____   _____
Date   Age of patient

vincing evidence" exists about a patient's wishes. Because this standard was not met, the Court did not allow removal of the feeding and hydration tube. Significantly, the Court implied that when clear and convincing evidence exists, the patient's wishes will be respected.

Two months after the Supreme Court ruling, the Cruzans petitioned the local court with new evidence. A Missouri judge granted them the right to remove Nancy's feeding and hydration tube. She died shortly thereafter. Publicity about Nancy Cruzan's legal ordeal heightened the awareness of millions of Americans about the need to plan ahead for critical medical decisions.

Freedom of religion

Jehovah's Witnesses may refuse treatment on the grounds of freedom of religion. Members of this sect oppose blood transfusions based on their interpretation of a biblical passage that forbids "drinking" blood. Some sect members believe that even a lifesaving transfusion given against their will deprives them of everlasting life. The courts usually uphold their right to refuse treatment because of the constitutionally protected right to religious freedom. In the case of *In re Osborne* (1972), for example, the court respected a Jehovah's Witness's right to refuse consent.

Most other religious freedom court cases involve Christian Scientists, who oppose many medical interventions, including medicines. For example, in *Winters v. Miller* (1971), a psychiatric patient claimed she involuntarily received treatment and medications at a New York state hospital. After her discharge, she sued for damages based on a violation of her religious freedom as a Christian Scientist. The trial court *dismissed* her complaint, but an appeals court ordered a new trial on the grounds that the unwanted treatment might have violated her rights.

Besides court rulings, most *patient's bills of rights* support the right to refuse treatment, starting with the bill of rights adopted by the American Hospital Association.

Right to die

Most states have enacted right-to-die laws (also called *natural death laws* or *living will laws*). These laws recognize the patient's right to choose death by refusing extraordinary treatment when he has no hope of recovery.

Whenever a competent patient expresses his wishes concerning extraordinary treatment, health care providers should attempt to follow them. If the patient is incompetent or unconscious, the decision becomes more difficult.

In some cases, the next of kin may express the patient's desires for him, but whether this is an honest interpretation of the patient's wishes is sometimes uncertain.

Written evidence of the patient's wishes provides the best indication of what treatment he would consent to if he were still able to communicate. This information may be provided through:
• a living will — this is an advance care document that specifies a person's wishes regarding medical care should he become terminally ill and incompetent or unable to communicate. (See *Living will.*) In some states, living wills don't address the issue of discontinuing artificial nutrition and hydration.

• a *durable power of attorney* — here the patient designates a person who will make medical decisions for him if he should become incompetent to do so. This differs from the usual form of *power of attorney,* which requires the patient's ongoing consent and deals only with financial issues. (See *Durable power of attorney,* pages 81 and 82.)

All states recognize living wills as legally valid, and most states have laws authorizing durable powers of attorney

Living will

The living will is an advanced care document that specifies a person's wishes with regard to medical care should he become terminally ill and incompetent or unable to communicate. The will applies to decisions that will be made by a person the patient has designated, only after the terminally ill patient has no reasonable possibility of recovery. The will is often used in combination with the patient's durable power of attorney.

All states and the District of Columbia have living will laws that outline documentation requirements. The sample document below is from Nebraska.

Nebraska Declaration

If I should lapse into a persistent vegetative state or have an incurable and irreversible condition that, without the administration of life-sustaining treatment, will, in the opinion of my attending physician, cause my death within a relatively short time and I am no longer able to make decisions regarding my medical treatment, I direct my attending physician, pursuant to the Rights of the Terminally Ill Act, to withhold or withdraw life-sustaining treatment that is not necessary for my comfort or to alleviate pain.

Other directions:

_____

_____

_____

_____

_____

_____

_____

_____

Signed this _____ day of _____

Signature _____

Address _____

_____

The declarant voluntarily signed this writing in my presence.

Witness _____

Address _____

_____

Witness _____

Address _____

_____

OR

The declarant voluntarily signed this writing in my presence.

_____

Notary Public

Courtesy of Choice in Dying, Inc.

for the purpose of initiating or terminating life-sustaining medical treatment.

Recent legislation

The Patient Self-Determination Act of 1990 requires that health care facilities ask whether the patient has completed an *advance directive.* This law includes the following requirements:

• Each patient must be given written information about his rights under state law to make decisions concerning medical care, including the right to accept or refuse medical or surgical treatment and to formulate advance directives.

• The patient's decision whether or not to execute an advance directive must be documented in the medical record.

• The facility must ensure that the patient's decision regarding the execution of an advance directive does not influence the provision of care. Nor can health care providers discriminate against a patient in any way based on this decision.

• The health care facility must provide education for the staff and community on issues concerning advance directives.

Challenging the patient's right to refuse treatment

There are two grounds for challenging a patient's right to refuse treatment: You can claim that the patient is incompetent, or you can claim that compelling reasons exist to overrule his wishes. (See *Overruling the patient,* page 83.)

The courts consider a patient incompetent when he lacks the mental ability to make a reasoned decision, such as when he's delirious.

Compelling circumstances

The courts also recognize several compelling circumstances that justify overruling a patient's refusal of treatment. These include:

• when refusing treatment endangers the life of another. For example, a court may overrule a pregnant woman's objection to treatment if it endangers her unborn child's life.

• when a parent's decision to withhold treatment threatens a child's life. For example, a court may overrule the parents' religious objections to their child's treatment when the child has a condition that endangers his life. When the child's life isn't in danger, the courts are more likely to respect the parents' convictions.

• when, despite refusing treatment, the patient makes statements indicating that he wants to live. For example, some Jehovah's Witnesses who oppose blood transfusions say or imply that they won't prevent the transfusions if a court takes responsibility for the decision. In *Powell v. Columbia-Presbyterian Medical Center* (1965), the court authorized transfusions when a Jehovah's Witness indicated that she wouldn't object to receiving blood, although she'd refused to give written consent.

• when the public interest outweighs the patient's right. For example, the law requires school-age children to receive a polio vaccine before they can attend classes.

Responding to the patient's request to stop treatment

When a patient plans to refuse treatment, you may be the person he tells first. Whether he tells you he's going to refuse treatment or he simply refuses to give consent, take the following steps:

• Stop preparations for any treatment at once.

• Immediately notify the doctor.

• Report your patient's decision to your supervisor.

Durable power of attorney

The durable power of attorney for health care is an extension of the traditional power of attorney concept.

The power of attorney allows a person to designate another to act or conduct legally binding transactions on his behalf. The power of attorney traditionally was used for managing property or financial assets, and it lapsed when the principal died or became mentally incapacitated. Many states created a "durable" power of attorney—one that would continue after the principal died or became incapacitated.

More recently, states have created a durable power of attorney specifically for health care decisions. Durable power of attorney for health care statutes enable competent patients to delegate the authority to consent or refuse health care treatment to other people. This helps a patient to ensure that his wishes will be carried out if he should become incompetent.

Each state with a durable power of attorney for health care law has specific requirements for executing a durable power of attorney. The durable power of attorney form shown below provides blank lines for the patient to specify his wishes about life-support measures and to list limitations or provisions if appropriate.

Durable Power of Attorney
for health care

I, _____,
hereby appoint:

Name _____
Home address _____
_____
Home telephone number _____
Work telephone number _____
as my agent to make health care decisions for me if and when I am unable to make my own health care decisions. This gives my agent the power to consent to giving, withholding, or stopping any health care, treatment, service, or diagnostic procedure. My agent also has the authority to talk with health care personnel, get information, and sign forms necessary to carry out those decisions.

If the person named as my agent is not available or is unable to act as my agent, then I appoint the following

persons to serve in the order listed below:

1. Name _____
   Home address _____
   _____
   Home telephone number _____
   Work telephone number _____

2. Name _____
   Home address _____
   _____
   Home telephone number _____
   Work telephone number _____

By this document I intend to create a power of attorney for health care which shall take effect upon my incapacity to make my own health care decisions and shall continue during that incapacity.

My agent shall make health care decisions as I direct below or as I make known to him or her in some other way.

(continued)

Durable power of attorney continued

(a) Statement of desires concerning life-prolonging care, treatment, services, and procedures:

_____
_____
_____
_____

(b) Special provisions and limitations:

_____
_____
_____
_____
_____
_____

By signing below I indicate that I understand the purpose and effect of this document.

I sign my name to this form on

_____
(date)

My current home address:

_____
_____
_____
(Sign here)

Witnesses

I declare that the person who signed or acknowledged this document is personally known to me, that he or she signed or acknowledged this durable power of attorney in my presence, and that he or she appears to be of sound mind and under no duress, fraud, or undue influence. I am not the person appointed as agent by this document, nor am I the patient's health care provider or an employee of the patient's health care provider.

First Witness

Signature: _____
Home Address: _____

Print Name: _____
Date: _____

Second Witness

Signature: _____
Home Address: _____

Print Name: _____
Date: _____
(At least one of the above witnesses must also sign the following declaration.)

I further declare that I am not related to the patient by blood, marriage, or adoption, and, to the best of my knowledge, I am not entitled to any part of his or her estate under a will now existing or by operation of law.

Signature: _____

I further declare that I am not related to the patient by blood, marriage, or adoption, and, to the best of my knowledge, I am not entitled to any part of his or her estate under a will now existing or by operation of law.

Signature: _____

Check requirements of individual state statute.

Overruling the patient

Even when a patient's decision to refuse treatment rests on constitutionally protected grounds, such as religious beliefs, the court will intervene in certain circumstances. Becoming familiar with court rulings in this area will help you to better cope if you ever get caught between a patient or his family and a court. Here are some delicate legal situations the courts have ruled on.

Incapacitated patient

If an adult patient becomes physically or mentally incapacitated, a relative can't always refuse treatment for him. The court reserves the right to overrule even a spouse on the patient's behalf if the decision seems to be medically unreasonable. For example, in *Collins v. Davis* (1964), the court overruled a wife's refusal of surgery for her unconscious husband.

Patient responsible for child

If a patient who's responsible for the care of a child refuses lifesaving treatment, the court may reverse the patient's decision. In *Application of the President and Directors of Georgetown College, Inc.* (1964), the court ordered a blood transfusion for a Jehovah's Witness who was the mother of an infant and who refused to give consent for her own transfusion. In the *Melideo* case (1976), the court said that it might have ordered a lifesaving transfusion for the patient if she had had a child.

Pregnant patient

If a patient who's pregnant refuses treatment, thereby threatening not only her own health, but also that of her unborn child, the court has reversed the patient's decision. In *Jefferson v. Griffin Spalding County Hospital Authority* (1981), the court awarded temporary custody of an unborn child to a state agency. The mother had a complete placenta previa but had refused to consent to a cesarean section. The court's custody award included full authority to give consent for a surgical delivery.

Patient who's a minor

If a patient is a minor, the court will allow his parents or legal guardian to consent to medical treatment, but not allow them to deny him lifesaving treatment. *In re Sampson* (1972) was such a case.

Never delay informing your supervisor, especially if a delay could be life-threatening. Any delay you're responsible for will greatly increase your legal risks.

The doctor and hospital have the responsibility to take action, such as trying to convince the patient to accept treatment or asking him to sign a release form. This form relieves the hospital and the health care team of liability for any consequences the patient suffers by refusing treatment. It does not, however, release the health team from its obligation to continue providing other forms of care.

Don't ignore the patient

Never ignore a patient's request to refuse treatment. A patient can sue you for battery — intentionally touching another person without authorization to do so — for simply following doctor's orders (see *Is the nurse liable?* page 84).

To overrule the patient's decision, the doctor or your hospital must obtain a court order. Only then are you legally authorized to administer treatment.

Is the nurse liable?

In the course of providing daily care, you may easily overlook the potential legal consequences of ignoring a patient who refuses treatment. Consider the fictional case described below.

A battle of wills

Albert Proxmire, age 69, is hospitalized with a gastrointestinal disorder. He's also depressed and uncooperative. His day-shift nurse, Bernice Bransted, reads on his chart that the doctor ordered an enema.

Disgruntled and surly, Mr. Proxmire has other ideas. He bluntly tells the nurse, "Leave me alone. I'm not getting an enema now!"

Despite his protests, Ms. Bransted insists. She gently turns him in his bed and administers the enema.

Later, Mr. Proxmire's son becomes angry when his father tells him what happened. The son confronts the nursing supervisor and warns her that he intends to pursue the matter.

A battle in the courts?

Does Mr. Proxmire have a case for battery against the nurse? Yes. As a conscious, coherent adult, even though depressed, Mr. Proxmire has the right to refuse treatment. After he—or any other adult patient—refuses any nursing treatment, giving it will make the nurse liable for battery.

If the doctor or hospital tries to convince the court to overrule the patient on the grounds that he's incompetent, they'll need proof that he lacks the mental ability to make a reasoned decision. Your documented observations about your patient's mental status may be used as evidence.

No matter how serious the patient's condition, refusing treatment does not constitute evidence of incompetence. In *Lane v. Candura* (1978), for example, a diabetic patient first agreed to have her leg amputated and then changed her mind and refused the surgery. The doctors applied for a court order, arguing that by changing her mind, the patient had shown incompetence. The court disagreed, and upheld the patient's right to withdraw her consent.

Right to refuse emergency treatment

A competent adult has the right to refuse emergency treatment. His family can't overrule his decision, and his doctor may not give the expressly refused treatment, even if the patient becomes unconscious.

If there are no grounds for overruling your patient's decision, you have an ethical duty to defend his right to refuse treatment in the face of all opposition, even his family's. Try to explain the patient's choice to family members. Emphasize that the decision is his as long as he's competent.

Patient's right to privacy

Obtaining highly personal information from a patient can be uncomfortable and embarrassing. Reassuring the patient that you will keep information confidential may help to put you both at ease. But stop to think about the legal complexities of this responsibility. What do you do when your patient's spouse, other health care professionals, the media, or public health agencies ask you to disclose confidential information?

Is there a constitutional right to privacy?

Privacy and confidentiality were first proposed as basic legal rights in 1890 in a *Harvard Law Review* article titled "The Right to Privacy."

The U.S. Constitution doesn't explicitly sanction a right to privacy. But in several cases, including *Roe v. Wade* (1973), the U.S. Supreme Court cited several constitutional amendments that imply the right.

The right to privacy essentially is the right to make personal choices without outside interference. In the landmark case of *Griswold v. Connecticut* (1965), for example, the Supreme Court recognized a married couple's right to privacy in contraceptive use. In *Eisenstadt v. Baird* (1972), the Supreme Court extended the right to privacy in contraceptive use to include unmarried people. In *Carey v. Population Services International* (1977), the Supreme Court said a state law that prohibited the sale of contraceptives to anyone under age 16 was unconstitutional.

The U.S. Department of Health and Human Services tried to modify the *Carey* ruling by publishing a regulation called "Parental Notification Requirements Applicable to Projects for Family Planning Services." Also known as the "squeal rule," this regulation proposed that any federally funded clinic or health agency that gave contraceptives to a minor be required to inform the minor's parents or guardian. A New York federal district court, however, declared that this regulation was unconstitutional. (See *Distributing contraceptives in public schools*, page 86.)

Right to privacy and abortion law

The Supreme Court ruling in *Roe v. Wade* (1973) protects a woman's right to privacy in a first-trimester abortion.

After the first trimester, a state may regulate abortion to protect the mother's health and prohibit an abortion if the fetus is judged viable.

Restrictions on the abortion right

Since *Roe v. Wade,* the Supreme Court has handed down more than 20 major opinions related to the abortion issue.

A 1989 Supreme Court decision, *Webster v. Reproductive Health Services,* placed certain aspects of *Roe v. Wade* into doubt. Although viability of the fetus remains the guideline, the Supreme Court appears more willing to allow states to regulate abortion.

In *Planned Parenthood of S.E. Pennsylvania v. Casey* (1992), the Supreme Court let stand Pennsylvania's Abortion Control Act of 1989. This act requires that a woman wait 24 hours between consenting to and receiving an abortion, except in narrowly defined medical emergencies. It also requires that a woman seeking an abortion be offered state-mandated information about fetal development and abortion.

However, in the same ruling the Supreme Court struck down a requirement in the Pennsylvania law that a married woman inform her husband of her intent to have an abortion. Overall, the ruling in *Planned Parenthood of S.E. Pennsylvania v. Casey* upholds a woman's right to obtain an abortion, but it also underscores the Court's willingness to allow states to regulate the abortion right.

In a 1991 ruling, the Court, in the case of *Rust v. Sullivan,* upheld federal regulations prohibiting health care workers at government-subsidized family planning clinics from providing information about abortion. Under the regulations, employees of a subsidized clinic were forbidden from advising a pregnant woman about abortion as a possible option. President Clinton, however, overturned these regulations in 1993.

Distributing contraceptives in public schools

Making contraceptive devices readily available in public schools has caused a political uproar. Advocates claim that school-based family planning services effectively counter high pregnancy rates and lower the incidence of sexually transmitted diseases (STDs) among teenagers. Consider these statistics:

- About 12 million (48%) adolescents in the United States are sexually active.
- By age 19, 75% of all American girls have had sexual intercourse.
- Girls ages 15 to 19 have the highest incidence of pelvic inflammatory disease.
- About 35% of sexually active teens do not use any form of birth control; those who do commonly use it incorrectly, providing inadequate protection against pregnancy and STDs.
- Twenty-six percent of all abortions are performed on teenagers.

In 1986, the National Academy of Sciences (NAS) recommended that adolescents not be forced to seek parental consent for abortion. The NAS also recommended that contraceptives be made available in the schools. These recommendations drew strong opposition. The National Right To Life Committee and then-Secretary of Education William J. Bennett argued that providing contraceptives in school would contribute to teenage promiscuity and abortion. Local initiatives have been opposed by parents and clergy, who argue that school-based family planning undermines the relationship between parents and adolescents.

Chicago: A case study

The first school-based health clinic to dispense contraceptives in Chicago opened in 1984. Anti-abortion activists picketed the facility; members of the clergy sued, unsuccessfully, to stop it; and conservative activist Phyllis Schlafly backed a bill to outlaw such clinics (the bill was vetoed by the governor of Illinois).

By 1990, three school-based clinics in Chicago were dispensing contraceptives without incident. To use these clinics, students need parental permission, and parents who don't want their children to receive contraceptives can say so.

Thus far, the Chicago clinics apparently haven't reduced pregnancy rates. In one Chicago high school with about 1,000 girls, 30 to 50 pregnancies continue to occur each year. Nevertheless, school officials believe that their clinics help control repeat pregnancies, and that they promote the overall health of the students. In fact, fewer than 20% of the visits to clinics have been for contraceptives. Most are for inoculations, basic medical care, and emergency first aid.

A mixed report

The Chicago experience is apparently not unusual. There are more than 170 school-based clinics in the United States. Many provide family planning services, as well as counseling on alcohol, smoking, and drug use. To date, school-based family planning services have not had the impact that advocates hoped for; they have also not had the effect that opponents feared. Studies by the Center for Population Options, an independent group, have shown that school-based clinics reduce students' use of alcohol and tobacco. They also find that making contraceptives readily available doesn't spur sexual activity. But studies also show that school-based clinics that provide contraceptives haven't had a significant effect on teenage pregnancy rates.

Abortion rights for minors

Roe v. Wade played an important role in extending abortion rights to minors. In *Planned Parenthood of Central Missouri v. Danforth,* the Supreme Court overruled a law that prevented first-trimester abortions for minors without parental consent. This decision was based on the *Roe v. Wade* ruling.

In *Bellotti v. Baird II* (1979), the Supreme Court acknowledged that the privacy rights of a minor are not equal to those of an adult. The Court held, however, that a state law requiring a minor to obtain parental consent for an abortion infringed on the minor's rights.

In *H.L. v. Matheson* (1981), the Supreme Court upheld a Utah law requiring a doctor to notify the parents of an unemancipated minor before an abortion. More recently, however, in *Hodgson v. Minnesota* (1990), the Court found unconstitutional a Minnesota statute that required notification of both biological parents before a minor's abortion, followed by a wait of at least 48 hours. The chief difference between the two cases is that the Utah law required notification of only one parent, where feasible; the Minnesota law required notification of *both* parents, even if they were divorced or separated. In *Hodgson,* the Supreme Court decreed that the rule requiring notification of both parents was too burdensome on the abortion right. The Court also stated that the 48-hour waiting period required under the Minnesota law would not, by itself, render the statute unconstitutional.

By letting stand Pennsylvania's Abortion Control Act in 1992, the Supreme Court allowed the state to require that one parent or guardian give consent in person for a minor seeking an abortion, unless the minor obtains a judicial waiver.

In *Hodgson* and *Ohio v. Akron Center for Reproductive Health* (1990), the Supreme Court set forth its position on so-called *judicial bypass statutes.* Judicial bypass statutes allow a minor to avoid notifying parents or obtaining consent for an abortion by going before a judge. The Court stated that judicial bypass satisfies the requirement that parents or other third parties cannot have an absolute veto over the minor's abortion decision.

State law and the right to privacy

The right to privacy has received even more attention at the state level. Ten states — Alaska, Arizona, California, Florida, Hawaii, Illinois, Louisiana, Montana, South Carolina, and Washington — have written a privacy provision into their constitutions. Nearly all states recognize the right to privacy through *statutory law* or *common law.*

Privilege doctrine

The state courts have been strong in protecting a patient's right to have information kept confidential. Even in court, your patient is protected by the *privilege doctrine.* People who have a protected relationship, such as a doctor and patient, can't be forced, even during legal proceedings, to reveal communication between them unless the person who benefits from the protection agrees to it. This means that the patient must agree before confidential information is revealed in court. The purpose of the privilege doctrine is to encourage the patient to reveal confidential information that may be essential to his treatment.

State law determines which relationships are protected by the privilege doctrine. Most states include husband-wife, lawyer-client, and doctor-patient relationships.

Nurse-patient relationships
Only a few states (including New York, Arkansas, Oregon, and Vermont) recognize the nurse-patient relationship as protected. But some courts have said that the privilege exists when a nurse is following doctor's orders. Whether the privilege applies to LPNs and LVNs as well is uncertain.

Extent of privilege
State laws also determine the extent of privilege in protected relationships. In *Hammonds v. Aetna Casualty and Surety Co.* (1965), the court reinforced the privilege doctrine by declaring that protecting a patient's privacy is a doctor's legal duty. It further ruled that a patient could sue for damages any unauthorized person who disclosed confidential medical information about him. Similarly, a patient can sue for invasion of privacy any unauthorized personnel, such as student nurses, who observe him without his permission. The only hospital personnel who have a right to observe a patient are those involved in his diagnosis, treatment, and related care.

Exceptions
In some states, a patient automatically waives his right to doctor-patient privilege when he files a personal injury or *workers' compensation* lawsuit.

A hospital or doctor cannot invoke the privilege doctrine if the motive is self-protection. In *People v. Doe* (1978), a nursing home was being investigated for allegedly mistreating its patients. The court ruled that the nursing home's attempt to invoke patient privilege was unjust, since the issue at hand was the patients' welfare.

Patient privilege and Canadian law
Canadian common law recognizes the privilege doctrine in doctor-patient relationships, but not in nurse-patient relationships. (Cases that suggest the doctor-patient privilege include *Dembie*, 1963; *Re SAS*, 1977; and *Geransky*, 1977.) The *Canadian Nurses' Association* and the provincial licensing authorities have adopted the International Council of Nurses Code of Ethics. The code requires you to keep confidential any personal information you receive from a patient during your nursing care. Consequently, although violation of a patient's right to privacy isn't subject to criminal prosecution in Canada, it is deemed professional misconduct. A nurse who violates a patient's right to privacy could lose her nursing license.

Your responsibilities in protecting patient privacy
Despite legal uncertainties regarding your responsibilities under the privilege doctrine, you have a professional and ethical responsibility to protect your patient's privacy, whether you're an RN, an LPN, or an LVN.

This responsibility requires more than keeping secrets. You may have to educate your patients about their privacy rights. Some of them may be unaware of what the right to privacy means, or even that they have such a right. Explain to the patient that he can refuse to allow pictures to be taken of his disorder and its treatment, for example. Tell him that he can choose to have information about his condition withheld from others, including family members. Make every effort to assure that the patient's wishes are carried out.

When you may disclose confidential information
Under certain circumstances, you may lawfully disclose confidential information about your patient. For example,

the courts allow disclosure when the welfare of a person or a group of people is at stake. Consider the patient who is diagnosed as an epileptic and asks you not to tell his family. Depending on the circumstances, you may decide that this isn't in the patient's and his family's best interest, particularly in terms of safety. In that situation, inform the patient's doctor; he may then decide to inform the family to protect the patient's well-being. In most states, the doctor is required to inform the Department of Motor Vehicles of uncontrolled epilepsy.

You're also protected by law if you disclose confidential information about a patient that's necessary for his continued care, or if your patient consents to the disclosure.

Be careful not to exceed the specified limit of a patient's consent. Taking pictures is the largest single cause of invasion of privacy lawsuits. In *Feeney v. Young* (1920), a woman consented to the filming of her cesarean delivery for viewings by medical societies. But the doctor incorporated the film into a generally released movie titled *Birth*. The court awarded damages to the woman under the state's privacy law.

Protecting the public

The courts have granted immunity to health care professionals who, in good faith, have disclosed confidential information to prevent public harm. In *Simonsen v. Swenson* (1920), a doctor who thought that his patient had syphilis told the owner of the hotel in which the patient was staying about the patient's contagious disease. The court ruled that doctors are privileged to make disclosures that will prevent the spread of disease.

A controversial California case established a doctor's right to disclose information that would protect any person whom a patient threatened to harm. In *Tarasoff v. Regents of the University*

of California (1976), a woman was murdered by a mentally ill patient who had told his psychotherapist that he intended to kill her. The victim's parents sued the doctor for failing to warn their daughter. The Supreme Court found the doctor liable because he did not warn the intended victim. The Court ruled similarly in *McIntosh v. Milano* (1979).

When you must disclose confidential information

In some situations, the law requires you to disclose confidential information.

Child abuse

All 50 states and the District of Columbia have *disclosure laws* for *child abuse* cases. Except for Maine and Montana, all states also grant immunity from legal action for a *good-faith* report on suspected child abuse. In fact, there may be a criminal penalty for failure to disclose such information.

Courts also may order you to disclose confidential information in cases of child custody and *child neglect.* One case involving such an order was *D. v. D.* (1969). Despite the doctor-patient privilege, the court ordered the doctor to turn the mother's *medical records* over to the court for a private inspection. The mother had a history of illness, and the court said that the inspection would help it to decide which parent should be granted custody. The courts made a similar ruling in the custody case of *In re Doe Children* (1978). The court stated that the children's welfare outweighed the parents' right to keep their medical records private.

Criminal cases

Some laws create an exemption to the privilege doctrine in criminal cases so that the courts can have access to all essential information. In states where neither a law nor an exemption to the law exists, the court may find an exemption to the doctrine in criminal cases.

Government requests

Certain government agencies can order you to reveal confidential information, including federal agencies such as the Internal Revenue Service, the Environmental Protection Agency, the Department of Labor, and the Department of Health and Human Services. State agencies that may order you to reveal confidential information include revenue, or tax, bureaus and public health departments. For example, most state public health departments require reports of all communicable diseases, births and deaths, and gunshot wounds.

Public's right to know

The newsworthiness of an event or person can make disclosure acceptable. In such circumstances, the public's need for information may outweigh a person's right to keep his medical condition private. For example, newspapers routinely publish the findings of the President's annual physical examination in response to the public's demand for information.

Even the First Lady's health may become a matter of public record. In 1990, when Barbara Bush underwent radiation therapy for Graves' disease, the media publicized many details of her treatment. Other events for which the public's right to know may outweigh the patient's right to privacy include product-tampering cases (for example, in 1991, the nation's media widely reported an incident in Washington state in which three persons who took Sudafed 12-Hour Capsules suffered acute onset of cyanide poisoning) and breakthroughs in medical technology (such as the first successful implantation of an artificial heart).

Even when the public has a right to know about a confidential matter, the courts will not allow the public disclosure to undermine a person's dignity. In *Barber v. Time, Inc.* (1942), *Time* magazine was sued by a woman whose name and photograph were published in an article that revealed she suffered from an illness that caused her to eat as much food as 10 persons could eat. The court ruled that publishing the patient's name and picture was an unnecessary invasion of her privacy, and that ethics required keeping such information confidential.

Doe v. Roe (1977) is a similar case. A patient sued a psychiatrist for publishing the patient's biography and thoughts verbatim. Even though the doctor didn't use the patient's name, the court stated that the patient was readily identifiable by the article. It found the doctor liable for violating the doctor-patient privilege.

When the patient demands his chart

Suppose your patient says to you, "I'm paying for the tests; I have a right to know the results." Does the patient have the legal right to know what's in his medical records?

Yes. And because patients increasingly want explanations about what's being done to them and why, know how to respond when your patient asks to see his medical records.

Disclosure debate

For years, health care experts have debated the merits of letting a patient see his medical records. Proponents argue that knowing the information helps the patient to better understand his condition and care and makes him a more cooperative patient.

Opponents, usually doctors and hospitals, argue that the technical jargon and medical abbreviations found in medical records may confuse or even frighten a patient. In addition, opponents claim that opening medical records to a patient will increase the risks of malpractice lawsuits. No evidence exists to support this contention.

The *right-to-access* issue has spawned an important legal debate. The first issue the courts had to answer involved ownership.

Determining ownership

The hospital owns the hospital medical records, and the doctor owns his office records, according to court decisions. Most courts have decided that a patient sees a doctor for diagnosis and treatment, not to obtain records for his personal use.

Right to access

The second issue the courts had to resolve involved access. While granting ownership of medical records to doctors and hospitals, the courts have expressed their own right to get the records anytime they need them for a case review.

For this reason, any patient in any state can file a lawsuit to *subpoena* his medical records. But some court decisions and some states' laws have given patients the right to direct access. Many states guarantee a patient's right to his medical information.

In *Cannell v. Medical and Surgical Clinic S.C.* (1974), the court ruled that a doctor had the duty to disclose medical information to his patient. The court also ruled, however, that doctors and hospitals needn't turn over the actual files to the patient. Instead, they need only show the complete medical record — or a copy — to the patient.

The court based the patient's limited right to access on two important concepts:
● A patient has a right to know the details about his medical treatment under common law.
● A patient has a right to the information in his records because he pays for the treatment.

Setting up roadblocks

Despite the laws and court decisions, hospitals don't always make access to records easy. Some hospitals discourage a patient from seeing his medical records by putting up bureaucratic barriers. For example, requiring the patient to have an attorney make the request can stifle a patient's attempt to gain access and encourage visits to malpractice lawyers.

Other hospitals charge high copying fees in an effort to discourage patient record requests. Some states, such as Pennsylvania, have passed laws that require reasonable copying fees.

How to respond to your patient's request

A patient's request should, first, make you question whether you and your colleagues have done enough to communicate with him. Assess why the patient wants to see his records. He may simply be curious, or his request may reflect hidden fears about his treatment.

Many hospitals have established policies that deal with this issue. These policies may include notifying your nursing supervisor that the patient has asked to see his medical records and notifying the *risk manager,* if your facility has one, to alert administrative staff and legal counsel, if necessary.

After your patient gets approval to see his records, stay with him while he reads them. Explain to him that state laws prohibit him from changing or erasing information on his records, even information he considers incorrect. Tell him to show you any information he considers incorrect. Offer to answer any of his questions you can; assure him that his doctor will answer questions, too. In fact, encourage the patient to write down specific questions for his doctor, and offer to contact his doctor for him.

While your patient reads, help him to interpret the abbreviations and jargon used in medical charting. One patient hospitalized for hypertension was greatly relieved when her nurse explained that the "malignant hypertension" notation on her chart had nothing to do with cancer.

Observe how the patient responds while he reads. If he becomes apprehensive, puzzled, or angry, try to provide him with calm, professional explanations about what he's read in his records. He may simply seem relieved: Some patients want to read their records just to be sure you and the doctors aren't hiding any information. For example, one patient who demanded to see her medical records merely flipped through the pages. The hospital's willingness to share information about her treatment apparently satisfied her.

When a relative requests medical records

A relative may see a patient's medical records under any of these conditions:
• The relative or next of kin is the patient's legal guardian, and the patient is incompetent.
• The relative has the patient's approval.

Patient discharge against medical advice

The patient's bill of rights and the laws and regulations based on it give a competent adult the right to refuse treatment for any reason without being punished or having his liberty restricted.

Some states have turned these rights into law. And the courts have cited the bills of rights in their decisions.

The right to refuse treatment includes the right to leave the hospital against medical advice (AMA) any time, for any reason. All you can do is try to talk the patient out of it.

Recognizing a potential patient walk-out

Because you have more contact with your patient than any other health care professional, you're likely to be the first person to suspect that a patient is contemplating leaving *AMA.*

Complaints or hostile behavior may indicate the patient's extreme dissatisfaction with hospital routine or with the care he's receiving. By carefully observing, listening, and talking with him, you may be able to resolve the problems by offering him a fresh perspective and perhaps change his mind about leaving.

If you discover that a specific problem has caused his dissatisfaction, try to resolve it. If the problem lies outside the scope of your practice, call the patient's doctor.

A patient may tell you that he's changed his mind about leaving just to divert your attention. If you suspect this, check on him more often and ask colleagues to do the same. Stay with him when you escort him to another part of the hospital.

When the patient insists on leaving

If your patient still insists on leaving AMA, and your hospital has a policy on managing the patient who wants to leave, follow it exactly. Following policy will help to protect the hospital, co-workers, and you from charges of unlawful restraint or false imprisonment. If your employer doesn't have such a policy, take these steps:

• Contact the patient's family (if the patient hasn't already called them), and explain that the patient is getting ready to leave. If you can't reach the family, contact the person listed in the patient's records as being responsible for him, or for his body and valuables if he should die.

• Explain the hospital's AMA procedures to the patient if hospital policy delegates this responsibility to you.

• Give the patient the AMA form to sign (see *Documenting a patient's decision to leave AMA,* page 94). His decision to leave is the same as a refusal of treatment. Inform the patient of his medical risks if he leaves the hospital, and explain the alternatives available at the hospital and at other locations, such as regular visits to the hospital's outpatient clinic or admission to another facility. His signature on the AMA form is evidence of his refusal of treatment. You should witness the signature.

• Provide routine discharge care. Even though your patient is leaving AMA, his rights to discharge planning and care are the same as those for a patient who's signed out with medical advice. So if the patient agrees, escort him to the door (in a wheelchair, if necessary), arrange for medical or nursing follow-up care, and offer other routine health care measures. These procedures will protect the hospital as well as the patient.

When the patient refuses to sign out

If the patient refuses to sign the AMA form, you should document his refusal in a note stating that all risks have been explained to the patient. One innovative nurse routinely told emergency department patients that if they refused to sign the form, she would like them to indicate their refusal to sign by signing the back of the form. Most patients complied with her request.

Dealing with an escape

If you discover that a patient is missing from the hospital, notify the nursing supervisor and security immediately. If the patient was in police custody or if he poses a threat to anyone outside the hospital, the administration should contact the police. The hospital administration subsequently may ask you to notify the patient's family or friends, collect the patient's belongings, and document the escape in the patient's medical chart and *incident report.*

False imprisonment

Never attempt to detain a competent adult who has a right to leave. Any attempt to detain or restrain him may be interpreted as unlawful restraint or false imprisonment, for which you can be sued or prosecuted.

Your hospital's policy should reflect state law. It should specifically answer such questions as:

• How long and for what reasons may a patient be detained?

• When can you use forcible restraints?

• Who may order the use of restraints?

• Who may apply the restraints?

Knowing the policies will reduce your liability exposure.

Documenting a patient's decision to leave AMA

An against-medical-advice (AMA) form is a medical record as well as a legal document. It's designed to protect you, your co-workers, and your institution from liability resulting from the patient's unapproved discharge or escape.

To document an AMA incident, begin by getting your institution's AMA form. The form may look like the one shown below. You'll notice the form clearly states that the patient:

• knows he's leaving against medical advice

• has been advised of and understands the risks of leaving

• knows he can come back.

Discuss this form with the patient and ask him to sign it. Don't try to force the patient to sign if he is unwilling to do so. You should sign it, too, as a witness.

Add the AMA form to the patient's medical chart. Then write a detailed description of how you first learned of the patient's plan to leave AMA, what you and the patient said to each other, and what alternatives to the patient's action were discussed.

Also, check your institution's policy concerning incident reports. If the patient leaves without anyone's knowledge, or if he refuses to sign the AMA form, you'll probably be required to file an incident report. Be sure to include the names of any other employees involved in the discovery of the patient's absence. Hospital administration or your head nurse also may want to solicit corroborating reports from other employees, including other registered nurses, licensed practical nurses, doctors, nurses' aides, orderlies, and clerical staff.

Responsibility release

This is to certify that I, _____,
a patient in _____,
am being discharged against the advice of my doctor and the hospital administration. I acknowledge that I have been informed of the risk involved and hereby release my doctor and the hospital from all responsibility for any ill effects that may result from such a discharge. I also understand that I may return to the hospital at any time and have treatment resumed.

_____   _____
(Patient's signature)   (Date)

_____   _____
(Witness's signature)   (Date)

RE: _____   Patient #_____
(Name of patient)

Court cases

Most courts disapprove of detaining a patient arbitrarily or for an unreasonably long time, which may be ruled false imprisonment. (For an example of a case in which the court found a health care institution guilty of false imprisonment, see *Patient or prisoner?*)

Court cases that involve false imprisonment charges have occurred when institutions threatened to hold patients or their personal belongings until bills were paid. In most such cases, the courts ruled against the institutions.

A hospital or nursing home can delay a patient's discharge, for a reasonable period of time, until routine paperwork is complete. *Bailie v. Miami Valley Hospital* (1966) was a case in which the court ruled in favor of a hospital.

An exception

In a few cases, because of extenuating circumstances, the courts have ruled against patients who sued on grounds of false imprisonment. The case of *Pounders v. Trinity Court Nursing Home* (1979) is one such example.

Mrs. Pounders, 75, was a disabled widow. When her niece and nephew no longer wanted her to live with them, the niece arranged for her to move to Trinity Court Nursing Home. Mrs. Pounders did not object.

During her 2 months at Trinity Court, Mrs. Pounders complained only once to a nurses' aide that she wanted to leave. Unfortunately, the aide failed to report the complaint to anyone in authority at the home.

Mrs. Pounders was finally released, through the aid of an attorney, into another niece's care. She eventually sued the nursing home.

But because Mrs. Pounders couldn't prove she'd been involuntarily detained, the court absolved the nursing home of the false imprisonment charges.

COURT CASE

Patient or prisoner?

The case of *Big Town Nursing Home v. Newman* (1970) provides a good example of how a health care institution may become vulnerable to charges of false imprisonment.

Mr. Newman, 67, had Parkinson's disease, arthritis, heart trouble, hiatal hernia, a speech impediment, and a history of alcoholism. Four days after his nephew signed him into a nursing home, Mr. Newman decided to leave.

No exit

Employees at the nursing home stopped Mr. Newman, locked away his suitcase and clothes, restricted his use of the phone, and restricted his right to visitors. When Mr. Newman tried to walk off the grounds, employees locked him in a wing with severely emotionally disturbed patients and patients addicted to drugs and alcohol. He made other unsuccessful escape attempts, so staff tied Mr. Newman to a chair for long periods. Twenty-two days after his admission, Mr. Newman escaped. Eventually, he sued.

The court ruled in favor of Mr. Newman. Despite his physical infirmities, Mr. Newman had not legally been declared incompetent and was, therefore, legally entitled to exercise his rights.

Lawful detention

The right to leave the hospital AMA isn't absolute. Certain patients who pose a threat to themselves or to others cannot legally leave the hospital. Restraint, when necessary, is lawful with psychiatric patients, prisoners, and violent patients.

Patients from psychiatric hospitals or prisons

If a patient transferred to your hospital for medical care from a prison or psychiatric hospital threatens to escape, notify the custodial institution immediately. They're responsible for sending personnel to guard the patient and for making new arrangements for his care. Restrain the patient only if his medical condition warrants it or if the police or psychiatric hospital authorities instruct you to do so.

If the prisoner or psychiatric patient escapes, you or your hospital or nursing administration should call the authorities at the custodial institution or the police.

Violent patients

If you suspect that a patient with a history of violence or violent threats is planning to leave AMA, notify hospital and nursing administrators immediately. If state law allows it, your hospital administrators may decide to get police assistance to restrain the patient.

If the violent patient has escaped, notify your nursing or hospital administration immediately. They will contact the police and mental health authorities. If the patient ever expressed an intention to harm a known person, the administration also should contact that person.

When a patient dies

When a patient dies, his rights don't end; they transfer to his estate. But in recent years, legally determining when death has occurred has become difficult. That, in turn, complicates your role.

How can you be sure a patient is legally dead? Who has the right to pronounce death? What are your responsibilities after the patient dies?

Controversy over the definition of death

Determining death used to be fairly simple. When a person's circulation and respiration stopped, he was dead. But advances in medical technology have made death pronouncements more complicated. Because medical equipment—such as ventilators, pacemakers, and intra-aortic balloon pumps—can maintain respiration and circulation, patients may continue to "live" even after their brains have died.

Criteria for brain death

To help doctors determine death in such cases, an *ad hoc committee* at Harvard Medical School published a report, in 1968, establishing specific criteria for brain death. These are:
• a failure to respond to the most painful stimuli
• an absence of spontaneous respirations or muscle movements
• an absence of reflexes
• a flat electroencephalogram (EEG).

The committee recommended that all these tests be repeated after 24 hours, and that hypothermia and the presence of central nervous system depressants, such as barbiturates, be ruled out.

In 1981, the American Medical Association, the American Bar Association, and the President's Commission for the Study of Ethical Problems in Medicine and Behavioral Research collaborated to derive a working definition of brain death. The result of this effort, the Uniform Determination of Death Act (UDODA), has gained wide acceptance among the health care and legal communities.

In general terms, the UDODA defines brain death as the cessation of all measurable function or activity in every area of the brain, including the brain stem. This definition excludes comatose patients as well as those in a persistent vegetative state. Current debate centers on whether to expand the definition to include certain patients who still have brain stem function, such as anencephalic infants.

Court cases

Several court decisions have been based on such definitions.

In the case of *State v. Brown* (1971), an Oregon court was among the first to recognize brain death. In this case of second-degree murder, the defendant argued that he hadn't caused the victim's death by inflicting a gunshot wound to the brain. Instead, he claimed, a doctor killed the victim by removing artificial life support. But the court ruled that the defendant caused the victim's death because the gunshot wound resulted in brain death.

In 1975, several New York hospitals initiated a lawsuit to get a legal ruling on the definition of death when the patient was a potential organ donor *(N.Y.C. Health and Hospitals Corporation v. Sulsona)*. Expert testimony showed that the common law definition of death (cessation of circulation and respiration) raised the failure rate of organ transplants. The incidence of renal failure in kidney recipients was about 88%. But, using the brain death standard, the incidence of renal failure in recipients was only about 15%. (Medical advances have since improved the success rate of almost all types of transplant surgery.)

The court ruled that it would recognize brain death in transplantation cases to encourage anatomic gifts, even though the state had no law defining brain death. Its ruling applied only to transplantation cases, however.

In 1979, a Colorado court also accepted the criteria for brain death. In *Lovato v. Colorado*, a mother was charged with abusing her child. The child was comatose, with a flat EEG and fixed and dilated pupils, and lacked spontaneous respirations or reflexes or responses to painful stimuli. The mother petitioned the court to keep the child on a ventilator. The court ruled that the child was dead because he met the criteria for brain death.

Know your state's law

In states without laws defining death or without judicial precedents, the common law definition of death (cessation of circulation and respiration) is still used. In these states, doctors are understandably reluctant to discontinue artificial life support for brain-dead patients. If you are likely to be involved with patients on life-support equipment, protect yourself by finding out how your state defines death.

Canadian law

In Canada, defining the moment of death has traditionally been left to medical professionals. Human tissue gift legislation states that death is determined by accepted medical practice.

Pronouncing death

Only a doctor or a *coroner* can legally pronounce a person dead. In some health care facilities, such as nursing homes, nurses pronounce death when a doctor isn't available. The state board must indicate that this is an appropriate nursing practice. If you work in such a facility, you should understand that pronouncing death typically isn't a nursing responsibility.

The attending doctor usually is responsible for signing the death certificate, unless the death comes under the jurisdiction of a medical examiner or coroner. State laws specify when this occurs. The coroner or medical examiner usually has jurisdiction over deaths with violent or suspicious circumstances. These include suspected homicides and suicides, and deaths after accidents.

Canadian law
The Canadian provincial laws on *autopsies* are similar. Any death that occurs in violent or suspicious circumstances comes under the jurisdiction of a medical examiner or coroner. Depending on the province, other types of death — including a prisoner's death, a sudden death, or a death not caused by a disease — also may come under the jurisdiction of a medical examiner or coroner.

Your responsibility when a patient dies

When a patient dies, you are responsible for accurately and objectively charting all his signs and any actions you take. For example, an appropriate entry in the *nurses' notes* would be: "Midnight. No respirations or pulses, pupils fixed and dilated. Notified Dr. York." Don't write a conclusion that borders on a medical diagnosis, such as "patient seems dead."

You're also responsible for notifying the doctor who can be reached most quickly. If this is the doctor on call, he should notify the patient's doctor, who should notify the family. Find out who will be notifying the family, and document it.

At the appropriate time, you should prepare the body for removal to the morgue, according to institutional procedure. When doing this, carefully identify the body. In *Lott v. State* (1962), a nurse mistagged two bodies, causing a Roman Catholic to be prepared for an Orthodox Jewish burial and an Ortho-

dox Jew to be prepared for a Roman Catholic burial. The court found her liable.

Obtaining consent for an autopsy

If a death comes under the jurisdiction of a medical examiner or coroner, the decision to perform an autopsy rests solely with him, despite the family's wishes. In all other cases, the patient's family has a right to give or withhold consent. In some states, the patient can give written consent to an autopsy before he dies.

When a doctor or other hospital representative seeks consent from a patient's family, you can help by explaining why the autopsy is needed and how autopsy arrangements are made.

Who may give consent
Most states have laws that specify who has the right to give consent to autopsies. Some laws simply list which relatives can give consent. Others list relatives in descending order, according to their relationship to the deceased. The usual order is spouse, adult children, parents, brothers or sisters, grandparents, uncles or aunts, and cousins. The person with the right to consent may withhold consent or impose limits on the autopsy. If the autopsy exceeds these limits, the consenting relative may sue.

The relative with the right to consent also may sue if an autopsy is performed without any consent. The grounds for such lawsuits usually are mental or emotional suffering.

Experimental procedures

The family has a right to give or withhold specific consent to practice medical procedures on a corpse. In teaching hospitals, residents and medical students practice procedures, such as intubation, on corpses. But if a hospital does not obtain proper consent, the family member responsible for consent may sue. In many states, the hospital may even face criminal charges.

Responsibility for burial

In the United States and in Canada, the family member who has the right to consent to autopsy usually has the responsibility to bury the body as well. In one Canadian case (*Hunter v. Hunter*, 1930), however, the court ruled that the deceased's son, who was the executor of the will, had this responsibility—not the wife, who was the next of kin.

If no one claims the body, despite the hospital's effort to contact the person responsible, a state or county official must dispose of it. Laws in many states direct this official to deliver unclaimed bodies to an appropriate educational or scientific institution, unless the person is a veteran or has died from a contagious disease. In these situations, the state pays for burial or cremation.

Canadian law

In Canada, the hospital must notify an appropriate official of an unclaimed body, and the body will be delivered to a medical school.

Selected references

"AIDS: When Your Patient Refuses HIV Testing," *American Journal of Nursing* 94(11):48-54, November 1994.

Althaus, F.A., et al. "The Effects of Mandatory Delay Laws on Abortion Patients and Providers," *Family Planning Perspectives* 16(5):228-31, 233, September-October 1994.

Anthony, J. "Who's Reading Your Medical Records?" *American Health: Fitness of Body and Mind* 12(9):54-58, November 1993.

Beck, M. "A Lesson In Dying Well," *Newsweek* 123(20):58, May 1994.

Brandt, M. "Confidentiality Today: Where Do You Stand?" *Journal of AHIMA* 64(12):59-64, December 1993.

Brody, H. "Causing, Intending, and Assisting Death," *Journal of Clinical Ethics* 4(2):112-17, Summer 1993.

Cassidy, J. "A Confidence Betrayed," *Nursing Times* 90(12):16-17, March 23-29, 1994.

Curtin, L.L. "Ethics in Management: A Sudden and Unexpected Discharge," *Nursing Management* 26(7):84, 86, July 1995.

Curtin, L.L. "Patient Privacy in a Public Institution," *Nursing Management* 24(6):26-27, June 1993.

Dewing, J., et al. *Journal of Clinical Nursing* 2(1):3-4, January 1993.

Franklin, K. "Letters: The Final Rule," *Nursing95* 25(7):4, 6, July 1995.

Frawley, K.A.."Confidentiality in the Computer Age," *RN* 57(7):59-60, July 1994.

Harvard Medical School, Ad Hoc Committee to Examine the Definition of Brain Death. "A Definition of Irreversible Coma," *JAMA* 205:337-40, August 1968.

Kemmett, V. "Fit to Consent?" *Nursing Times* 89(24):40-2, June 1993.

Krynski, M.D., et al. "How Informed Can Consent Be? New Light on Comprehension Among Elderly People Making Decisions About Enteral Tube Feeding," *Gerontologist* 34(1):36-43, February 1994.

"Legal Questions. Discharge AMA: Premature Checkout," *Nursing95* 25(8):20, August 1995.

Milholland, D.K. "Privacy and Confidentiality of Patient Information: Challenges for Nursing," *Journal of Nursing Administration* 24(2):19-24, February 1994.

Nussbaum, W., et al. "Perioperative Challenges in the Care of the Jehovah's Witness: A Case Report," *AANA Journal* 62(2):160-64, April 1994.

Pierson, V.H. "Missouri's Parental Consent Law and Teen Pregnancy Outcomes," *Women and Health* 22(3):47-58, 1995.

Rosen, L.F. "Legal Issues Involving the Treatment of Minors," *Today's OR Nurse* 17(2):39, March-April 1995.

Salladay, S.A. "Patient Confidentiality: On the Spot," *Nursing94* 24(8):29-30, August 1994.

Salladay, S.A. "Patient Self-determination: Assessing Competence," *Nursing94* 24(9):22, September 1994.

Sanchez-Sweatman, L. "What is Informed Consent?" *Canadian Nurse* 89(9):49-50, October 1993.

Siegel, D.M. "Consent and Refusal of Treatment," *Emergency Medical Clinics of North America,*" 11(4):833-40, November 1993.

Stewart-Amidei, C. "Is There Really Such a Thing as Informed Consent?" *Journal of Neuroscience Nursing* 26(3):131, June 1994.

Sulmasy, D.P., et al. "Patients' Perceptions of the Quality of Informed Consent for Common Medical Procedures," *Journal of Clinical Ethics* 5(3):189-94, Fall 1994.

Warren, S.D., and Brandeis, L.D. "The Right to Privacy," *Harvard Law Review* 4:193, 1890.

Weiler, K. "The Elements of Informed Consent," *Journal of Gerontology Nursing* 20(8):48, August 1994.

Weinstein, L.B. "Home Care: The Right to Refuse Treatment," *American Journal of Nursing* 95(8):52-53, August 1995.

Wenning, K. "Long-term Psychotherapy and Informed Consent," *Hospital and Company Psychiatry* 44(4):364-67, April 1993.

3

Legal risks and responsibilities on the job

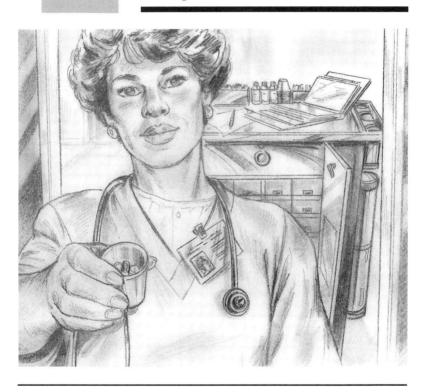

Harried and tense, you're struggling through your shift in a critical care unit. You're already caring for more patients than one nurse can possibly handle, when the emergency department calls and says two more patients will be arriving soon. You know that there's no way you can provide safe care. Your supervisor turns down your pleas for additional staff. Your first impulse is to walk out. How can you remedy this situation?

You're caring for a patient with a criminal record and a reputation in the community for narcotics dealing. You're nervous enough as it is, but the situation gets worse when a stranger stops you in the hallway, flashes a detective's badge, and asks for articles of the patient's clothing and a blood sample. He says that you are legally obligated to turn over this evidence. Should you do what he tells you?

A prestigious civic leader and candidate for local political office has recently made several trips to the emergency department. She has brought her daughter, whom she calls "Miss Clumsy." The child has had multiple bruises and hematomas. You think it *might* be *child abuse.* Fearful of wrongfully damaging the woman's reputation, you hesitate to make a report. What should you do?

Your patient has told you repeatedly that he doesn't want any "heroic measures" taken or "extraordinary means" used to preserve his life if there is no reasonable chance of recovery. However, one evening after the patient has experienced a massive stroke, five members of his family march into your office demanding that everything be done to preserve his life. Should you fight to have the patient's wishes respected?

The situations described above are examples of the complex legal dilemmas you may encounter in daily practice. As the nursing profession grows and you take on greater responsibilities, you will inevitably face increased legal vulnerability. Hardly any aspect of nursing practice is untouched by legal risk. (See *Taking steps to prevent lawsuits.*)

Reading this chapter will enable you to thoroughly understand the legal responsibilities and risks of your profession. You'll find information on the legal consequences of violating your hospital's policies and "legally safe" steps to take to help you cope with understaffing. You'll read about your responsibilities for witnessing and signing documents, maintaining patient safety, administering drugs (one of the riskiest aspects of nursing practice), and upholding a patient's *living will.* You'll learn about your responsibility under the law when you encounter victims of child abuse, are forced to use restraints on a psychologically disturbed patient, or are asked by police to turn over a patient's belongings or blood samples for evidence. This chapter also covers the special legal risks incurred when working in the emergency department, operating room, *intensive care unit,* and other special care units. Becoming fa-

miliar with your legal duties will not restrict your patient care options but instead will free you to give your patients the best care possible.

Basic standards

Whether you're an *RN,* an *LPN,* or an *LVN,* you're always legally accountable for your nursing actions. In any practice setting, your care must meet baseline legal *standards.* And your care should:
• reflect the scope of your *nurse practice act*
• measure up to established practice standards
• consistently protect your patient's rights.

Upholding these standards should provide a base for sound legal practice no matter where you practice nursing.

Hospital policies

Every hospital and other health care institution has *policies* — a set of general principles by which it manages its affairs. If you work for a hospital, you're obligated to know those policies and to follow the established procedures that flow from them.

But never do this blindly. As a nurse, you're also obligated to maintain your professional standards, and these standards may sometimes conflict with your employer's policies and procedures. At times, you may be forced to make decisions and take actions that risk violating those policies and procedures. At times like these, you need help balancing your *duty* to your patient with your responsibility to your employer. Your best help is a well-prepared nursing department policy manual, coupled with high standards of performance. This combination is the mark of a successful nursing department —

Taking steps to prevent lawsuits

Any time that you provide care that consistently falls short of current legal and nursing standards, you make yourself a target for a malpractice lawsuit.

In most situations, you can prevent this from happening to you by following the guidelines below in your daily practice.

Defend the patient

Your first duty is to protect your patient, not his doctor. If your judgment says your patient's condition warrants a call to his doctor, don't hesitate – in the middle of the day or in the middle of the night. If your judgment says to question a doctor's order because you can't read it, don't understand it, think it's incomplete, or think it may harm your patient, don't hesitate.

If your hospital doesn't already have a policy covering nurse-doctor communications, ask for one and keep asking until you get one. Meanwhile, for your own protection, carefully record all contacts with doctors, including the date and time.

Stay current

Here are some effective ways to stay up to date on nursing practices: read nursing journals, attend clinical programs, attend inservice programs, and seek advice from nurse specialists. If your hospital doesn't offer needed inservice programs, ask for them.

Remember, ignorance of new techniques is no excuse for substandard care. If you're ever sued for malpractice, your patient care will be judged by current nursing standards.

Use the entire nursing process

Taking shortcuts risks your patient's well-being and your own. If you're charged

with malpractice, and the court finds out you took a dangerous patient care shortcut, the court may hold you liable for causing harm to your patient.

Document thoroughly

Document every step of the nursing process for every patient. Chart your observations immediately, while facts are fresh in your mind; express yourself clearly; and always write legibly. If you're ever involved in a lawsuit, a complete patient care record could be your best defense.

Audit your nursing records

Audit your records consistently and comprehensively, using specific criteria to evaluate the effectiveness of patient care. Ask for a charting class – or start one yourself – to encourage staff nurses to chart patient care correctly and legibly. Use problem-oriented charting (to be sure you're documenting all parts of the nursing process) and flow sheets (to record large volumes of data). Encourage other nurses to use these documenting aids.

Use what you know

Use your nursing knowledge to make nursing diagnoses and give clinical opinions. You have a legal duty to your patient not only to make a nursing diagnosis, but also to take appropriate action to meet his nursing needs. Doing so helps protect your patient from harm and you from malpractice charges.

Delegate patient care wisely

Know the legal practice limits of the people you supervise, and caution them to act only within those limits. If your delegation of skilled tasks to an unskilled

(continued)

Taking steps to prevent lawsuits continued

person harms a patient, you can be held liable for breaching your nurse practice act.

Know your nursing department policy manual

Review the policies at least yearly. If you think new policies are needed, ask for them. If you're ever involved in a malpractice lawsuit, a well-prepared manual and your knowledge of nursing policies could be important in your defense.

Show kindness and respect

Treat your patient's family, as well as your patient, with kindness and respect. When you help relatives cope with the stress of the patient's illness and teach them the basics of home care, they'll more likely remember you with a thank-you card than with a legal summons.

one whose first concern is to deliver high-quality patient care.

Qualities of a good nursing department manual

Although manuals will differ, most good ones will do the following:
• show how general hospital policies and procedures apply to the nursing department
• outline the nursing department's roles and responsibilities, both internally and in relation to other hospital departments
• identify the expected limits of nursing action and practice
• offer guidelines for handling emergency situations
• contain procedures that show compliance with state or federal laws, such as *patient anti-dumping laws*
• give *standing orders* for nurses who work in special areas, such as the intensive care unit (ICU) or the *coronary care unit* (CCU)
• show the steps to be taken before — and after — arriving at nursing care decisions. These steps provide the basis for the institution's nursing care standards. The manual itself can be used as evidence in *malpractice* cases.

Today, hospitals are rapidly revising and expanding their basic policies and procedures. Any good nursing department manual should be undergoing regular revision. Some of these procedure and policy changes result from efforts to streamline and standardize patient care. Others result from efforts to comply with new state, provincial (Canada), and federal regulations or to implement recommendations of the *Joint Commission on Accreditation of Healthcare Organizations (JCAHO).*

How hospital policies affect court decisions

Policies aren't *laws,* but courts have generally ruled against nurses who violated their employers' policies. Courts have also held hospitals *liable* for poorly formulated — or poorly implemented — policies.

Legally, if you practice within the scope of your job description and are sued for malpractice, the hospital will have to assume secondary responsibility. Whether you've acted properly is ordinarily determined, in court, by the patient's condition on admission and the hospital's nursing service policy.

How policy is applied in court

In *Utter v. United Health Center* (1977), nurses failed to report a patient's deteriorating condition to the department chairman and so caused a critical 24-hour delay in the patient's treatment. A provision in the hospital's nursing manual said that if the doctor in charge — after being notified — did nothing about adverse changes in a patient's condition or acted ineffectively, the nurse was to "call this to the attention of the Department Chairman."

The judge told the jury that it could label the nurses' failure to follow this provision as the ***proximate cause*** of the patient's injury. Because they failed to follow hospital policy, the nurses shared blame for the doctor's inaction.

How laws affect hospital policies

Many hospital policies and procedures are mandated by state or provincial licensing laws or by such federal regulations as the conditions for participation in ***Medicare.***

Many such mandatory requirements exist. In the United States, for instance, the Civil Rights Act of 1964 compels any hospital receiving federal funds to adopt policies against discrimination based on race, creed, color, national origin, handicap, or sex. (These requirements mainly refer to admitting patients, not to giving bedside care.) The Freedom of Information Act requires hospitals to give consumers and patients access to certain data previously considered privileged. And the Department of Health and Human Services' regulations require that hospitals observe strict guidelines when using patients in research studies.

Canadian law

In Canada, each province has its own laws governing hospitals, both public and private. According to the Ontario Public Hospitals Act, certain classes of hospitals receiving provincial aid must, with few exceptions, admit patients needing treatment.

The provincial legislatures also pass laws governing hospitalization in psychiatric facilities. Matters of criminal law, however, are in the hands of the federal parliament, so hospital policymakers look to the federal parliament for guidance on issues such as narcotics and abortions.

Comparing U.S. and Canadian policy

Hospital policies in the United States and Canada generally show more similarities than differences. One difference involves control at the federal level. Federal agencies in the United States exert more power than their Canadian counterparts do.

Under English ***common law,*** people are usually not obligated to help each other — not even in emergencies. However, where hospitals are concerned, Canadian provincial legislatures have departed from this tradition. For example, the Public Hospitals Act of Nova Scotia states that when a qualified medical practitioner makes application for a patient and the (publicly funded) hospital has room, it must admit the patient — even if he can't pay for his care. (Private hospitals, however, needn't do this.)

In the United States, if an uninsured patient tries to get emergency treatment in a hospital but is turned away, the hospital subsequently can be found negligent if the patient's condition becomes significantly worse. *Hunt v. Palm Springs General Hospital* (1977) involved a patient who died from brain damage caused by prolonged seizures after one hospital refused to admit him because he hadn't paid past-due bills. He wasn't treated until another hospital admitted him, 4 hours later.

Recent federal legislation

In 1986 Congress amended the Social Security Act to prevent hospitals from turning away uninsured or financially strapped patients. Called patient anti-dumping legislation, these amendments require that hospitals participating in Medicare provide screening and stabilizing treatment for anyone who has an emergency condition or is in labor. What's more, the Act gives guidelines and requires *documentation* for transfers or for hospital discharge. Failure to comply can lead to fines, loss of Medicare provider status, or both. This legislation has expanded regularly since 1989 and is called the Emergency Treatment and Active Labor Act, or EMTALA.

How hospital policies affect your job

Hospital administrators write policies to guide workers in the hospital's daily operations. Policies stem from the hospital's philosophy and objectives and are part of the hospital's planning process. So they affect your job directly.

If you're considering employment at a hospital, study its policies carefully. If they're well defined, they may give you an indication of how satisfied and secure you can expect to be in your job.

If you're working in a specialized nursing area, such as the ICU or CCU, give special attention to any policies that directly or indirectly apply to you. Make sure your specialty is clearly defined in keeping with your state or provincial nurse practice act—and with the standards recommended by accrediting agencies and professional medical and nursing associations.

Besides reading policies—the general principles by which a hospital is guided in its management—read the hospital's *rules,* too. These describe the actions that employees should or should not take in specific situations. "No smoking in the patient's room," for example, is a rule that should be enforced without exception.

If you feel reasonably comfortable with the hospital's philosophy, objectives, policies, rules, and quality of care, you'll probably feel comfortable on the job. But if the hospital's policy calls for nursing procedures that conflict with your personal nursing standards or ethics, then you should consider looking elsewhere for employment.

When hospital policy and your nurse practice act conflict

You must refuse to follow hospital policy when it conflicts with your nurse practice act. Any willful violation of rulings passed by the board of nursing, even with your hospital's knowledge and encouragement, could result in suspension or revocation of your license.

The case of *O'Neill v. Montefiore Hospital* (1960) illustrates the dilemma a nurse faces when she must choose between hospital policy and her professional standards. This case involved a nurse who, following hospital policy, refused to admit a patient because he belonged to an insurance plan her hospital didn't accept. The man returned home and died. Although the trial court ruled in favor of the nurse, the New York Supreme Court reversed the decision and ruled the hospital nurse negligent for refusing to admit the patient.

Hospital policies that apply to LPNs and LVNs

In general, LPNs and LVNs should not be required to exceed limits that law and education place on their practice. Exceptions to this rule do exist. Both state law and national health commissions have recognized the rights of LPNs to perform in an expanded role—

for example, to administer I.V. drugs — if the LPN is properly trained for the task and it's one that other LPNs perform in the hospital.

Get it in writing

Be careful to protect yourself. Make sure the conditions for your doing this work are included in your hospital's written policies. And make sure the policies have been established by a committee representing the medical staff, the nursing department, and the administration. The written version should be available to all medical and nursing staff members. If, for example, the policy that allows LPNs to administer I.V. drugs isn't stated in writing, you'd better not administer I.V. drugs. If you're sued on this basis and can't back up your actions with written hospital policy, you may be found liable.

Changing hospital policy

When seeking to bring nursing policy problems to your hospital administration's attention, you can involve your health-team colleagues by discussing policy problems at committee meetings, conferences, and interdepartmental meetings. Alternatively, you can communicate directly with your hospital administration via the *grievance procedure*, counseling, attitude questionnaires, and formal and informal unit management committees.

Legal risks caused by understaffing

Understaffing occurs when the hospital administration fails to provide enough professionally trained personnel to meet the patient population's needs. If you're like most nurses, you're familiar with understaffing and the problems it can cause.

A number of court cases have addressed this issue, suggesting not only that understaffing is widespread but also that it results in substandard bedside care, increased mistakes and omissions, and hasty documentation — all of which increase nurses' (and their employers') liability. For example, if during hospitalization a patient is harmed and can demonstrate that the harm resulted from the hospital's failure to provide sufficient qualified personnel, the hospital may be held liable.

What constitutes adequate staffing?

You won't find many legal guidelines to help you answer this question. Determining whether your unit has too few nurses or too few specially trained nurses may be difficult. The few guidelines that do exist vary from state to state and are limited mainly to specialty care units (such as intensive care). Even the JCAHO offers little help. The 1995 JCAHO staffing standard sets no specific nurse-patient ratios. It just states generally that "The organization provides an adequate number of staff whose qualifications are commensurate with defined job responsibilities and applicable licensure, law and regulation, and certification."

In the absence of well-defined staffing guidelines, the courts have had no reliable standard for ruling on cases of alleged understaffing. Each case has been decided on an individual basis.

Important court rulings

The decision in the landmark case *Darling v. Charleston Community Memorial Hospital* (1965) was based partly on the issue of understaffing. A young man broke his leg while playing football and was taken to Charleston's emergency department, where the on-call doctor set and cast his leg. The patient began to complain of pain almost immediately.

Later, his toes grew swollen and dark, then cold and insensitive, and a stench pervaded his room. Nurses checked the leg only a few times a day, and they failed to report its worsening condition. When the cast was removed 3 days later, the necrotic condition of the leg was apparent. After making several surgical attempts to save the leg, the surgeon had to amputate below the knee.

After an out-of-court settlement with the doctor who'd applied the cast, the court found the hospital liable for failing to have enough specially trained nurses available at all times to recognize the patient's serious condition and to alert the medical staff.

Since the *Darling* case, several similar cases have been tried (for example, *Cline v. Lund,* 1973; *Sanchez v. Bay General Hospital,* 1981; and *Harrell v. Louis Smith Memorial Hospital,* 1990). Almost every case involved a nurse who failed to continuously monitor her patient's condition — especially his vital signs — and to report significant changes to the attending doctor. In each case, the courts have emphasized:

• the need for sufficient numbers of nurses to continuously monitor a patient's condition

• the need for nurses who are specially trained to recognize signs and symptoms that require a doctor's immediate intervention.

Hospital liability

Courts hold hospitals primarily liable in lawsuits in which nursing understaffing is the key issue. A hospital can be found liable for patient injuries if it accepts more patients than its facilities or nursing staff can accommodate. The hospital controls the purse strings and, in the courts' view, is the only party that can resolve the problem.

Defending understaffing

Hospitals accused of failing to maintain adequate nursing staffs have offered various defenses. Some have argued they acted reasonably because their nurse-patient ratio was comparable to other area hospitals. This argument fails if any applicable rules and regulations contradict it.

Other hospitals have defended understaffing by arguing that no extra nurses were available. The courts have hesitated to accept this defense, however, especially when hospitals have knowingly permitted an unsafe condition to continue for a long period. One possible future scenario — a hospital may be held liable for failing to use the nursing personnel available from temporary-nursing service agencies or **nurses' registries.**

Still other hospitals have excused understaffing by pleading lack of funds. The courts have repeatedly rejected this defense.

Emergency defense

Hospital liability for understaffing isn't automatic. If the hospital couldn't have provided adequate staff by any reasonable means — because, for example, a nurse suddenly called in sick and no substitute could quickly be found — the hospital may escape liability. This is known as a **sudden emergency exception** when used as a defense during a trial. The emergency could not have been anticipated — in contrast to chronic understaffing.

Except for the sudden emergency exception defense, a hospital has only two alternatives for avoiding liability for understaffing: either hire sufficient personnel to staff an area adequately or else close the area (or restrict the number of beds) until adequate staff can be found.

Charge nurse's liability

Any nurse who's put in charge of a unit, even temporarily, may find herself liable in understaffing situations, including the following:

• She knows understaffing exists but fails to notify the hospital administration about it.

• She fails to assign her staff properly and then also fails to supervise their actions continuously. (See *When coworkers put you at risk*.)

• She tries to perform a nursing task for which she lacks the necessary training and skills.

Court cases

In *Horton v. Niagara Falls Memorial Medical Center* (1976), the charge nurse, one LPN, and one nurses' aide were responsible for 19 patients on a unit. During their shift, one patient became delirious and tried to climb down from a balcony off his room. The attending doctor, when notified, ordered that someone stay with the patient at all times to keep him from going out on the balcony again.

The charge nurse, instead of calling for additional help from within the hospital or notifying the administration, called the patient's wife and summoned her to the hospital. The wife agreed to send her mother but said it would take time before her mother could arrive. During the interim, the charge nurse provided no supervision of the patient, who went out on the balcony again, jumped, and sustained injuries. In the lawsuit that followed, the court held the charge nurse liable.

In *Norton v. Argonaut Insurance Co.* (1962), a temporary staff shortage led the assistant director of nurses to volunteer her nursing services on a pediatric floor. Because she had been an administrator for several years and was unfamiliar with pediatric care, she proceeded to give a newborn 3 ml of Lan-

---

QUESTIONS ABOUT THE LAW

When co-workers put you at risk

To help you steer clear of legal dangers when working with the health care team, here are some questions and answers to clarify legal responsibilities.

Can I be held liable for mistakes made by a student nurse under my supervision?
Yes, if you have primary responsibility for instructing the student and correcting her mistakes.

If a student nurse performs tasks that only a licensed nurse should perform, and does so with my knowledge but without my supervision, am I guilty of breach of duty?
Yes, because as a staff nurse, you should know that a student nurse can perform nursing tasks only under the direct supervision of a nurse licensed to perform those tasks.

What should I do if I see another health team member perform a clinical procedure incorrectly?
If the incorrect procedure can harm the patient, you have a legal duty to stop the procedure—tactfully, when possible—and immediately report your action to your nursing supervisor. If the incorrect procedure doesn't threaten to harm the patient, don't stop the procedure—but report your observation to your supervisor.

Can I face legal action if I ask a hospital volunteer to help me give patient care and she does something wrong?
Yes. Don't ask a volunteer to participate in any task she isn't trained and professionally qualified to perform.

oxin (digoxin) in injectable rather than elixir form. The infant died of cardiac arrest, and the court held the assistant director liable.

Viable defenses

A charge nurse is not automatically liable for mistakes made by a nurse on her staff. Most courts will not hold the charge nurse liable unless she knew, or should have known, that the nurse who made the mistake:

• had previously made similar mistakes
• wasn't competent to perform the task
• had acted on the charge nurse's erroneous orders.

And remember, the *plaintiff*-patient has to prove two things: that the charge nurse failed to follow customary practices, thereby contributing to the mistake; and that the mistake actually caused the patient's injuries.

Coping with a sudden overload

Like other nurses, you're probably all too familiar with understaffing. You begin your shift and suddenly you find yourself assigned more patients than you can reasonably care for. What can you do to protect yourself?

First, make every effort to protest the overload and get it reduced. Begin by asking your supervisor or director of nursing services to supply relief. If they can't or won't, notify the hospital administration. If no one there will help either, write a memorandum detailing exactly what you did and said and the answers you got. Don't walk off the job (you could be held liable for abandonment); instead, do the best you can. After your shift is over, prepare a written report of the facts and file it with the director of nursing.

Filing a written report isn't guaranteed to absolve you from liability if a patient is injured during your shift. You may still be found liable, especially if you could have foreseen and pre-vented the patient's injury. But a written report will impress a jury as a sincere attempt to protect your patients. And the report could provide you with a defense if the alleged malpractice involves something you should have done, but didn't because of understaffing.

Refusing to work

If conditions become intolerable and you refuse to work, you may be suspended from duty without pay. (See *Floating: Understanding your legal responsibility.*) Consider the Canadian case *Re Mount Sinai Hospital and Ontario Nurses Association* (1978).

This case involved three nurses in the hospital's ICU. Because they were already caring for many critically ill patients, they refused to accept still another from the emergency department. The nurses argued that admitting the new patient would endanger the patients already under their care. The hospital disagreed and suspended them for three shifts without pay.

The case was settled in favor of the hospital, on the premise that a hospital is legally obligated to provide care for patients it admits and can insist that certain instructions be carried out. If the hospital had to defer to its employees' opinions, the decision stated, it would be placed in an intolerable legal position.

Chronic understaffing

Chronic understaffing, if it occurs on your unit, presents you with a dilemma. On the one hand, your conscience tells you to try your best to help every patient. On the other hand, you feel compelled to protect yourself from liability.

Collective action

The best protection, as you might expect, is prevention — action taken to remedy the understaffing situation. Try to work with your institution to develop creative, workable solutions.

If you and your colleagues act responsibly and collectively to try to bring about institutional change, the law will protect you in several important ways.

A case in point is *Misericordia Hospital Medical Center v. N.L.R.B.* (1980), which involved a charge nurse who was discharged from her job because her employer found her activities "disloyal."

She belonged to a group of hospital employees called the Ad Hoc Patient Care Committee. The committee was formed after the JCAHO, which intended to survey the hospital, had invited interested parties — including hospital staff — to submit at a public meeting information on whether accreditation standards were being met. One *complaint* lodged by the nurse and her committee was insufficient coverage on many shifts — a situation the hospital had failed to remedy.

Even though the JCAHO examiners approved the hospital, the nurse was fired shortly afterward. When the National Labor Relations Board (NLRB) ordered the hospital to reinstate the nurse, the hospital appealed. The appeals court upheld the NLRB order, citing a U.S. Supreme Court ruling that employees don't lose protection "when they seek to improve terms and conditions of employment or otherwise improve their lot as employees through channels outside the immediate employee-employer relationship."

This decision offers nurses considerable protection in conflicts with employers, especially those in which working conditions directly affect the care given patients.

Be sure you follow the appropriate channels of communication. If you can't get help to remedy a dangerous understaffing situation, first go through all hospital channels, up to and including the board of trustees. Simply report

Floating: Understanding your legal responsibility

For many nurses, an order to float to an unfamiliar unit triggers worry and frustration. It may cause worry about using skills that have grown rusty since nursing school, or frustration at being pulled away from familiar or enjoyable work.

A necessary evil

Unfortunately, floating is necessary. Hospitals must use it to help solve their understaffing problems. And the courts sanction it as being in the public's best interests.

Exceptions

Legally, you can't refuse to float simply because you fear that the skills you need for the assignment have diminished or because you're concerned about legal risks in the assigned unit. You'll have to go along with an order to float unless:

• you have a union contract that guarantees you'll always work in your specialty

• you can prove you haven't been taught to do the assigned task.

Tell your supervisor if you haven't been taught a task she has assigned you. Usually, she'll accommodate you by changing your assignment. But if she insists that you perform the task you don't know how to do, refuse the assignment. If the hospital reprimands or fires you, you may be able to appeal the action taken against you in a court of law.

what the problem is, the number of hours you've been forced to work without relief, the number of consecutive days you've been forced to work, and any other relevant facts. Then, if you still can't get help, and if your complaint involves an alleged *unfair labor practice,* consider contacting the NLRB.

Witnessing and signing documents

As a nurse, you may be asked to *witness* the signing of documents, such as deeds, bills of sale, *powers of attorney,* contracts, and wills. You may also participate in witnessing oral statements made by patients and others that may have legal significance. Your actions at these times can influence whether what you witnessed has the force of law, and they can also expose you to legal consequences. Later, you may have to testify in court about the signing and the circumstances surrounding it.

Significance of your signature

When you sign as a witness, you're usually certifying only that you saw the person, known to you by a certain name, place his signature on the document. You're not certifying the primary signer's *mental competence* (although you should not sign if you believe he's incompetent), nor are you certifying the presence or absence of duress, undue influence, *fraud,* or error.

If you are called to testify about the signing, don't underestimate the importance of your testimony. A court looking into charges of fraud or undue influence used in executing a document will usually give great weight to a nurse's perception. You may be asked about the patient's physical and mental condition at the time of the signing, and the court may ask you to describe his interactions with his family, his attorney, and others.

Relevant laws

In the United States and Canada, nurse practice acts establish nurses' scope of professional and legal accountability. When you witness a document, other laws also apply. For example, all states have laws setting out the legal requirements for written and oral wills, dying declarations, living wills, powers of attorney, and gifts *causa mortis* (in expectation of death).

Wills

State laws establish requirements for wills, including:
• format requirements
• the number of witnesses needed
• who can be a witness
• what makes a will valid or invalid
• how to make a will inoperative
• how to contest a will.

Usually an individual must be age 18 or older and have two witnesses present to make a valid will. In about two thirds of all states, the will may be handwritten — such a document is called a holographic will.

In many states, your signature on a will certifies that:
• you witnessed the will signing
• you heard the maker of the will declare it to be his will
• all witnesses and the maker of the will were actually present during the signing.

By attesting to the last two facts, you help ensure the authenticity of the will and the signatures. Your signature doesn't certify, however, that the maker of the will is competent.

Precautions
If a patient asks you to serve as a witness when he draws up his will, follow these precautions:
• Don't forget to notify the patient's doctor and your supervisor before you act as a witness.

- Don't give the patient any legal advice.
- Don't offer to assist him in phrasing the document's wording.
- Don't comment on the nature of his choices.
- Don't forget to document your actions in your *nurses' notes.*

The laws also cover dying declarations and gifts *causa mortis,* specifying when they're valid and when they aren't.

In the case of a living will, your state law may prohibit you from acting as a witness.

Your liability

You can be held liable and in violation of the prevailing **standard of care** if the signature you witness is false or if you sign knowing the patient is incompetent or has given uninformed consent. You can also be held liable if you knowingly allow a **minor,** nonguardian, or other ineligible person to sign a document.

If you're the only person who informs a patient about a planned medical procedure and you then witness his signature, you can be liable for practicing outside your nurse practice act, for **practicing medicine without a license,** or both. And your hospital may be liable for negligence under the doctrine of **respondeat superior.** If you give the patient false information in an attempt to deceive him, you may be guilty of fraud or **misrepresentation.**

Read before you sign

Before you sign any document, read at least enough of it to make sure it is the type of document the primary signer represents it to be. Usually you won't have to read all the text, and legally that isn't necessary for your signature to be valid. But always examine the document's title and first page, and give careful attention to what's written immediately above the place for your signature. (The place for your signature should be clearly labeled.)

How to sign

When signing a document, write legibly and use your full legal name. When signing on hospital forms, add your title. On other documents the title is optional, but adding it will establish why you're in the hospital.

When to sign

When you're asked to sign as a witness, do so only if you believe the patient to be both mentally and physically competent. Legally, you don't need to have knowledge of exactly what's contained in the documents you witness. But professionally you should be aware of the content, just as you should be aware of the content when witnessing the patient's signature to an **informed consent** form.

When to refuse

Here are some instances when you shouldn't witness a document:
- when the patient is not legally able to give consent — for example, when he's a minor or a nonguardian
- when the patient is not who he says he is, or you can't be sure
- when the patient has no power of free choice — for example, when he's being blackmailed or otherwise pressured into signing
- when the patient is uninformed about what he's consenting to because he has been given misleading information, doesn't understand the information given, or hasn't been told of the risks involved
- when a patient is obviously incompetent — for example, when he's suffering from advanced dementia and is being pressured to sign a deed trans-

ferring a real estate title to someone else

• when you feel uncomfortable about signing. Keep in mind that you have no legal obligation to witness a will or other document.

In such situations, simply explain that you choose not to act as a witness. Then record the incident in your nurses' notes, using a chronologic format. Chart the setting, the patient's mental and physical condition, the reason for the refusal, what you saw and heard, and what happened after your refusal (for instance, that someone else witnessed or someone else gave consent).

Finally, report the incident to other concerned staff members — for example, your supervisor and the patient's doctor.

Writing the nurses' notes

When you record in your notes that you've witnessed a patient's signature on any type of document, always include something about his apparent perceptions of his health and general circumstances.

When you witness a *written will,* document that it was signed and witnessed, who signed it, who else was present, what was done with it after signing, and what the patient's condition was at the time.

When you witness *oral statements* such as dying declarations or oral wills, document the names of other witnesses, the patient's physical and mental condition at the time, and the patient's reaction to the statements afterwards. Make your notes carefully: remember, they could be used in court for ***probating*** the will, for resolving creditors' claims, or for prosecuting alleged criminals. The notes will also refresh your memory if you're called to testify in court.

Canadian procedures

Formalities of signing and witnessing documents in the United States and Canada may differ. Both countries, however, have legal systems based primarily on English common law, and both have essentially the same rules governing how a witness should sign legal documents.

Legal risks in special care units

In special care units, such as the emergency department (ED), operating room (OR), postanesthesia care unit (PACU), ICU, and CCU, nurses regularly perform tasks that only doctors used to perform. Here, patient care offers exciting nursing challenges, increased nursing responsibilities — and extra risk of liability.

For example, if you're an ED nurse, you'll have to employ triage — classifying patients according to the seriousness of their medical problems. If you make a mistake and a patient's treatment is needlessly delayed, you may be liable.

If the PACU, ICU, or CCU is your assignment, you know you must watch your patients for signs and symptoms of adverse anesthetic effects, of postoperative cardiac and pulmonary complications, and of shock caused by hypoxia, hemorrhage, or infection. In these units, you may also have to administer sophisticated drugs or perform sophisticated procedures, such as operating an intra-aortic balloon pump. In any of these special care units, the patient's survival may depend on your judgment.

Self-protection for nurses working in special care units

If you're working in a special care unit of a hospital – the emergency department, intensive care unit, operating room, or postanesthesia care unit – your expanded responsibilities make you especially vulnerable to malpractice lawsuits. To protect yourself, take the following precautions.

Know your role

Request a clear, written definition of your role in the hospital. Your hospital should have an overall policy and an individual, written job description for you that specifies the limits of your nursing role. You'll be better protected if guidelines for advanced nursing competencies are formally established.

Document thoroughly

Document everything you do, so there's no question later about your actions. Your nurses' notes, of course, should reflect the nursing process: Document your assessment of the patient, your care plan, your actual care, and your evaluation of the plan's effectiveness.

Maintain skills

Make sure of your own competence. If your role expands, your skills have to grow too. If that requires advanced courses and supervised clinical experience, make sure you get both.

Insure yourself

Damages awarded to patients can be very high, and high legal fees may mean you can't afford even to win a lawsuit. If you don't have your own professional liability insurance, and your hospital doesn't help defend you against a lawsuit, you could face a startling bill even after all claims against you are proven groundless and dropped. (You might never even get to court – but you could still find yourself with a large bill for legal consultation.)

Where you stand legally

If you work in a special care unit, take your increased liability seriously. Remember, even though hospital policy requires that you perform certain tasks, or you perform them under doctor's orders as a doctor's ***borrowed servant*** or ostensible agent, your individual liability continues. If a patient sues for malpractice, all the persons involved can be held separately and jointly liable. That suggests that you carefully evaluate the jobs you're asked to do. If any task is beyond your training and expertise, don't attempt it. And even if you can do it, make sure you're permitted to do it according to hospital policy and your state or provincial nurse practice act. (See *Self-protection for nurses working in special care units.*)

Role expansion and the law

In general, a nurse can't legally make a medical diagnosis or prescribe medical, therapeutic, or corrective measures, except as authorized by the hospital and the state where she's working. This means that if you intubate a patient with an endotracheal tube while working on a postoperative orthopedic floor, you may be liable for performing a medical function, especially if you could have called a doctor. But you probably wouldn't be liable if you had been trained in advanced cardiac life support and performed endotracheal intubation in the ED during a disaster.

In Canada, several provinces, including Ontario and Quebec, have passed medical practice acts that permit the delegation of specific medical functions to nurses. Some provinces require that a nurse obtain special training or *certification* to perform these functions. In the United States, however, current laws provide little guidance for nurses who daily face situations like these.

Suppose, for example, you're working in an ICU and so must often act on standing orders and without a doctor's supervision. How can you be sure when you perform quasi-medical functions, even with standing orders, that you're not violating your nurse practice act?

You can't be sure, of course, because nurse practice acts don't provide specific guidelines. Treating patients on the basis of standing orders is a matter of judgment. In such situations, be sure you're qualified to recognize the problem; then follow established medical protocol.

How nursing standards apply

In general, a nurse working in a special care unit is subject to the same general rule of law as her staff nurse colleagues: she must meet the standard of care that a reasonably well-qualified and prudent nurse would meet in the same or similar circumstances.

However, in a malpractice lawsuit, when deciding whether a specialty nurse has acted reasonably the court won't consider what the average LPN, LVN, or RN would have done. Instead, the court will seek to determine the standard of care that an LPN, LVN, or RN specifically trained to work in the special care unit would have met. Thus, the law imposes a higher standard of conduct on persons with superior knowledge, skill, or training.

Courts' view of standards
Hunt v. Palm Springs General Hospital (1977) illustrates how the courts evaluate the reasonable person standard in light of prevailing practices.

The patient, Mr. Hunt, was rushed to the ED with seizures. Once he was examined, his doctor concluded that Mr. Hunt, a known drug addict, was experiencing seizures because he'd gone without drugs for several days. The doctor advised the hospital administration that the patient's condition wasn't critical, but he nevertheless requested hospitalization.

The hospital refused to admit Mr. Hunt because of a history of unpaid bills. During the next 4 hours, Mr. Hunt waited in the ED while the doctor tried to find hospitalization for him elsewhere in the city. Eventually, Mr. Hunt was admitted to a neighboring hospital. He lived for 26 hours before dying of brain damage caused by prolonged seizures.

During the lawsuit that followed, the court examined the practice of ED nurses elsewhere and found that the Palm Springs General Hospital nurses had acted unreasonably. Their duty was to monitor Mr. Hunt's condition periodically while he awaited transfer to another hospital. If this duty had been carried out, the court concluded, the nurses would have noted his elevated temperature — a clear indication that he needed immediate hospitalization.

Similarly, in *Cline v. Lund* (1973), the patient, Ms. Cline, was sent to a coronary care step-down unit when problems developed after she underwent a hysterectomy on July 10. Except for one bout with nausea, she appeared to be making satisfactory progress. At about 2:30 p.m. on July 11, a nurse dangled Ms. Cline's legs from the side of her bed. The nurse charted that the patient tolerated the dangling well. By 3:30 p.m., Ms. Cline was unresponsive, her blood pressure was rising, and she was vomiting.

At 9:00 p.m., when Ms. Cline's blood pressure reached 142/90, the attending nurse notified her supervisor, who at

9:40 p.m. notified the attending doctor. He came to the hospital, examined the patient, and — suspecting an internal hemorrhage — ordered blood work and vital signs taken every 30 minutes. At 11:45 p.m., the patient's blood pressure was 160/90. Her arms and legs were stiff, her fists clenched.

Instead of summoning the doctor again, the attending nurse once more notified her supervisor. At 12:15 a.m. on July 12, when Ms. Cline's blood pressure had reached 230/130, the doctor was called. The patient stopped breathing at 12:40 a.m., suffered a cardiac arrest at 12:45 a.m., and died at 4:45 a.m.

In the ensuing lawsuit, the court found the nurse liable, stating that her care had fallen below that of a *reasonably prudent nurse* in the same or similar circumstances. "Nurses," the court decision said, "should notify the doctor of any significant change or unresponsiveness."

How Canadian nursing standards apply

A Canadian nurse's performance is also measured against the appropriate standard of care. For example, in *Laidlaw v. Lions Gate Hospital* (1969), the court held that both the PACU nurse who left for a coffee break and the supervisor who permitted her to leave should have anticipated an influx of patients from the OR.

When the nurse left for her break, only two patients and the nurse supervisor were in the PACU. In a short time, however, three more patients arrived — including the plaintiff, Mrs. Laidlaw. Because only one nurse was on duty to care for five patients, Mrs. Laidlaw did not receive appropriate care and suffered extensive, permanent brain damage as a result of anesthesia-related hypoxia.

When the resulting lawsuit came to trial, another nursing supervisor testified that usually two nurses were present in the PACU and that nurses weren't permitted to take breaks after new patients arrived. Other testimony revealed that PACU nurses should know the OR schedule and thereby anticipate when new patients will arrive.

The court found the nurse who left, and her supervisor, negligent in leaving only one nurse on duty in the PACU.

Staying within nursing practice limits

When you work in special care units, you mustn't presume that your increased training and broadened authority permit you to exceed nursing's legal limits. That's especially important in an area such as medical diagnosis, in which you can easily cross the legal boundary separating nursing from medicine.

One place where this sometimes happens is in the ED, where an on-call doctor may refuse to see a patient himself, instead ordering care based on a nurse's observations of the patient. In another common ED situation, a patient asks an ED nurse for advice over the telephone. In such a case, she should respond carefully, telling the patient to come to the ED or see his doctor if he has questions or his symptoms persist. Similar situations may occur in the PACU, ICU, and CCU, where split-second patient care decisions are sometimes made on the basis of nurses' phone calls to attending doctors.

Keep in mind that all state and provincial nurse practice acts prohibit you from medically diagnosing a patient's condition. You can tell the doctor about signs and symptoms you've observed. You cannot decide which medical treatments to administer. If you do, you'll be practicing medicine without a license. And you'll be held at least partly liable for any harm to the patient that results.

In *Methodist Hospital v. Ball* (1961), a young man, Mr. Ball, was brought to the ED with injuries sustained in an automobile accident. Because of a sudden influx of critically ill patients, the ED staff was unable to care for him immediately. While lying on a stretcher in the hospital hallway, Mr. Ball became boisterous and demanded care. Apparently, the attending nurse decided he was drunk. Instead of being treated, Mr. Ball was put into restraints and transported by ambulance to another local hospital. There, 15 minutes after arriving, he died from internal bleeding.

An *autopsy* revealed no evidence of alcohol in Mr. Ball's system. In the resulting lawsuit, the court found the attending nurse and medical resident negligent because they failed to diagnose Mr. Ball's condition properly, to give supportive treatment, and to alert personnel at the second hospital about Mr. Ball's critical condition.

A few precautions

If you practice in a special care unit, be sure you know — and follow — hospital policies and procedures. Know your own limitations too — never perform a procedure you feel unsure about. Remember, admitting to inexperience is never wrong. But performing a procedure that may exceed your capabilities could be, especially if it results in injury or death.

If you're an LPN or LVN working in a special care unit, the same precaution applies. As you help RNs care for acutely ill patients and carry out doctors' orders, remember that you assume a significant legal risk when you perform a task ordinarily assigned to an RN. If you injure the patient in the process and he sues you for malpractice, your care will be measured against what a reasonably competent RN would do in the same or similar circumstances.

If you work in an ED, remember to reassess the patient after treatment. It is both sound nursing care and a requirement of the JCAHO to note and document a patient's response to care. If the patient has not had the expected response to treatment, you will also need to document your subsequent intervention.

Legal responsibility for patient safety

One of your most important responsibilities is your patient's physical safety. To prevent falls, for example, you have to make sure bed side rails are up for a debilitated, elderly, confused, or medicated patient. You also have to help a weak patient walk, use proper transfer methods when moving a patient, and sometimes use restraining devices to immobilize a patient.

In the interest of patient safety, you also have to keep an eye on your hospital's facilities and equipment. If you spot loose or improperly functioning side rails, water or some other substance on the unit floor, or an improperly functioning ventilator, you have a duty to report the problem and call for repairs or housekeeping assistance. Failure to do so may not only endanger patients, but also make you — and the hospital — liable if injuries occur.

Patient-safety standards of care

In any malpractice lawsuit against a nurse, she's judged on how well she performed her duty as measured against the appropriate standards of care. The court will analyze whether the *defendant*-nurse gave the plaintiff-patient care equal to that of a reasonably well-qualified and prudent nurse in the same or similar circumstances.

With regard to patient safety, your duty includes anticipating foreseeable risks. For example, if you're aware that the floor in a patient's room is dangerously slippery, you must report the condition to the appropriate hospital department and place caution signs on the floor to warn of the dangers. If you don't, and a patient falls and is injured, you could be held liable.

In fact, you might be held liable even if you didn't know the floor was slippery. Using accepted standards of care, a court might reason that part of your duty as a reasonable and prudent nurse was to check the floor of your unit regularly and report any patient hazard immediately.

The standards of care that you meet will vary with your job and the training you've had. A staff nurse's actions, for example, will be measured against staff nurse standards, and a gerontologic nurse's actions will be measured against standards that gerontologic nurses must meet.

Special safety concerns

In your practice, you need to recognize special safety concerns, such as patient falls, the use of restraints, the prospect of suicide attempts, the safety of equipment, and the risk of transmitting disease.

Patient falls
Almost anything can cause a patient to fall, particularly if he's elderly or receiving medication. Elderly patients are, in many instances, confused, disoriented, and weak. Medications can cause or increase confusion and lessen a patient's ability to react in situations in which he might fall. Here are some ways to protect your patient from falls:
• Make sure his bed's side rails are kept up, when indicated.
• Orient him to where he is and what time it is, especially if he's elderly.

• Monitor him regularly — continually, if his condition makes this necessary.
• Offer a bedpan or commode regularly.
• Provide adequate lighting and a clean, clutter-free environment.
• Make sure that someone helps and supports him whenever he gets out of bed and that he wears proper shoes when walking.
• Make sure adequate staff are available to transfer him, if necessary.

Elderly patients and patients taking medications that cause orthostatic hypotension, central nervous system depression, or vestibular toxicity need special nursing care when doctors' orders require them to be "up in chair for 15 minutes × 3 daily" or "up in chair for meals." If you can't supervise such a patient while he's sitting up, at least make sure another member of the health care team is available.

Restraints
Usually prescribed to ensure a patient's safety, restraints unfortunately can also endanger the patient. When a doctor prescribes a restraining device, keep in mind that such devices don't remove your responsibility for the patient's safety. In fact, they increase it.

For example, when a patient wears a restraining belt, you have to make sure he doesn't undo it or inadvertently readjust it; if he does, it could choke or otherwise injure him. You also have to make sure the belt fits properly; if it's too tight, it could restrict the patient's breathing or irritate his skin. You may have to decide when the belt is no longer necessary. If you fail to do this, you may be accused of *false imprisonment.*

Suicide prevention
Preventing suicides is another important aspect of patient safety. Keep in mind that self-destructive, suicidal patients are found in medical as well as psychiatric wards.

Your first obligation is to provide close supervision. A suicidal patient may require one-on-one, 24-hour-a-day supervision until the immediate threat of self-harm is over. Take from him all potentially dangerous objects, such as belts, bed linens, glassware, and eating utensils. And make sure he swallows pills when you give them; otherwise, he may retain them in his mouth, to save them for later.

Assess the hospital environment carefully for possible dangers. If he can easily open or break his room windows, or if escape from your unit would be easy, you may have to transfer him to a safer, more secure place — if necessary, to a seclusion room.

Remember, whether you work on a psychiatric unit or a medical unit, you'll be held responsible for the decisions you make about a suicidal patient's care. If you're sued because he's harmed himself while in your care, the court will judge you on the basis of:
• whether you knew (or should have known) that the patient was likely to harm himself
• whether, knowing he was likely to harm himself, you exercised reasonable care in helping him avoid injury or death.

Safety of equipment
You are responsible for making sure that the equipment used for patient care is free from defects. You also need to exercise reasonable care in selecting equipment for a specific procedure and patient and then help to maintain the equipment. Here again, your patient care must reflect what the reasonably well-qualified and prudent nurse would do in the same or similar circumstances. This means that if you know a specific piece of equipment isn't functioning properly, you must take steps to correct the defects and document the steps you took. If you don't, and a patient is injured because of the defective equipment, you may be sued for malpractice.

Selecting proper equipment and maintaining it also means making sure it's not contaminated. When cleaning equipment, always follow hospital procedures strictly, and document your actions carefully. That will decrease the possibility that you could be held liable for using contaminated equipment.

You can also be held liable for improper use of equipment that's functioning properly. This liability frequently occurs with equipment that can cause burns — for example, diathermy machines, electrosurgical equipment, and hot-water bottles. When using such equipment, carry out the procedure or therapy carefully, observe the patient continually until finished, and ask the patient frequently (if he's awake) whether he's experiencing any pain or discomfort.

Disease transmission
Be careful not to cause contamination or cross-infection of patients. In *Widman v. Paoli Memorial Hospital* (1989), the hospital was found negligent because a preoperative patient was assigned to the same room as a patient infected with the *Klebsiella* organism. The court found that the hospital did not make sure that personnel assigned to care for the patient followed established infection-control procedures.

Hospital's responsibility for patient safety
Your hospital shares responsibility for the patient's safety. This institutional responsibility for patient safety rests on the two most frequently used doctrines of malpractice liability.

The first doctrine, *corporate liability*, holds the hospital liable for its own wrongful conduct — for any breach of its duties as mandated by *statutory law*, common law, and applicable rules and regulations. The hospital's duty to keep patients safe includes the duty to provide, inspect, repair, and maintain reasonably adequate equipment for diagnosis and treatment. The hospital also has a duty to keep the physical plant reasonably safe. Thus, if a patient is injured because the hospital alone breached one of its duties, the hospital is responsible for the injury.

In recent years, the courts have expanded the concept of an institution's liability for breaching its duties. In a landmark case, *Darling v. Charleston Community Memorial Hospital* (1965), the Illinois Supreme Court expanded the concept of hospital corporate liability to include the hospital's responsibility to supervise the quality of care.

In *Thompson v. The Nason Hospital* (1991), the courts went even further and discussed four general areas of corporate liability. These include:
• a duty to use reasonable care in the maintenance of safe facilities and equipment
• a duty to staff the hospital with only competent doctors
• a duty to oversee all individuals practicing medicine within the hospital
• a duty to develop and enforce policies and procedures designed to ensure quality patient care.

The second doctrine of institutional malpractice liability is *respondeat superior*. Under this doctrine, the liability for an employee's wrongful conduct is transferred to the institution. This means that both the employee and the institution can be found liable for a breach of duty to the patient — including the duty of ensuring his safety.

Determining liability

In a lawsuit involving failure to ensure patient safety, the hospital alone may be held liable or the nurse may share in the liability. The outcome depends on the facts involved.

If, for example, a court can determine that the duty to monitor patient care equipment and to repair any discovered defects rests with the hospital and the nurse, then both could be held liable for a breach of that duty. In *May v. Broun* (1972), the plaintiff-patient sued the hospital, the circulating nurse, and the doctor for burns she sustained when an electric cautery machine's electrode burned her during a hemorrhoidectomy.

Although the machine had been used successfully earlier in the day, when the doctor began to use it on the plaintiff, he noticed that its heat was not sufficient to cauterize blood vessels. So he asked the circulating nurse to check the machine. She did, and after that it apparently worked properly. Nevertheless, the plaintiff was burned where the electrode had touched her body. She later sued the hospital, the circulating nurse, and the doctor.

Because the hospital and the nurse settled with the plaintiff out of court, the doctor was the only one to stand trial. The court held the doctor not liable for the patient's injuries because the hospital had the duty to monitor the equipment and to provide trained personnel to operate it. This meant that the hospital had to bear responsibility for the defective equipment and any wrongful conduct by the nurse. In this case, the hospital and the nurse were liable for the plaintiff's injury.

In *Story v. McCurtain Memorial Management, Inc.* (1981), the outcome was different. This case involved the delivery of one twin by the mother herself when she was left unattended in a shower room. The patient continuously called for help, but her calls went unanswered and the baby that the mother delivered died.

The mother sued both the hospital and the nurse on duty at the time. The court found the nurse not liable, but it held the hospital liable (under the doctrine of corporate liability) for failing to provide safeguards in the shower room and adequate supervision on the unit. Here, then, the hospital alone was liable for breaching its duty to protect patients from harm.

Decreasing your liability

As a nurse, you have an important duty to ensure your patients' safety. Remember, all your actions directed toward patient safety must be in line with your hospital's policies and procedures, so be sure you know what these are. If no policies exist, or if they're outdated or poorly drafted, bring this to your supervisor's or head nurse's attention. Consider volunteering to help write or rewrite the policies. By getting involved in efforts to improve patients' safety, you may reduce your potential liability and, at the same time, improve the quality of patient care.

Legal risks when administering drugs

Administering drugs to patients continues to be one of the most important—and, legally, one of the most risky—tasks you perform.

Over time, nurses' responsibilities with regard to drug administration have increased. For many years, U.S. and Canadian nurses were only permitted to give drugs orally or rectally. Today nurses give subcutaneous and intramuscular injections, induce anesthesia, and administer I.V. therapy. In some states, nurses may even prescribe drugs, within certain limitations.

Both U.S. and Canadian laws continue to strictly limit the nurse's role in drug administration. Within this limited scope, however, the law imposes exceptionally high standards.

Five rights formula
When administering drugs, one easy way to guard against malpractice liability is to remember the long-standing "five rights" formula:
- the right drug
- to the right patient
- at the right time
- in the right dosage
- by the right route.
  And you'd be wise to add a sixth right to this checklist:
- by the right technique.

Drug-control laws

Legally, a drug is any substance listed in an official state, provincial, or national formulary. A drug may also be defined as any substance (other than food) "intended to affect the structure or any function of the body... (or) for use in the diagnosis, cure, mitigation, treatment, or prevention of disease" (N.Y. Educ. Law).

A *prescription drug* is any drug restricted from regular commercial purchase and sale. A state, provincial, or national government has determined that this drug is, or might be, unsafe unless used under a qualified medical practitioner's supervision.

Federal laws
Two important federal laws governing the use of drugs in the United States are the Comprehensive Drug Abuse Prevention and Control Act and the Food, Drug, and Cosmetic Act. The Comprehensive Drug Abuse Prevention and Control Act (incorporating the Controlled Substances Act) categorizes drugs by how dangerous they are and regulates drugs thought to be most subject to abuse. The Food, Drug, and Cosmetic Act restricts interstate shipment of drugs not approved for human use and outlines the process for testing and approving new drugs.

State laws

At the state and provincial level, pharmacy practice acts are the main laws affecting the distribution of drugs. These laws give pharmacists (in Canada, sometimes doctors as well) the sole legal authority to prepare, compound, preserve, and dispense drugs. *Dispense* refers to taking a drug from the pharmacy supply and giving or selling it to another person. This contrasts with administering drugs—actually getting the drug into the patient. Your nurse practice act is the law that most directly affects how you administer drugs.

Most nursing, medical, and pharmacy practice acts include:
• a definition of the tasks that belong uniquely to the profession
• a statement saying that anyone who performs such tasks without being a licensed or registered member of the defined profession is breaking the law.

In some states and provinces, certain tasks overlap. For example, both nurses and doctors can provide bedside care for the sick and, in Canada, both doctors and pharmacists can prepare medicines.

In many states, if a nurse prescribes a drug, she's practicing medicine without a license; if she goes into the pharmacy or drug supply cabinet, measures out doses of a drug, and puts the powder into capsules, she's *practicing pharmacy without a license.* For either action, she can be prosecuted or lose her license, even if no harm results. In most states and Canadian provinces, to practice a licensed profession without a license is, at the very least, a *misdemeanor.*

Court case

In *Stefanik v. Nursing Education Committee* (1944), a Rhode Island nurse lost her nursing license in part because she'd been practicing medicine illegally: She'd changed a doctor's drug order for a patient because she didn't agree with what had been prescribed. No one claimed she had harmed the patient. But to change a prescription is the same as writing a new prescription, and Rhode Island's nurse practice act didn't consider that to be part of nursing practice.

Lawsuits related to medication errors

Unfortunately, lawsuits involving nurses' drug errors are common. The court determines liability based on the standards of care required of nurses when administering drugs. In many instances, if the nurse had known more about the proper dose, administration route, or procedure connected with giving the drug, she might have avoided the mistake that resulted in the lawsuit. (See *Documenting spoken drug orders,* page 124.)

In *Derrick v. Portland Eye, Ear, Nose and Throat Hospital* (1922), an Oregon nurse gave a young boy a pupil-contracting drug when the doctor had ordered a pupil-dilating drug. As a result, the boy lost his sight in one eye, and the nurse and the hospital were found negligent.

A diagnostic drug can also prompt a lawsuit. In a 1967 case in Tennessee, *Gault v. Poor Sisters of St. Francis Seraph of Perpetual Adoration, Inc.,* a nurse was supposed to give a patient a saltwater gastric lavage in preparation for undergoing a gastric cytology test. Instead, she gave the patient dilute sodium hydroxide, which caused severe internal injuries. The hospital lost the verdict and also an appeal.

Getting the dose right is also important. In a Louisiana case, *Norton v. Argonaut Insurance Co.* (1962), a nurse inadvertently gave a 3-month-old infant a digoxin overdose that resulted in the infant's death. At the malpractice trial

Documenting spoken drug orders

When a doctor writes a drug order for his patient and signs it—or when another health care professional writes an order and the doctor countersigns it—the courts usually will not question the legality of the order. But if a doctor gives you a verbal drug order—either in person or by telephone—protect yourself legally, as follows:

• Write down the order *exactly* as he gives it, the date, and the time.
• Repeat the order back to him so that you're sure you heard the doctor correctly.

Documentation guidelines

Once you've given the drug to the patient, make sure you document all necessary information:

• Record *in ink* the type of drug, the dosage, the time you administered it, and any other information your institution's policy requires.
• Sign or initial your notes.

• Be sure the doctor co-signs the drug order as soon as possible.

If your institution keeps drug orders in a special file, make sure that you transfer the doctor's drug order, which you wrote on the patient's chart, to that file.

If a doctor orally gives a drug order during an emergency, your first duty is to carry it out at once. When the emergency is over, document what you did.

The danger of poor documentation

Here's what can happen if you don't document drug orders:

• You could face disciplinary measures for failing to document.
• You could damage your defense or your hospital's in any malpractice lawsuit.
• Other nurses, not knowing what drugs have been given, may administer other drugs that could result in harmful interactions.

---

that followed, the nurse was found liable, along with the hospital and the attending doctor.

Similarly, in *Dessauer v. Memorial General Hospital,* a 1981 New Mexico case, an ED doctor ordered 50 mg of lidocaine for a patient. But the nurse, who normally worked in the hospital's obstetrics ward, gave the patient 800 mg. The patient died, the family sued, and the hospital was found liable.

In *Moore v. Guthrie Hospital,* a 1968 West Virginia case, a nurse made a mistake in the administration route, giving the patient two drugs intravenously rather than intramuscularly. The patient suffered a seizure, sued, and won.

When reviewing these cases, one point becomes clear: The courts will

not permit carelessness that harms the patient.

Dispensing drugs: When you can't escape liability

In rare instances, a nurse may have to administer a drug that isn't available on the unit. If she's working on the night or weekend shift and no pharmacist is available, she may have to dispense the drug herself. If a lawsuit results, the nurse cannot escape liability.

Emergency doses

Some hospitals and nursing homes have written policies that permit a nurse under special circumstances to go into the pharmacy and dispense an emergency drug dose. In the ED, doctors frequently write emergency orders for one to three doses — just enough to hold the patient until he can go to the pharmacy and have his prescription filled. If there is no pharmacist on duty, hospital policy may allow the nurse to obtain the required drug, bottle it, and label it.

Regardless of whether her institution has such a policy, a nurse who dispenses drugs is doing so unlawfully — unless her state's pharmacy practice act specifically authorizes her actions. If she makes an error in dispensing the drug and the patient later sues, the fact that she was practicing as an unlicensed pharmacist can be used as evidence against her.

Your options

If you need to dispense an emergency drug dose, you may choose to disregard the laws that govern your practice for the benefit of your patient's well-being. But you do so at your own risk. And even if you don't harm your patient, you can still be prosecuted and you can still lose your license. When ethics and the law conflict, and you have to weigh concern for your patient's life or health against concern for your license — you must make up your own mind about what action to take.

If your hospital policy requires you to dispense emergency medications and is in clear violation of your state's nurse practice act, consider taking steps to have your hospital policy changed. Start by approaching your nurse-manager with a copy of the nurse practice act and relevant hospital policies. Point out the inconsistencies and the professional risk nurses in the ED are taking. Then offer to accompany your nurse-manager when she approaches *nursing administrators* and the policy and procedure committee. Hospital administrators may designate an ED pharmacist, hire additional pharmacy staff, or prevail upon pharmacists on staff to take greater responsibility for distribution of ED medications.

Your role in drug experimentation

At times, you may participate in administering experimental drugs to patients or administering established drugs in new ways or at experimental dosage levels. Your legal duties do not change. But if you have any questions, you'll get your answers from the experimental *protocol*, not your usual sources, such as books or package inserts. You'll also need to make sure no drug is given to a patient who hasn't consented to participate. (Note that if it's a federally funded experiment, consent should be in writing.)

Your responsibility for knowing about drugs

Once you have your nursing license, the law expects you to know about any drug you administer. If you're an LPN or LVN, you assume the same legal responsibility as an RN once you've taken a pharmaceutical course or obtain authorization to administer drugs. More specifically, the law expects you to:

• know a drug's safe dosage limits, toxicity, potential *adverse reactions,* and indications and contraindications for use

• refuse to accept an illegible, confusing, or otherwise unclear drug order

• seek clarification of a confusing order from the doctor and not to try to interpret it yourself.

Increasingly, judges and juries expect nurses to know what the appropriate observation intervals are for a patient receiving any type of medication. They expect you to know this even if the doctor doesn't know or if he doesn't write an order stating how often to check on the newly medicated patient. A case that was decided on this basis is *Brown v. State,* a 1977 New York case. After a patient was given 200 mg of chlorpromazine (Thorazine), the nurses on duty left him largely unobserved for several hours. When someone finally checked on the patient, he was dead. The hospital and the nurses lost the resulting lawsuit.

Questioning a drug order

If you question a drug order, follow your hospital's policies. Usually they'll tell you to try each of the following actions until you receive a satisfactory answer:
• Look up the answer in a reliable drug reference.
• Ask your charge nurse.
• Ask the hospital pharmacist.
• Ask your nursing supervisor or the prescribing doctor.
• Ask the chief nursing administrator, if she hasn't already become involved.
• Ask the prescribing doctor's supervisor (service chief).
• Get in touch with the hospital administration and explain your problem.

When you must refuse to administer a drug

All nurses have the legal right not to administer drugs they think will harm patients. You may choose to exercise this right in a variety of situations:
• when you think the dosage prescribed is too high
• when you think the drug is contraindicated because of possible dangerous interactions with other drugs, or with substances such as alcohol
• because you think the patient's physical condition contraindicates using the drug.

In limited circumstances, you may also legally refuse to administer a drug on grounds of conscience. Some states and Canadian provinces have enacted *right-of-conscience laws.* These laws excuse medical personnel from the re-

quirement to participate in any abortion or sterilization procedure. Under such laws, you may, for example, refuse to give any drug you believe is intended to induce abortion.

When you refuse to carry out a drug order, be sure you do the following:
• Notify your immediate supervisor so she can make alternative arrangements (assigning a new nurse, clarifying the order).
• Notify the prescribing doctor if your supervisor hasn't done so already.
• If your employer requires it, document that the drug wasn't given, and explain why.

Protecting yourself from liability

If you make an error in giving a drug, or if your patient reacts negatively to a properly administered drug, protect yourself by documenting the incident thoroughly. Besides normal drug-charting information, include information on the patient's reaction and any medical or nursing interventions taken.

In the event of error, you should also file an incident report. Identify what happened, the names and functions of all personnel involved, and what actions were taken to protect the patient after the error was discovered.

LPN's role in administering drugs

Most nurse practice acts now permit LPNs and LVNs *with the appropriate educational background or on-the-job training* to give drugs under the supervision of an RN, a doctor, or a dentist. What constitutes appropriate training or educational background? No clear-cut definitions exist, but most courts probably would be satisfied if an LPN or LVN could prove that her supervising RN or doctor had watched her administer drugs and had judged her competent. (Note, however, that some states prohibit LPNs and LVNs from inserting I.V. lines.)

Patient teaching and the law

Anytime you give a patient information about his care or treatment, you're involved in patient teaching — a professional nursing responsibility and a potential source of liability.

Patient teaching has taken on increased significance, largely because patients are routinely discharged much earlier from hospitals. Patients and their families need more understanding of patients' illnesses and how to manage them at home.

Patient teaching may be formal or informal. You teach *formally* when, for example, you prepare instructions on stoma care for a colostomy patient. When giving the patient this detailed information, you should follow these steps:

• assessing what the patient wants or needs to know
• identifying goals that you and the patient want to reach
• choosing teaching strategies that will help reach the goals
• evaluating how well you've reached the goals.

You teach *informally* when, for example, you calm a patient's fears by explaining an upcoming diagnostic test or when you answer a friend's questions about how to treat her child's fever.

For best results, patient teaching should include the family and others involved in the patient's care. If family members understand the reason for a patient's treatment, they will be more willing to provide emotional support.

Patient-teaching standards

Most nurse practice acts in the United States and Canada contain wording about promoting patient health and preventing disease or injury. But they don't specify a nurse's responsibility for patient teaching. Nurses can find this information in the practice standards developed by professional organizations, in nursing *job descriptions,* and in statements about nursing practice from national commissions.

The JCAHO requires that the "patient and his or her family be provided with appropriate education and training to increase the knowledge of the patient's illness and treatment needs and to learn skills and behaviors that promote recovery and improve function." The Commission requires that patient teaching be done in an interdisciplinary manner, considering the patient's ability to learn and any cultural or emotional factors or any cognitive or physical limitations that would impact his or her ability to learn.

Patient teaching should be a dynamic process that changes to meet the patient's and the family's needs. It should include instruction in how to adapt to the illness as well as how to prevent future problems.

Patient's right to health care information

Both statutory law and common law support the patient's right to have information about his condition and treatment. In fact, when a patient is admitted to a hospital, he may be handed a *patient's bill of rights* that clearly outlines his rights. The doctrine of informed consent further supports the patient's right to know.

Despite RNs' deep involvement in patient teaching, the courts have rarely addressed nurses' liability in this area of patient care. But some legal experts believe that as nurses take on greater patient-teaching responsibilities, they will increasingly become the target of lawsuits dealing with the patient's right to information.

A court faced with a question involving a nurse's responsibility for patient teaching will probably examine the question under the general category of a patient's right to know (*Gerety v. Demers*, 1978; *Canterbury v. Spence*, 1972). Health care requires the patient's participation and cooperation; therefore, the right to know is an inherent part of successful treatment. When the right to know becomes critical to the patient's health, a court is likely to view patient teaching as a health care provider's legal duty.

Suppose you're sued for malpractice, and your alleged wrongful act involves patient teaching. The court will consider whether patient teaching was your legal duty to the patient and whether you met or breached it.

Court case

Kyslinger v. United States (1975) addressed the nurse's liability for patient teaching. In this case, a veterans hospital sent a hemodialysis patient home with an artificial kidney. He eventually died (apparently while on the machine), and his wife sued the federal government — because a veterans hospital was involved — alleging that the hospital and its staff had failed to teach either her or her late husband how to properly use and maintain a home hemodialysis unit.

After examining the evidence, the court ruled against the patient's wife, as follows:

"During those 10 months that plaintiff's decedent underwent biweekly hemodialysis treatment on the unit (at the VA hospital), both plaintiff and decedent were instructed as to the operation, maintenance, and supervision of said treatment. The Court can find no basis to conclude...that the plaintiff or plaintiff's decedent were not properly informed on the use of the hemodialysis unit."

If the patient doesn't want to be taught

Suppose you begin teaching a patient about the medications he's taking, only to hear him say, "Oh, just tell my wife; she gives me all my pills." When something like this happens, be sure to document the incident. Include the patient's exact words; then describe what you taught his wife, and how.

LPN's role in patient teaching

Unlike RNs, LPNs and LVNs aren't taught the fundamentals of patient teaching as part of their school curriculum — nor is patient teaching included in their *scope of practice*. RNs are primarily responsible for patient teaching and may delegate to LPNs or LVNs only the responsibility to reinforce what has already been taught. For example, if an RN is preparing a patient for a barium enema, she could ask an LPN to tell the patient about the X-ray room and what to expect. The RN could add to the information as necessary.

Cooperating with colleagues

Doctors, nurses, and other health team members sometimes disagree about how patient teaching should be done and who should do it. To avoid conflict, always consult doctors and other appropriate health team members when you're preparing routine patient-teaching protocols. A team approach to patient teaching not only decreases conflicts, but also ensures continuity in teaching — and a better-educated patient.

You can also avoid conflicts by listening to the instructions that doctors, respiratory therapists, dietitians, and others give the patient. Then you'll know exactly what's already been said to him, and you can structure your teaching accordingly.

Candor and diplomacy, of course, also help reduce conflict. Everyone profits when health-team members share their patient-teaching approaches and work together to achieve patient-teaching goals.

Incident reports

An *incident* is an event that is inconsistent with the hospital's ordinary routine, regardless of whether injury occurs. In most health care institutions, any injury to a patient requires an *incident report.* Besides patient injuries, incident reports are required for patient complaints, medication errors, and injuries to employees and visitors.

An incident report serves two main purposes:
• to inform the hospital administration of the incident so that it can monitor patterns and trends, thereby helping to prevent future similar incidents (risk management)
• to alert the administration and the hospital's insurance company to the possibility of liability claims and the need for further investigation (claims management).

Even when the incident isn't investigated, the report serves as a contemporary, factual statement of it. The report also helps identify witnesses if a lawsuit is started months or even years later.

To be useful, an incident report must be filed promptly, thoroughly, and factually.

Your duty to report patient incidents

Whether you're an RN, an LPN or LVN, an aide, a staff nurse, or a nurse-manager, you have a duty to report any incident of which you have first-hand knowledge. Not only can failure to report an incident lead to your being fired, but it can also expose you to personal liability for malpractice — especially if your failure to report the incident causes injury to a patient.

If you're the staff member who knows the most about the incident at the time of its discovery, you should complete the incident report. When you do so, include only the facts: what you saw when you came upon the incident or what you heard that led you to believe an incident had taken place. If information is second-hand, place it within quotation marks and identify the source. After completing the incident report, sign and date it. You should complete it during the same shift the incident occurred or was discovered.

What to include

An incident report should include only the following information:
• the names of the persons involved and any witnesses
• factual information about what happened and the consequences to the person involved (supply enough information so the hospital administration can decide whether the matter needs further investigation)
• any other relevant facts (such as your immediate actions in response to the incident, for example, notifying the patient's doctor).

What not to include

Never include the following types of statements in an incident report:
• opinions (such as your opinion of the patient's prognosis)

• conclusions or assumptions (for example, about what caused the incident)
• suggestions of who was responsible for causing the incident
• suggestions of how to prevent the incident from happening again.

Including this type of information in an incident report could seriously hinder the defense in any lawsuit arising from the incident.

Remember, the incident report serves only to notify the administration that an incident has occurred. In effect, it says, "Administration: Note that this incident happened, and decide whether you want to investigate it further." Such items as detailed statements from witnesses and descriptions of remedial action are normally part of an investigative follow-up; don't include them in the incident report itself.

Potential pitfalls

Be especially careful that the hospital's reporting system does not lead to improper incident reporting. For example, some hospitals require nursing supervisors to correlate reports from witnesses and then to file a single report. And some incident report forms invite inappropriate conclusions and assumptions by asking, "How can this incident be prevented in the future?" If your hospital's reporting system or forms contain such potential pitfalls, alert the administration to them.

Reporting an incident

An incident report is an administrative report and therefore doesn't become part of the patient's *medical record.* In fact, the record shouldn't even mention that an incident report has been filed because this serves only to deflect the medical record's focus. The record should include only factual clinical observations relating to the incident. (Again, avoid value judgments.)

Entering your observations in the nurses' notes section of the patient's record doesn't take the place of completing an incident report. Nor does completing an incident report take the place of proper documentation in the patient's chart.

An incident report, once it's filed, may be reviewed by the nursing supervisor, the doctor called to examine the patient, appropriate department heads and administrators, the hospital attorney, and the hospital's insurance company. (See *Filing an incident report: Chain of events.*) The report may be filed under the involved patient's name or according to the type of injury, depending on the hospital's policy and the insurance company's regulations. Reports are rarely placed in the reporting nurse's employment file.

If you're asked to talk with the hospital's ***insurance adjuster*** or attorney about an incident, be cooperative, honest, and factual. Fully disclosing what you know early on will help the hospital decide how to handle any legal consequences of an incident. And it preserves your testimony in case you're ever called to testify in court.

Using incident reports as courtroom evidence

Controversy exists over whether a patient's attorney may "discover" (request and receive a copy of) an incident report and introduce it into evidence in a malpractice lawsuit. The law on this issue varies from state to state. To avoid ***discovery,*** the hospital may send copies of the incident report to its attorney, or the hospital attorney may write a letter stating that the report is being made for his use and benefit only.

Concern about incident report discovery should be minimal if an incident report contains only properly reportable material. The information in a

Filing an incident report: Chain of events

The chart below provides a comprehensive overview of incident report routing.

Patient incident

Record significant medical and nursing facts in patient's chart.

Write incident report during the shift on which the incident took place or is discovered.

Give incident report to supervisor.

Unit supervisor forwards report to appropriate administrator within 24 hours.

Administrator reviews report.

Administrator forwards pertinent information from the report to the appropriate department for follow-up action.

Incident reports are collected and summarized to detect patterns and trends and to highlight trouble spots.

Administrator reviews patterns and trends, using this information in continuous quality improvement projects for a single nursing unit or a multidisciplinary committee.

Refer information to existing quality improvement teams.

Use information as the basis for establishing new quality improvement projects.

properly completed incident report is readily available to the patient's attorney through many other sources. Only when an incident report contains second-hand information, opinions, conclusions, accusations, or suggestions for preventing such incidents in the future does discovery of the incident report become an important issue for attorneys and the courts.

Reporting your own error

If an incident results from your error, you still have the duty to file an incident report immediately. Making a mistake is serious and may invite corrective action by your hospital, but the potential consequences of attempting to cover it up are worse.

For one thing, the likelihood that an incident report will be used against you is slight. A hospital wants its nurses to report incidents and to keep proper records. Nurses may not do this consistently if they're always reprimanded for even small errors. Most hospitals, in fact, will reprimand a nurse for not filing an incident report if injury is done to the patient.

If an incident results from your act of *gross negligence* or irresponsibility or is one of a series of incidents in which you've been involved, then the hospital may take action against you. And that possibility increases if the patient sustains an injury because of your error.

Reporting a co-worker's error

If a fellow employee's error causes a reportable incident, your duty to your patient and your hospital requires that you report your observations. If corrective action is taken, remember that the person who made the error is responsible, not the person who filed the incident report. Be factual and objective in your report. This will minimize any potential liability if the employee brings a civil suit for *libel*.

Here's another point to remember: Most states have laws granting "qualified privilege" to those who have a duty to discuss or evaluate their co-workers, employees, or fellow citizens. This privilege means that no liability for libel exists unless the person giving the information knows it's false or has acted with a reckless disregard for the truth.

Risk management strategy

How can you minimize the chances that a patient will sue after an incident? And how can you protect yourself and your hospital in case he does? The best way is to follow the "three Rs" of risk management strategy: rapport, record, and report.

Maintain rapport with the patient

Answer his questions honestly. Don't offer any explanation if you weren't personally involved in the incident; instead, refer the patient to someone who can supply answers. If you try to answer his questions without direct knowledge of the incident, inconsistencies could arise and the patient could interpret these as a cover-up.

If you feel uncomfortable talking to the patient or family, ask your supervisor, the hospital patient-relations specialist, or an administrator for advice on how to answer questions or to participate and help you provide answers. Remember that patients generally respond favorably if they know you are being honest and you show that you care about their well-being.

Don't blame anyone for the incident. If you feel someone was at fault, tell your charge nurse or supervisor — not the patient.

If an incident necessarily changes the way you care for the patient, tell the patient about it and clearly explain the reasons for the change.

Record the incident

Be sure to note the incident in the medical record. Remember, truthfulness is the best protection against lawsuits. If you try to cover up or play down an incident, you could end up in far more serious trouble than if you'd reported it objectively. Never write in the medical record that an incident report has been completed. An incident report is not clinical information; it's an administrative tool.

Report every incident

Some nurses think incident reports are more trouble than they're worth and, furthermore, that they're a dangerous admission of guilt. That's false. Here's why incident reports are important:

• Incident reports jog our memories. Much time may pass between when an incident occurred and when it comes to court. So we simply can't trust our memories—but we can trust an incident report.

• Incident reports help administrators act quickly to change the policy or procedure that seems to be responsible for the incident. An administrator can also act quickly to talk with families and offer assistance, explanation, or other appropriate support. Sometimes helpful communication with an injured patient and his family can be the balm that soothes a family's anger and prevents a lawsuit.

• Incident reports provide the information hospitals need to decide whether restitution should be made. When a patient is injured instead of helped during his hospital stay, the hospital sometimes decides it has a moral obligation to **compensate** the patient. In fact, this moral obligation is another reason (besides protection against having to pay damages awarded in a lawsuit) that hospitals carry **professional liability insurance.**

Caring for a minor

A minor is any person under the **age of majority,** which is usually 18 or 21, depending on state or provincial law. When you care for a minor, you should keep in mind the way minors' legal rights are structured. The legal rights of a minor depend largely on his age. He may also have special legal status.

Minor's rights

A minor's rights fall into three categories:

• *Personal rights that belong to everyone from birth.* Examples include the right to **privacy** and the right to protection against crimes.

• *Rights that can be exercised as a minor matures.* These fall into two groups. The first includes the right to drive a car, to work at a paying job, and to have sexual relations—as long as both partners are of legal age. These rights are granted at certain ages, according to state laws, whether or not the minor is mature enough to exercise the right intelligently.

The second group includes rights granted by the courts rather than by statutory law. These are given to any minor who shows the mental and emotional ability to handle them.

• *Rights that belong to adults and can be exercised only by adults and by **emancipated minors.*** Examples include many financial and contractual rights, such as the right to consent to medical treatment.

The law provides special protection for minors so that they may exercise certain rights after reaching the age of majority. For example, because a minor cannot sue in court, most states give minors a **grace period** after they reach the age of majority to bring to court any lawsuit relating to when they were minors. This includes suing persons their parents could have sued earlier on the minors' behalf but chose not to. Because this can include a lawsuit for medical malpractice, the law generally requires that hospitals keep the records of pediatric patients longer than the records of adults.

Mature minor

A mature minor is a nonemancipated minor in his middle to late teens who shows clear signs of intellectual and emotional maturity. A mature minor may be able to exercise certain adult rights, depending on laws in his state.

Becoming emancipated

Emancipation is the legal process whereby children may obtain freedom from the custody, care, and control of their parents before the age of majority. Under most state statutes, an emancipated minor loses his right to financial support from his parents in exchange for the ability to govern his own affairs. Emancipation may also enable a minor to enter into binding contracts and to sue and be sued in his own name. Some statutes also give an emancipated minor the ability to consent to medical, dental, or psychiatric care without parental consent.

Depending on the jurisdiction, emancipation may be addressed by common law or statutory law. Most states require a hearing in emancipation cases.

Standards for emancipation may include:
• *Best interests of the minor.* Many state statutes contain a provision allowing judges to use the best interest of the child as a standard for emancipation.
• *Ability to manage financial affairs.* Many state statutes have a provision requiring that a minor demonstrate the ability to manage financial affairs before becoming emancipated.

• *Living separate and apart from parents.* Many statutes require that minors who wish to be emancipated live separate and apart from their parents. Some require parental consent for separate living arrangements.
• *Parental consent.* Many states require parental consent for an emancipation petition.
• *Age.* Most states require that children be at least age 16 before initiating emancipation proceedings.

Restrictions on rights

Even an emancipated minor may not exercise certain rights. If he's 18 and the drinking age in his state is 21, he still can't legally buy an alcoholic beverage. Some states set a minimum age for making a will (usually the age of majority). In those states, even if the minor is married or has a child, any will he draws up won't be valid.

Guardians *ad litem*

A *guardian ad litem* is a person appointed by the court to protect a minor's interests in a legal proceeding. A guardian *ad litem* may be appointed when these two conditions coexist:
• A decision is needed for the minor.
• A "diversion of interest" exists; that is, the court possesses evidence that the interests of the minor's parents or *legal guardians* probably don't coincide with those of the minor.

The court may appoint a guardian *ad litem* even if one or both parents are still living and interested in the minor's welfare or if the minor already has a guardian.

Obtaining consent

By far the most common problem with minors is obtaining proper consent for their medical care. Although the doctor bears the legal responsibility for this, you'll commonly be involved in the process. Here are 11 different situations you may face in helping to obtain a minor's consent.

Nonemancipated minor

If the minor isn't emancipated, his mother, father, or legal guardian has the right to refuse or consent to treatment for him. Whenever possible, consent should be obtained from both parents or both guardians when joint guardians have custody of the minor.

If the parents are divorced or separated, the policy is to obtain consent from the parent who has custody. If the minor's parents are incompetent or dead and he has no legal guardian, the court will usually appoint a legal guardian for him. The guardian can consent or refuse, just as if he were a parent.

Mature, nonemancipated minor

In Canada, mature, nonemancipated minors can consent to medical treatment themselves. In the United States, nonemancipated but mature minors' rights are not as broad. In some jurisdictions, however, parental consent is no longer necessary for various types of medical and psychiatric care. In California, for example, nonemancipated minors age 15 and older, who live separate from their parents and manage their own finances, may consent to their own medical care. Ask your hospital attorney to check your state's statutes in this area.

In its rulings on abortion and contraception, the U.S. Supreme Court has indicated that mature minors have certain rights of consent and privacy.

Emancipated minor

An emancipated minor can usually refuse or consent to treatment himself. But if he's unable to do so (for example, because he's unconscious after an accident), you have to try to find someone who can give consent for him. Possibilities, in descending order of preference, include his spouse, parents or guardians, and nearest living relative. You may waive this requirement for consent only in an emergency situation, when your failure to treat a minor immediately could result in further injury or in death.

When parents or joint guardians disagree

Problems can arise when parents (whether married, divorced, or separated) or joint guardians disagree about consenting to treatment for a nonemancipated minor. The hospital's only recourse may be to go to court, where a judge either makes the decision himself or assigns responsibility to one parent or guardian. You may find yourself caught in a situation in which a minor's parents or guardians can't agree on consenting to his treatment. When this happens, tell the hospital administrators immediately so they can talk to the parents or guardians and, if necessary, alert the hospital's attorney.

When a minor needs emergency care

The legal rule to follow when a minor needs emergency care is the same as that for adults: Treat first and get consent later. Some courts have held that any mature minor, emancipated or not, may give valid and binding consent to emergency treatment. For example, in *Younts v. St. Francis Hospital and School of Nursing* (1970), a nonemancipated but mature 17-year-old was found able to consent to surgical repair of a severed fingertip.

When a minor requests an abortion

Recent U.S. Supreme Court rulings, including *Ohio v. Akron Center for Reproductive Health* (1990) and *Hodgson v. Minnesota* (1990) indicate that state laws can't prevent a minor from seeking and obtaining a *legal abortion;* however, states can impose conditions on consent. The law in some states may require a minor seeking an abortion to notify her parents or to bypass this consent requirement by going before a judge (judicial bypass).

For the rules your state requires you to follow when verifying consent for a minor's abortion, check with your hospital's attorney.

When a minor asks for a contraceptive

In *Carey v. Population Services International* (1977), the U.S. Supreme Court ruled unconstitutional a state law prohibiting the sale of contraceptives to anyone under age 16. The court held that the decision to bear a child is a fundamental right and that state interference can only be justified if it protects a compelling state interest. As a result, a minor can obtain contraceptives without parental consent.

Again, consult the hospital's attorney if you have questions regarding restrictions on distributing contraceptives to minors. For example, your state may require you to notify a parent or guardian about the matter.

When a minor needs treatment for a communicable disease

Most states and Canadian provinces have laws that permit minors to consent to treatment for serious communicable diseases, including sexually transmitted diseases, without parental approval.

If you must deal with a minor who's refusing diagnosis or treatment for a communicable disease, check your state's laws. Most states permit public health authorities to deal with a nonconsenting minor as an adult, including deciding whether he should be quarantined.

When a minor needs treatment for drug abuse

State and federal laws generally permit minors to consent to take part in *drug-abuse* treatment and rehabilitation programs just as though they were adults. Like adults, minor patients in drug treatment programs are entitled to have their records kept confidential.

When religious beliefs conflict with a minor's treatment

If your patient or his parents or guardians are Jehovah's Witnesses or Christian Scientists, you may have special problems getting consent to treatment.

Although competent adults or emancipated minors may refuse treatment for religious reasons, nonemancipated minors may not. In most states in which the question has come before the courts, judges have ruled that parents and guardians can't stop a hospital from treating their child solely on religious grounds, if a reasonable chance exists that the treatment will help the patient.

Note, however, that in this situation a court will have to appoint a guardian *ad litem* for the sick minor. This may take some time, so to avoid delaying the minor's treatment unnecessarily, notify your hospital administration as quickly as possible.

When a minor seeks or receives mental health care

Minors, like adults, may be treated at private and state-run mental health facilities. When the minor and his parents agree to seek such treatment for the minor, the facility will follow its normal medical guidelines and procedures in deciding whether to admit him. This usually involves informing the patient and his parents or guardian of their rights and then obtaining their informed consent for admission.

The U.S. Supreme Court, in *Parham v. J.R.* (1979) and in *Secretary of Public Welfare v. Institutionalized Juveniles*

(1979), held that nonconsenting minors can be admitted to state-run mental health facilities at the request of either or both parents. Such minors, however, always have the right to have a psychiatrist or other trained fact finder review the request at or before admission and periodically thereafter. The fact finder may be the facility's regular admissions officer.

In many states, however, the rules controlling admission of minors to *inpatient* mental health facilities are more rigorous. The rules may call for a full-scale hearing, with attorneys present, within a set time after admission (if not concurrent with admission).

Caring for an abused patient

In the course of your career, you're likely to encounter both adult and child victims of abuse. Sometimes abuse is physical battering, such as when a son regularly beats his aging father. At other times, abuse involves verbal, sexual, or emotional attack; neglect; or abandonment.

Profile of the abuser

People who abuse others come from all socioeconomic levels and all ethnic groups. No specific psychiatric diagnosis encompasses the abuser's personality and behavior. However, many abusers have a history of being abused themselves when young or of having witnessed abuse of parents or siblings. (Such childhood experiences are usually profound and can influence a person's behavior throughout his adult life.) In many cases, abusive persons lack self-esteem and the security of being loved — qualities that help nonabusive persons cope with stress.

In times of crisis, abusers resort to the behavior learned in childhood. They abuse just as they were abused — all in an attempt to restore their own feelings of self-control and self-esteem. After all, if abuse was an acceptable behavior for their parents, why can't it be the same for them now?

Abusers are usually unable to tolerate personal failure or disapproval from spouses, children, or friends. When an abuser's self-esteem is low, he expects rejection and will act in ways that cause others to reject him. Rejection in turn provokes the abuser to commit further verbal or emotional abuse.

Abusers commonly have unrealistic expectations of the people they abuse. When an individual fails to live up to these expectations, the abuser feels a strong compulsion to control, mortify, reject and, if necessary, physically injure that individual.

Cycle of abuse

Low self-esteem may prompt an abuser to choose a partner much like himself. Each will then feed into the other's forms of abuse. If the couple has children, in many cases they become targets of their parents' abusive behavior. And what the children witness and suffer begins another cycle of abused child to child abuser.

Child abuse

Children, especially between the ages of 4 months and 3 years, are commonly abused. (See *Responding to child abuse,* page 138.) Children with behavior problems are particularly vulnerable to abuse, as are malformed or developmentally disabled children and children born prematurely or born to unmarried parents. From the abusive parent's perspective, such a child represents an unplanned disruption or a

Responding to child abuse

Suppose you're on duty in the emergency department when Mrs. Firth comes in with her son Billy, age 4. She tells you, "Billy was riding in a friend's car and they had an accident. I didn't think he was hurt at first, but later on his knee swelled up. I decided I'd better have a doctor look at it."

You examine Billy closely for head and neck injuries. You don't see any, but you do notice some bruises on his left arm and on his legs that look several weeks old. You question Mrs. Firth about the accident, but she offers few details. Then, when you ask her about Billy's injuries, she gets defensive. Although his injuries look painful, Billy sits quietly while you examine him.

How to respond

You suspect Billy has been abused. What should you do next? Follow these guidelines:

• Tell the doctor that you suspect child abuse and ask him to order a total-body X-ray. If he resists your request, talk directly with the radiologist; he can do it on his own authority. Don't hesitate to take this action into your own hands. Also, inform your supervisor of the situation.

• If you suspect the child has been forced to ingest drugs or alcohol, get an order for toxicology studies of the child's blood and urine.

• If the child is severely bruised, get an order for a blood coagulation profile.

• If X-rays or other studies suggest the child has been abused, talk with the doctor about confronting the parents. Ask how you might help him do this.

• If a parent admits to abusing the child and appears to want help, supply the address and telephone number of a local group, such as a local chapter of Parents Anonymous, and encourage the parent to call.

• Whether or not the parent admits to abusing the child, report all suspected abuse to the state-designated agency empowered to investigate the situation. Keep in mind that in many states, failure to report suspected abuse is a crime.

---

stress-producing crisis. If the child has mental or physical defects, the parent may see this as reaffirming his own inadequacy and weakness. If the child has severe defects, the parent may be unable to accept that the child is his: He may pour on abuse in an effort to be rid of the child.

Parents may also view children as extensions of persons they hate. Sometimes this results from similarities in physical appearance or similarities in behavior. If a child resembles a spouse who deserted the family, he may be blamed for the spouse's failures and abused accordingly.

Adult abuse

Spouses and elderly parents or relatives are the most common victims of adult abuse.

The abused spouse in many cases suffers from lack of self-esteem. An abused spouse's parents may have abused each other, or one parent may have abused the other. Having witnessed these attacks as a child, the present-day abused spouse accepts that she too will be abused. By behaving passively, spouses make it easy for their partners to abuse them repeatedly without fear of retaliation.

Like children, adults can become abuse victims if they're viewed as too dependent, too sickly, or too much like a hated person. Ill or elderly persons who make financial, emotional, or personal demands in many cases will end up injured when the stress they create becomes intolerable for their abusers. (See *Elder abuse,* page 140.)

Among abusers of adults, men who abuse women predominate, but sometimes the opposite happens. Abused men, married or not, in most cases show the same low self-esteem and passivity as abused women. Sometimes an abused man is the less aggressive and more subservient member of the relationship and accepts a certain level of abuse in the hope that it won't get worse. At other times, he may be so ashamed by his inability to provide adequately that he invites abuse to give himself a feeling of atonement.

Abuse and the law

In 1874, grossly battered "Mary Ellen," age 9, was found chained to her bed in a New York City tenement. Etta Wheeler, a church worker, tried to find help for Mary Ellen, but she quickly discovered that New York had no laws to protect children. Her only recourse was the American Society for the Prevention of Cruelty to Animals, which agreed to intervene on Mary Ellen's behalf.

A year after Mary Ellen's case reached the courts, New York state adopted the country's first child-protection legislation. This gave child-protection agencies a legal base, and it proved a breakthrough for other disadvantaged groups as well.

Since then, child abuse has gained increasing attention from the public, from legislators, and from concerned health care professionals. In 1946, for

example, radiologists reported that subdural hematomas and abnormal X-ray findings in the long bones were commonly associated with early childhood traumatic injuries. In 1961, an American Academy of Pediatrics symposium on child abuse introduced the term "battered child."

The first statutory laws calling for mandatory reporting of child abuse resulted from a 1963 report by the Children's Bureau of the U.S. Department of Health, Education, and Welfare (now the Department of Health and Human Services). Most states, using the model in the report, developed protective legislation by the early 1970s. Unfortunately, the diversity of these laws makes uniform interpretation impossible.

To help remedy this, Congress passed the Child Abuse Prevention and Treatment Act in 1973. This act requires states to meet certain uniform standards in order to be eligible for federal assistance in setting up programs to identify, prevent, and treat the problems caused by child abuse. The act also established a national center on child abuse and *child neglect.*

The act was amended in 1984 in response to "Baby Doe" cases. These cases involved parents who refused life-saving treatment for mentally and physically handicapped infants. The amendments require the states to respond to reports of a child's medical neglect. States must respond to reports that medically indicated treatment (including appropriate nutrition, hydration, and medication) has been withheld from an infant. The law allows three exceptions whereby treatment may be withheld:

• when the infant is chronically ill and irreversibly comatose

• when treatment would only prolong dying

• when treatment itself would be inhumane and futile in terms of survival.

Elder abuse

Elder abuse has reached alarming proportions. Estimates range from 700,000 to 1 million cases of mistreatment annually in the United States alone. Perhaps 1 in 10 of all dependent elderly persons are abused or neglected by family members or other caregivers each year; probably only 1 in 14 cases of mistreatment is reported.

The greater an elderly person's disabilities, the more vulnerable he is to abuse or neglect by caregivers – usually his relatives. Family members provide about 80% of all care given to older people. And about 85% of all reported abuse involves a family member's behavior.

Defining abuse and neglect

Nearly every state has laws mandating that suspected elder abuse be reported to the authorities. But not all states define elder abuse. Instead they leave its diagnosis to health care professionals. One definition of abuse and neglect goes as follows:

• *Elder abuse* is destructive behavior that's directed at an older adult, carried out in a context or relationship of trust, and occurring intensely or frequently enough to produce harmful physical, psychological, social, or financial suffering and a decreased quality of life.

• *Elder neglect* is harm cause by failure to provide prudently adequate and reasonable assistance to meet the elderly person's basic physical, psychological, social, and financial needs.

Detecting abuse

As a nurse – especially if you're in an outpatient or acute care setting – you have more contact with patients than most other members of the health care team. You may be the first to notice or suspect mistreatment of an elderly patient. In fact, in hospitals with special Elder Assessment Teams, most abuse referrals are generated by nurses – especially those in the emergency department. If you suspect elder abuse, report it according to hospital or agency policy.

Signs and symptoms

Detecting abuse in a frail, elderly person with multiple health problems can challenge your assessment skills. A situation or condition that suggests mistreatment may actually represent the progression of disease. For example, you may suspect that an elderly woman covered with bruises is battered when in fact she has a coagulation disorder caused by the medication she takes for heart disease.

The following signs and symptoms, though not definitive of abuse, call for further investigation and reporting:

• unexplained bruises, fractures, or burns
• poor hygiene or nutritional status
• pressure sores or other evidence of skin breakdown or infection
• dehydration
• fear of family member or a caregiver
• indications of overmedication or undermedication, such as grogginess or decreased level of consciousness
• unusual listlessness or withdrawal.

According to interpretive guidelines to the regulations (which do not have the force of law), even when one of these exceptions is present, the infant must still receive appropriate nutrition, hydration, and medication.

State law

Two common features characterize most state child abuse legislation:
• empowering of a social welfare or law enforcement bureau to receive and in-

vestigate reports of actual or suspected abuse

• granting of legal *immunity from liability,* for defamation or invasion of privacy, to any person reporting an incident of actual or suspected abuse.

Laws protecting abused spouses are still being written. Although many domestic relations laws exist, additional legislation is required to help protect victims of domestic violence.

Your legal duty to report abuse

As a nurse, you play a crucial role in recognizing and reporting incidents of suspected abuse. While caring for patients, you can readily note evidence of apparent abuse. When you do, you must pass the information along to the appropriate authorities. In many states, failure to report actual or suspected abuse constitutes a crime.

Protection from liability

If you've ever hesitated to file an abuse report because you fear repercussions, remember that the Child Abuse Prevention and Treatment Act protects you against liability. If your report is bona fide (that is, if you file it in good faith), the law will protect you from any suit filed by an alleged abuser.

Filing a report

Make your report as complete and accurate as possible. Be careful not to let your personal feelings affect either the way you make out a report or your decision to file the report.

Abuse cases can raise many difficult emotional issues. Remember, however, that not filing a report can have more serious consequences than filing one that contains an unintentional error. It is better to risk error than to risk breaching the child abuse reporting laws — and, in effect, perpetuating the abuse.

Recognizing abuse

Learn to recognize both the events that trigger abuse and the signs and symptoms that mark the abused and the abuser. Early in your relationship with an abused patient, you'll need to be adept at spotting the subtle behavioral and interactional clues that signal an abusive situation.

Examine the patient's relationship with the suspected abuser. For example, abused people tend to be passive and fearful. An abused child usually fails to protest if his parent is asked to leave the examining area. An abused adult, on the other hand, usually wants his abuser to stay with him.

Abused persons may react to hospital procedures by crying helplessly and incessantly. And they tend to be wary of physical contacts, including physical examinations.

Many hospitals have a policy, procedure, or protocol that establishes criteria to help nurses and other health care providers make observations that will help identify possible victims of abuse. Learning these criteria will make spotting victims of abuse more objective and prevent cases from going unrecognized.

Assessing the abuser

Sometimes the abuser will appear overly agitated when dealing with hospital personnel; for example, he'll get impatient if they don't carry out procedures instantly. At other times, he may exhibit the opposite behavior: a total lack of interest in the patient's problems.

Patient history

When you take an abuse victim's history, he may be vague about how he was injured and tell different stories to different people. When you ask directly about specific injuries, he may answer evasively or not at all. Sometimes he'll minimize or try to hide his injuries.

Physical examination

Look for characteristic signs of abuse. In most cases, you'll find old bruises, scars, or deformities the patient can't or won't explain. X-ray examinations may show many old fractures.

Documenting abuse

Always document your findings objectively; try to keep your emotions out of your charting. One way to do this is to use the *SOAP* technique, which calls for these steps:

• In the subjective (S) part of the note, record information in the patient's own words.

• In the objective (O) part, record your personal observations.

• Under assessment (A), record your evaluations and conclusions.

• Under plan (P), list sources of hospital and community support available to the patient after discharge.

Offering support services

Many support services have become available for both abusers and their victims. For example, if a female victim is afraid to return to the scene of her abuse, she may find temporary housing in an established women's shelter. If no shelter is available, she may be able to stay with a friend or family member.

Social workers or community liaison workers may also be able to offer suggestions for shelter. Another possibility is a church, synagogue, or mosque, which may have members willing to take the patient in. If no shelter can be found, the patient may have to stay at the hospital to provide for her safety.

Alert the patient to state, county, or city agencies that can offer protection. The police department should be called to collect evidence if the patient wants to press charges against the abuser. If the patient is a child, the law will probably require filing a report with a government family-service agency.

Help for the abuser

You need to evaluate the abuser's ability to handle stress. He'll probably pose a continued threat to others until he gets help in understanding his behavior and how to change it. In such a situation, your responsibility is to attempt to refer him to an appropriate local or state agency that can offer help.

For abusive fathers or mothers, a local chapter of *Parents Anonymous (PA)* may be helpful. (See *Help for the abused and the abuser.*) PA, a self-help group made up of former abusers, attempts to help abusive parents by teaching them how to deal with their anger.

Besides helping to short-circuit abusive behavior, a self-help group takes abusive parents out of their isolation and introduces them to other parents who understand their feelings. The group also can help in a crisis and prevent an abusive incident.

Telephone hot lines to crisis intervention services give abusers someone to talk with in times of stress and crisis and may help prevent abuse. Commonly staffed by volunteers, telephone hot lines provide a link between those who seek help and trained counselors.

These and other kinds of help are also available through family-service agencies and hospitals. By becoming familiar with national and local resources, you will be able to respond quickly and authoritatively when an abuser or his victim needs your help.

Teaching the public

Besides your duty to report abuse, you also have a duty to teach the public about abuse. The Child Abuse Prevention and Treatment Act encourages health care institutions to develop programs to identify, report, and ultimately prevent abuse. You can help reduce the incidence of abuse by teaching people about its signs and symptoms, diagnosis, and treatment.

Caring for the mentally ill or developmentally disabled patient

Despite his usually dependent condition, a mentally ill or developmentally disabled patient has most of the same rights as other members of society. In fact, usually the law covers such a patient's rights in extra detail to ensure that he receives proper care and treatment. If you violate these rights, even unwittingly, you could face serious legal complications.

Much of today's concern for the rights of the mentally ill and developmentally disabled stems from attempts to correct past abuses. Under the U.S. Constitution, a person's rights can't be limited or denied merely because of his mental status. Many health care professionals still don't realize that the courts have generally interpreted the Constitution to mean that mentally ill and developmentally disabled persons have a right to fair and humane treatment, including during hospitalization. Under most circumstances, such a patient can't be kept in a hospital against his will, for example. Nor can he be denied the right to refuse treatment or to receive information so he can give informed consent to proposed surgery.

Government action

State governments have tried to assure the rights of this special population by enacting legislation specifically addressing the problems of the mentally ill and developmentally disabled. This legislation describes and authorizes specific services and provides the necessary funding.

The federal government also provides for the mentally ill and developmentally disabled. The Rehabilitation Act of 1973, for example,

Help for the abused and the abuser

These organizations offer support and counseling for the abuse victim and the abuser. Also check the "Guide to Human Services" section of your phone directory under "Abuse" and "Child & Youth" for local or state agencies.

Child Help USA/I.O.F.
(800) 4-A-CHILD

National Clearinghouse on Marital and Date Rape
(510) 524-1582

National Coalition Against Sexual Assault
(717) 232-7460

National Committee for Prevention of Child Abuse
(312) 663-3520

Parents United International
(408) 453-7616

earmarked funds specifically for rehabilitative programs. It provides cash assistance for persons who, because of their disabilities, aren't able to provide adequately for themselves or their families. The act also outlines 14 patient's rights to ensure high standards of health care. Facilities that participate in Medicare must comply with these 14 rights and make sure that the patient, his guardian, *next of kin,* or sponsoring agency knows about them, too.

The Americans with Disabilities Act of 1990 (P.L. 101-336) further ensures a disabled citizen's rights by providing a "national mandate for the elimination of discrimination against individuals with disabilities." This act addresses discrimination in employment, public accommodations, and public services, programs, and activities.

Canada makes similar provisions for mentally ill and developmentally disabled persons. As in the United States, Canadian legislation seeks to prevent maltreatment and to fund programs that help these persons to function successfully in society.

Establishing legal responsibility

When a mentally ill or developmentally disabled child is admitted to a hospital, legal responsibility for him must be established immediately. If the patient is accompanied by a parent, usually the parent will be legally responsible.

If the child has been institutionalized before entering the hospital, the institution may have responsibility. However, this is true only if the parents have waived responsibility and the institution has written evidence to prove it.

If the courts have found the parents unfit or unable to care for the child, a legal guardian will have been appointed. This person has the legal right to assume responsibility for the child.

When no guardian has been appointed for the child, the state may act as a guardian under the doctrine of *parens patriae.* This doctrine also applies to mentally ill or developmentally disabled adults.

Adult guardianship

If your mentally ill or developmentally disabled patient is an adult, check his chart to see if he requires a legal guardian and to establish who it is. The guardian may be a parent or, if the patient is married, the patient's spouse.

Sometimes an adult patient and his guardian will seriously disagree about the patient's care. When this happens,

get clarification by going through proper hospital channels.

Remember, you have no right to control the life of a mentally ill or developmentally disabled patient. Restricting his liberty for any reason is almost never legally permissible, except when he may otherwise harm himself or others. You must analyze each situation carefully to determine at what point the patient needs help in managing his affairs.

Obtaining informed consent

When consent is required from a patient who's mentally ill or developmentally disabled, consider the following three questions:

• Can consent for treatment or a special procedure be obtained the same way it is from any other patient?

• Does the patient fully understand the procedure that he's to undergo, including the risks and alternatives?

• Does the patient have the authority to give his own consent, or must someone else give it?

The answers to these questions will vary with each patient. Clearly, if the patient is of unsound mind and can't understand the nature, purpose, alternatives, and risks of the proposed treatment, he can't legally consent. In such a case, consent must be obtained from the patient's legal guardian.

If the legal guardian is unavailable, a court authorized to handle such matters may authorize treatment.

Questioning a patient's ability to give consent

Sometimes a doctor or nurse may doubt a patient's capacity to consent, even though he hasn't been judged incompetent. This commonly happens during an illness that causes temporary incompetence. In such a situation, the nearest relative's consent must be obtained or, if none can be found, the court must authorize treatment.

In the New York case of *Collins v. Davis* (1964), a hospital administrator sought a court order to permit surgery on an irrational adult whose life was considered to be in danger. The patient's wife had previously refused to give consent, allegedly for reasons she felt served the patient's best interest. The court, after considering the entire situation — especially the patient's prognosis if surgery wasn't performed — agreed that the hospital and the doctor had only two choices: either let the patient die, or perform the operation against his wife's wishes. The court overruled the wife's refusal, holding that the patient had sought medical attention and that treatment normally given to a patient with a similar condition should be provided.

Nurse's role

You can best protect the mentally ill or developmentally disabled patient's legal rights to informed consent by making sure that a doctor has provided him or his guardian with information. Find out if the patient's and guardian's questions have been answered to their satisfaction.

Unless your absence would place the patient in danger, you should refuse to assist with procedures on a patient whose informed consent hasn't been obtained. If you do participate, you can be held liable along with the doctor and hospital. In fact, if your patient is a minor, you could face double liability: his parents could sue you now, and he could sue you when he comes of age.

Forced hospitalization and use of restraints

Mentally ill or developmentally disabled persons may be involuntarily kept in hospitals if they're at risk of taking their own lives or if they pose a threat to other persons' property or lives. However, mental illness alone is not a sufficient legal basis for detaining a patient. The U.S. Supreme Court, in *O'Connor v. Donaldson* (1975), held that a state cannot constitutionally confine a patient, without treatment or without the rehabilitation necessary to reintegrate him into society, "who is capable of surviving safely in freedom by himself or with the help of willing and responsible family members or friends."

Similar restrictions apply to physical restraint of patients. Most states require a doctor to write the restraint order and place it in the patient's medical record before restraints can be applied.

Restraint (or seclusion) may be used only to prevent a patient from seriously injuring himself or others — and only when all other physical and psychological therapies would likely fail to prevent such injuries. Whenever possible, use minimal restraint — only that amount necessary to protect the patient and safeguard the staff and others. Restraint should never be used for punishment, for the convenience of staff, or as a substitute for treatment programs. Use of restraints is usually limited to a specific period of time (see *Caring for a patient in restraints or seclusion*, page 146).

If you make a decision to apply restraints, you should immediately request that a doctor examine the patient and write an order to restrain him. In an emergency situation — such as a violent outburst with actual or potential harm to persons or property — any person may apply restraints to the patient. But obtain an order for the restraint as soon as possible, and document the incident carefully.

Potential liability

As a nurse, you may be held liable in a lawsuit if you can't verify that — in your judgment — a patient needed to be

Caring for a patient in restraints or seclusion

Before you can keep a patient in restraints or in seclusion, you must get an order from the patient's doctor authorizing it. The 1995 standards issued by the Joint Commission on Accreditation of Healthcare Organizations (JCAHO) are specific regarding restraint and seclusion.

Authorization

The JCAHO requires that before restraints or seclusion are used:
● documentation shows that such interventions are clinically justified
● less restrictive interventions have been attempted
● the patient's current condition is considered.

Orders are to be time limited. They are to be written for a specific episode, with start and end times, rather than for an unspecified time in the future. Established policy should specify the maximum length of time that each intervention may be used.

In an emergency, specially trained staff may initiate the use of restraints or seclusion and obtain the doctor's order within a specified time (as established by the institution's policy).

Care requirements

When you are caring for a patient in restraints or seclusion, periodic monitoring and observation are essential (as required by your institution's policy).

For patients who require frequent or prolonged restraint or seclusion, the treatment team should meet to consider alternatives and changes in the care plan. Generally, 72 hours of continuous restraint or more than four episodes in 7 days is considered prolonged or frequent.

Document such items as the patient's hydration, feeding, toileting, range-of-motion, and condition of limbs.

---

restrained, and that he was restrained only as long as necessary. If you restrain or seclude a patient simply for shouting obscenities, for example, you risk a lawsuit for false imprisonment.

You should also be sure you know how to use restraining devices safely and effectively. You made be held liable if your restraints do not prove effective and the patient is injured as a result. (See *Use of restraints and nursing liability*.)

If a competent patient makes an informed decision to refuse restraint, the hospital may require the patient to sign a release that would absolve the hospital of liability should injury result from the patient's refusal to be restrained.

How to apply restraints

When applying restraints, follow these guidelines:
● Restraint is a form of imprisonment, so it should only be used as a last resort. Before restraining a patient, consider alternatives, such as constant observation or walking with the patient.
● Take care to avoid undue force; otherwise, you may invite a lawsuit for *battery*. Even threatening to use force may be sufficient cause for legal action.
● When a doctor isn't immediately available, you're responsible for seeing that restraints and seclusion are used only to the extent necessary to prevent injury. Make sure the staff contacts the doctor as soon as possible.

COURT CASE

Use of restraints and nursing liability

Improperly restraining a patient can leave the nurse vulnerable to a host of legal charges, such as negligence, professional malpractice, false imprisonment, or battery. The case discussed below provides an example of nurses who failed to use restraints effectively.

The patient who escaped

In *Rohde v. Lawrence General Hospital* (1993), the patient was brought into the hospital at 1 a.m. by police, following an automobile accident. The patient assaulted a clinician in the emergency de-partment (ED) and was diagnosed as having an "acute psychotic episode." The doctor ordered leather restraints.

Around 6 a.m., the patient escaped from four-point restraints, went into the parking lot, found a car that had been left running, and drove off. He crashed the car and was seriously injured.

The patient sued the hospital, the ED doctor, and two nurses for medical malpractice, claiming that the staff did not supervise him properly and that his restraints were not securely fastened.

• Most states follow the *least restrictive principle,* which holds that no more restraint should be used than necessary. For example, a restraining vest shouldn't be used when simple wrist restraints will suffice.
• To avoid allegations of false imprisonment, document carefully the decision-making process that led to the use of restraints, and review the continuing need for restraints on a regular basis.
• Bed side rails are a form of restraint and shouldn't be raised indiscriminately. The patient's age alone isn't a justification for raising the side rails.
• Tranquilizing drugs may provide an alternative to restraints. However, use them sparingly, with caution, and only with a doctor's order. The patient's right to the least restrictive treatment or to an open-door policy that allows him to move about "freely" means little if drugs substitute for restraints.

Right to privacy

The law has tried to protect all citizens from unwarranted intrusion into their private lives. Unfortunately, mentally ill and developmentally disabled patients' rights to privacy are easily violated. A good definition of privacy, first presented at the International Commission of Justice in 1970, reads: "Privacy is the ability to lead one's life without anyone:

A. interfering with family or home life
B. interfering with physical or mental integrity or moral and intellectual freedom
C. attacking honor and reputation
D. placing one in a false light
E. censoring or restricting communication and correspondence, written or oral
F. disclosing irrelevant or embarrassing information
G. disclosing information given or received in professional confidence.

Remember this definition, and try to protect the privacy of all your patients.

Right to writ of *habeas corpus*

Institutionalization may, at times, breach a patient's rights, giving him cause to petition for a *writ of habeas corpus.* This writ seeks to ensure the timely release of any person who claims that he's being detained illegally and deprived of his liberty.

Right to treatment

In *Wyatt v. Stickney* (1972), the court upheld the legal right of a mentally ill person hospitalized in a public institution to receive adequate psychiatric treatment. This decision suggests that when a patient is involuntarily committed because he needs treatment, his rights are violated if he does not receive proper care. Furthermore, if the underlying reason for a patient's commitment is danger to himself or others, treatment must be provided to make him less dangerous.

In the *Wyatt* decision, the court outlined a complete bill of rights for the mentally ill patient. Among the key points, the court said treatment should be given as follows:
● by adequate staff
● in the least restrictive setting
● in privacy
● in a facility that ensures the patient a comfortable bed, adequate diet, and recreational facilities
● with the patient's informed consent, prior to unusual treatment
● with payment for work done in the institution, outside of program activities
● according to an individual treatment plan.

If possible, you must ensure that any mentally ill or developmentally disabled patient knows what treatment he needs and how he will get it. You must know what his major problems are and what he can do for himself — or what others must do for him — to help him get ready for discharge. You should also involve him in formulating his treatment plan, unless you have a documented reason why he can't or won't be involved.

Sexual rights

Many questions remain regarding the sexual rights of mentally ill and developmentally disabled patients. For example, should developmentally disabled persons be given sex education? Should they be allowed to reproduce, practice contraception, or undergo voluntary sterilization? Although the general inclination is to let guardians make these decisions, the issue of the individual's right to make his own decisions will not go away. If good care can be given to both the developmentally disabled and their offspring, who's to say that they should be denied the opportunity to enjoy the same satisfactions others do?

The U.S. Supreme Court has upheld the rights of mentally ill or developmentally disabled patients:
● to marry
● to have children
● to employ contraception, abortion, or sterilization, if desired
● to follow a life-style of their own choosing.

Several cases, such as *Sengstack v. Sengstack* (1958), *Wyatt v. Stickney* (1972), and *O'Connor v. Donaldson* (1975), have used the U.S. Supreme Court decisions as a basis for their rulings.

Involuntary sterilization

Involuntary sterilization of developmentally disabled patients isn't employed today as in the past. Although the U.S. Supreme Court upheld the constitutionality of involuntary sterilization in *Buck v. Bell* (1927), if a similar case were to come before the Supreme Court today, the precedent would likely be overturned.

In *Buck v. Bell,* the court held that the state has the right to sterilize a developmentally disabled or mentally ill person provided that:
● the sterilization isn't prescribed as punishment

• the policy is applied equally to all
• a potential child's interest is sufficient to warrant the sterilization.

Courts will authorize such a procedure only within specific guidelines or not at all. Generally, it must be shown that sterilization is the only workable means of contraception. In some cases, the court orders a separate, independent presterilization review of the case. (In New York state, for example, an independent medical review board must review and approve every planned involuntary sterilization before it can be performed.) Even though the patient's guardian has requested sterilization, if the patient refuses to submit to surgery, the court may call for use of a less permanent birth control method.

Participation in research

Another troublesome area involves using mentally ill and developmentally disabled persons as subjects for medical or other research — especially if risks are involved. Guidelines for consent to experimentation and drastic, questionable, or extreme forms of treatment are complicated and raise many unresolved questions. The so-called Willowbrook decision (*N.Y. State Association for Retarded Children, Inc. v. Carey,* 1977), however, decreed that both voluntary and involuntary residents of an institution have the constitutional right to be protected from harm. The proper authority (usually an institutional review board) should allow the patient to participate in the research only if it's relevant to his needs and the needs of others like him and its potential benefits outweigh its potential risks. For example, a depressed patient shouldn't be asked to participate in research involving anxiety and schizophrenia.

Strict federal regulations guide how experimental treatment can be carried out. Such treatment must be given with extreme caution to mentally ill or developmentally disabled patients.

Responding to patient requests

"Ordinary" requests made by mentally ill or developmentally disabled patients may require special consideration.

For example, a patient may demand to smoke a cigarette *now.* His doctor hasn't written an order for the request. If the patient should smoke only under supervision because of the danger of fire, you may decide to stay with him while he does so. But if you have a duty to be elsewhere, you should refuse his request, explaining why and telling him when he'll be able to smoke. Or, if you know a refusal will agitate and anger him, you can ask another nurse to supervise the patient while he smokes.

Perhaps the patient is well aware that he's violating the hospital's no-smoking policy and his request is really a challenge to authority. If so, you may decide to refuse the request, explaining the need to follow the hospital's social and safety policies.

If the patient's behavior is part of a pattern that includes, for example, refusing to shower, refusing to go to bed by a certain time, and demanding to make an immediate phone call, then you need to refer the situation to the treatment team for a well-thought-out decision — one that serves the best interests of both the patient and the hospital. Once it's made, ask all the health team members to enforce this decision consistently.

Caring for a suspected criminal

Suppose you're asked to care for an injured suspect who's accompanied by police. Because the police need evidence, they ask you to give them the patient's belongings and also a sample of his blood. Should you comply? The answer to this question isn't simple. If you are ignorant of the law and fail to follow proper protocol, the evidence you turn over to police may not be admissible in court. Worse still, later on, the patient may be able to sue you for invasion of privacy.

Constitutional rights

The Fourth Amendment to the U.S. Constitution provides that "the right of the people to be secure in their persons, houses, papers and effects, against unreasonable searches and seizures shall not be violated, and no warrants shall issue, but upon probable cause." This means that every individual, even a suspected criminal, has a right to privacy, including a right to be free from intrusions that are made without search warrants. However, the Fourth Amendment doesn't absolutely prohibit all searches and seizures, only unreasonable ones.

Under constitutional law, when a magistrate issues a warrant authorizing a police officer to conduct a search, the warrant must be specific about the places to be searched and the items to be seized.

The *exclusionary rule* is probably the most common rule affecting nurses in relation to suspected criminals and their victims. This rule stems from the Fourth Amendment's prohibition of unreasonable searches and seizures. In the landmark case of *Mapp v. Ohio* (1961), the U.S. Supreme Court held that evidence obtained through an unreasonable or unlawful search cannot be used against the person whose rights the search violated.

Searches without a warrant

Under the following circumstances, a police officer may lawfully conduct a

search and obtain evidence without a warrant:

• If an accused person consents to a search, any evidence found would be considered admissible in court (*Schneckloth v. Bustamonte,* 1973).

• A search incidental to an arrest may be conducted without a warrant. Usually, such a search should not extend beyond the accused person's body or an immediate area where he could reach for a weapon. However, in *Maryland v. Buie* (1990), the U.S. Supreme Court ruled that a search incidental to an arrest can extend to adjoining rooms and closets of a private residence from which an accomplice could attack. Police may even conduct a sweep of an entire area if they have reason to think they may be in danger. Although this case dealt with searches in a private home, the ruling could apply to searches conducted in a hospital.

• In *Horton v. California* (1990), the U.S. Supreme Court ruled that police could seize any evidence in plain view as long as they are lawfully in a position to see the object. Thus, when looking for persons who pose a danger, police can seize incriminating items in plain view.

• Police may search an area, even out of arms reach, to recover a weapon that could pose a threat to their safety (*New York v. Class,* 1985).

• Police may enter a private area and seize any items in plain view if they are in "hot pursuit" of a criminal suspect (*Warden v. Hayden,* 1967).

Evidence obtained as part of a blood test

Opinions differ as to whether a blood test, such as a blood alcohol test, is admissible in court if the person refused consent for the test. In *Schmerber v. California* (1966), the U.S. Supreme Court said that blood extracted without a warrant, incidental to a lawful arrest, is not an unconstitutional search and seizure and is admissible evidence.

Many courts have held this to mean that a blood sample must be drawn *after* the arrest.

Furthermore, the blood sample must be drawn in a medically reasonable manner. In *People v. Kraft* (1970), a suspect was pinned to the floor by two police officers while a doctor drew a blood sample. In *State v. Riggins* (1977), a suspect's broken arm was twisted while a policeman sat on him to force consent to a blood test. In both cases, the courts ruled the test results inadmissible. The courts have also ruled as inadmissible — and as violating **due process rights** — evidence gained by the forcible and unconsented insertion of a nasogastric tube into a suspect to remove stomach contents (*Rochin v. California,* 1952).

Courts have admitted blood tests as evidence when the tests weren't drawn at police request but for medically necessary purposes, such as blood typing (*Commonwealth v. Gordon,* 1968). Some courts have also allowed blood work to be admitted as evidence when it was drawn for nontherapeutic reasons and voluntarily turned over to police.

Be careful, though. A doctor or nurse who does blood work without the patient's consent may be liable for committing battery, even if the patient is a suspected criminal and the blood work is medically necessary.

Blood alcohol tests and drunk driving arrests

Many states have enacted so-called implied-consent laws as part of their motor vehicle laws. These laws hold that by applying for a driver's license, a person implies his consent to submit to a blood alcohol test if he's arrested for drunken driving. Many of these laws state specifically that if an individual refuses to submit to the chemical test, it may not be given, but the driver then forfeits his license. Check to see whether such laws exist in your state.

Evidence obtained during a surgical procedure

A Massachusetts case, *Commonwealth v. Storella* (1978), involved a bullet that a doctor removed during a medically necessary operation. After the operation, the doctor turned the bullet over to the police. The court allowed the bullet to be admitted as evidence because the doctor was acting according to good medical practice, and not as a state agent, in removing the bullet.

In 1985, the U.S. Supreme Court ruled that the constitutionality of such court-ordered surgery to acquire evidence must be decided on a case-by-case basis. The interest in individual privacy and security must be weighed against the societal interest in collecting evidence. Therefore, you should be wary if asked to assist in a highly invasive procedure to help the state obtain evidence if the suspect does not consent. If necessary, consult an attorney.

Swallowed contraband

Drug couriers have been known to carry contraband by swallowing it in small balloons, which can be recovered during elimination. As a nurse, you may become involved in efforts to detect and recover swallowed contraband. In *United States v. Montoya de Hernandez* (1985), the U.S. Supreme Court ruled that the police can lawfully detain drug couriers until swallowed items can be recovered and seized.

Searches by a private party

In *Burdeau v. McDowell* (1921), the U.S. Supreme Court said that Fourth Amendment protections applied only to governmental (such as police) action and not to searches conducted by private parties. Although several courts have criticized this rule, it has been repeatedly upheld.

In *State v. Perea* (1981), a nurse took a suspect's shirt for safekeeping, then turned it over to the police even though they hadn't requested it. A New Mexico court allowed the shirt to be admitted as evidence. The reason: Because no governmental intrusion was involved, the suspect's Fourth Amendment right wasn't violated.

The case of *United States v. Winbush* (1970) produced a similar result. In this case, the court ruled that evidence found during a routine search of an unconscious patient's pockets was admissible because the purpose of the search was to obtain necessary identification and medical information.

Evidence in plain view
As a nurse, if you find a gun, knife, drug, or other item that the suspect could use to harm himself or others, you have a right to remove it. You should, however, notify the hospital administration immediately and maintain control over the evidence until you can give it to an administrator or a law enforcement official.

When the suspect may sue
In general, searches that occur as part of medical care don't violate a suspect's rights. But searches made for the sole purpose of gathering evidence — especially if done at police request — very well may. Several courts have said that a suspect subjected to an illegal private search has a right to seek remedy against the unlawful searcher in a civil lawsuit. One such case was *Stone v. Commonwealth* (1967). (See *Conducting a drug search.*)

Canadian law
The major difference between U.S. and Canadian law regarding searches is that, in Canada, evidence obtained during an illegal search is still admissible in court. However, a police officer properly should have a search warrant before searching a suspected criminal to protect his rights.

A word of caution
The laws of search and seizure are complex and subject to change by new legal decisions. Consult with the hospital administration or an attorney before complying with a police request to turn over a patient's personal property. Some state laws require that police obtain a warrant before they are legally entitled to this evidence.

Documenting your actions

Be careful and precise in documenting all medical and nursing procedures when you care for a suspected criminal. Note any blood work done, and list all treatments and the patient's response to them.

If you turn anything over to the police or administration, record what it was and the name of the person you gave it to. Record a suspect's statements that are directly related to his care. If a suspect says, "I shot a cop in the arm tonight," that's not related to his care. But if he says, "I think I was shot in the leg by a cop," that relates directly to his medical care.

Safeguarding evidence

Before any evidence can be admissible in court, the court must have some guarantee of where, and how, it was gathered. Someone must account for evidence from the moment you collect it until it appears in court: a continuum known as the *chain of custody.* You can't leave evidence unattended where it might be tampered with.

If you discover evidence, use your hospital's chain-of-custody form. First used when evidence is taken from the patient, this form should remain with the evidence until the trial. It documents the identity of each person handling the evidence as well as the date and times it was in their possession. In effect, the form should serve as an

Conducting a drug search

If you suspect your patient is abusing drugs or alcohol, you have a duty to do something about it. If such a patient harms himself or anyone else, and a lawsuit results, the court may hold you liable for his actions.

When you know about drug abuse

Suppose you know for certain that a patient is abusing drugs—if you're an emergency department nurse, you may find drugs in a patient's clothes or handbag while looking for identification. Your hospital's policy may obligate you to confiscate the drugs and take steps to see that the patient doesn't acquire more.

When you suspect drug abuse

When a patient's erratic or threatening behavior makes you suspect he's abusing drugs or alcohol, your hospital's policy may require that you conduct a search. Is your search legal? As a rule of thumb, if you strongly believe the patient poses a threat to himself or others, and you can document your reasons for searching his possessions, you're probably safe legally.

Guidelines for searches

Before you conduct a search, review your hospital's guidelines on the matter. Then follow those guidelines carefully. Most hospital guidelines will first direct you to contact your supervisor and explain why you have legitimate cause for a search. If she gives you her approval, next ask a security guard to help you. Besides protecting you, he'll serve as a witness if you do find drugs. When you're ready, confront the patient, tell him you intend to conduct a search, and tell him why.

Depending on your hospital's guidelines, you can search a patient's belongings as well as his room. If you find illegal drugs during your search, confiscate them. Remember, possession of illegal drugs is a felony. Depending on your hospital's guidelines, you may be obligated to report the patient to the police.

If you find alcoholic beverages during your search, hospital guidelines may require you to take them from the patient. Explain to the patient that you'll return them when he leaves the hospital.

Maintaining written records

After you've completed your search, tell the patient's doctor about it and record your findings in your nurses' notes and in an incident report. Your written records will be an important part of your defense (and your hospital's) if the patient decides to sue.

---

uninterrupted log of the evidence's whereabouts.

If your hospital doesn't have a chain-of-custody form, keep a careful record of exactly what was taken, by whom, and when. Give this information to the hospital administrator when you deliver the evidence. Until such time as the evidence can be turned over, it should be kept in a locked area.

When a suspect dies, most states provide that the *coroner* can claim the body. Police are free to gather any evidence that will not mutilate the body. A dead body has no constitutional rights, so no rights are violated by a search.

Nursing behind bars

Even after conviction, an individual doesn't forfeit all constitutional rights. Among those retained is the Eighth Amendment's proscription against cruel and unusual punishment. This implies that prison officials and health care workers must not deliberately ignore a prisoner's medical needs.

The U.S. Supreme Court, in *Estelle v. Gamble* (1976), stated that the Eighth Amendment prohibits more than physically barbarous punishment. The amendment embodies "broad and idealistic concepts of dignity, civilized standards, humanity, and decency against which we must evaluate penal measures."

Right to medical care

The state has an obligation to provide medical care for those it imprisons. The Supreme Court has concluded that "deliberate indifference to serious medical needs of prisoners constitutes the unnecessary and wanton infliction of pain proscribed by the Eighth Amendment. This is true whether the indifference is manifested by prison doctors in response to a prisoner's needs or by prison personnel in intentionally denying or delaying access to medical care or intentionally interfering with the treatment once prescribed."

In *Ramos v. Lamm* (1980), the court outlined several ways in which prison officials show deliberate indifference to prisoners' medical needs:

• preventing an inmate from receiving recommended treatment

• denying access to medical personnel capable of evaluating the need for treatment

• allowing repeated acts of negligence that disclose a pattern of conduct by prison health staff

• allowing such severe deficiencies in staffing, facilities, equipment, or procedures to exist that inmates are effectively denied access to adequate medical care.

Providing care

Working daily with prisoners is difficult and demanding, both profession-ally and emotionally. Along with exhibiting a host of other unpleasant behaviors, prisoners can be abusive, manipulative, and angry. In spite of this, health care professionals can't forget their ethical and legal duty to provide quality care.

Nurses working in a prison setting should be aware that the doctrine of *respondeat superior* does not apply to prison cases. The nurse supervisor or manager cannot be held responsible for accusations of "cruel and unusual punishment" unless she has personally acted to deprive the prisoner of medical care (*Vinnedge v. Gibbs,* 1977).

When a prisoner refuses treatment

Several courts have stated that individuals have a constitutional right to privacy based on a high regard for human dignity and self-determination. That means any competent adult may refuse medical care, even lifesaving treatments. For instance, in *Lane v. Candura* (1978), an **appellate court** upheld the right of a competent adult to refuse a leg amputation that would have saved her life.

A suspected criminal may refuse unwarranted bodily invasions. However, an arrested suspect or convicted criminal does not have the same right to refuse lifesaving measures. In *Commissioner of Correction v. Myers* (1979), a prisoner with renal failure refused hemodialysis unless he was moved to a minimum security prison. The court disagreed, saying that although the defendant's imprisonment did not divest him of his right to privacy or his interest in maintaining his bodily integrity, it did impose limitations on those constitutional rights.

As a practical matter, inform your hospital administration anytime a patient refuses lifesaving treatments. In the case of a suspect or prisoner, notify law enforcement authorities as well.

Upholding a patient's living will

When a legally competent person draws up a living will, he declares the steps he wants or doesn't want taken when he's incompetent and no longer able to express his wishes. The will applies to decisions that will be made after a patient is incompetent and has no reasonable possibility of recovery. Generally, a living will authorizes the attending doctor to withhold or discontinue certain lifesaving procedures under specific circumstances.

The will is called *living* because its provisions take effect before death. By clearly stating his wishes regarding lifesaving procedures, the patient also helps relieve any guilt his family and the health care team might otherwise feel for discontinuing life support.

All states and the District of Columbia have living will laws. In each state, a living will is considered a legal statement of the patient's wishes. Living will laws help guarantee that the patient's wishes will be carried out.

A patient may also choose to execute a durable power of attorney for health care. Should the patient become incompetent, this document designates a surrogate decision maker with full authority to carry out the patient's wishes regarding health care decisions. Most states have laws authorizing durable power of attorney for the purpose of initiating or terminating life-sustaining medical treatment. (See *Living will laws*, pages 156 to 177.)

Content of living will laws

Generally, living will laws include provisions such as:
- who may execute a living will
- immunity from liability for following a living will's directives

- witness and *testator* requirements
- documentation requirements
- instructions on when and how the living will should be executed
- under what circumstances the living will takes effect.

When living wills don't apply

When the patient's condition is such that the living will is not applicable, or in cases where the patient has not drawn up a living will, the patient's surrogate will need to make decisions regarding the removal of life support systems and treatment.

The Supreme Court's ruling in *Cruzan v. Director, Mo. Dept. of Health* (1990) may influence future court rulings in this area. In this ruling, the Court held that the state of Missouri has the constitutional right to refuse to permit termination of life-sustaining treatment unless "clear and convincing evidence" exists about a patient's wishes. The Court implied that when clear and convincing evidence exists, the patient's wishes will be respected. Since states differ on what they consider "clear and convincing evidence," consult your hospital's ethics committee or attorney in cases of this type.

Interpreting the will

A doctor may also face real difficulties in determining when a living will should apply. The wording in many living wills is vague. What, for example, is a "reasonable expectation of recovery?" And what is a "heroic" or "extraordinary" measure? When a patient becomes comatose, it may be difficult to precisely interpret the intentions expressed in his living will. That is one reason why legislatures have been slow to make living wills binding.

Patients should be encouraged to review their living wills with their families and doctors so that unclear areas can be discussed. Living wills also need

(Text continues on page 176.)

Living will laws

All 50 states and the District of Columbia have adopted living will laws. The chart below summarizes the provisions of each state's living will law at the time of this writing. Specific provisions may change over time. For information on changes to the law, contact Choice in Dying, 200 Varick Street, 10th Fl., New York, NY 10014-4810, or call (212) 366-5540.

Note that a *testator* refers to an individual who makes and executes a living will. Also be aware that some state living will laws allow the testator to name a *proxy.* If the patient executing the living will becomes incapacitated, the proxy will have the authority to make health care decisions for him. Other state living will laws do not include a provision for a proxy. Even if a proxy isn't authorized by statute, the testator may have a state common law right to name a proxy for health care decisions.

STATE LIVING WILL DOCUMENT	TESTATOR REQUIREMENTS	WITNESS REQUIREMENTS
● Alabama Declaration ● Alabama Durable Power of Attorney for Health Care	Adult of sound mind	● Declaration requires two witnesses age 19 or older who personally know the patient and believe him to be of sound mind, excluding relatives by blood or marriage, anyone who signs the declaration on the patient's behalf, heirs, or anyone who is financially responsible for the patient. ● Durable Power of Attorney must be signed in the presence of a notary public.
● Alaska Declaration ● Alaska Durable Power of Attorney for Health Care	Age 18 or older	● Declaration requires two witnesses age 18 or older (excluding relatives by blood or marriage) who personally know the patient and believe he voluntarily signed the document; or state this in the presence of a notary public or U.S. postmaster. ● Durable Power of Attorney must be signed in the presence of a notary public.
● Arizona Health Care Power of Attorney ● Arizona Living Will	Age 18 or older and of sound mind	● Living will requires two witnesses who personally know the patient, excluding relatives by blood or marriage, heirs, those responsible for the patient's medical costs, and claimants against the patient's estate; or have the will notarized. ● Power of Attorney can be witnessed in the same manner as the Living Will.
Arkansas Declarations (The Terminal Condition Declaration and the Permanently Unconscious Declaration)	Age 18 or older	● Declarations require two witnesses who show that the patient voluntarily signed the documents.

MEDICAL REQUIREMENTS	ADDITIONAL INFORMATION
Attending doctor and one other doctor must examine the patient and subsequently certify in writing that death is inevitable, with or without life-sustaining treatments, and that such treatments artificially prolong dying.	• A pregnant patient's declaration will not be honored. • Nutrition and hydration are mentioned in the act. • Alabama law is unclear about whether the doctor is required to follow the agent's instructions concerning withholding or withdrawing medical care.
Patient is unable to make or communicate treatment decisions, and the attending doctor (and one other doctor, when available) confirms that the patient is suffering from a progressive, incurable, or irreversible disorder that will shortly cause death, unless life-sustaining treatments are undertaken.	• Act authorizes withholding or withdrawal of tube feedings. • Pregnant patient's declaration will not be honored. • Durable Power of Attorney allows the patient to name a guardian or conservator with limited powers.
Attending doctor and one other doctor confirm that the patient's condition is terminal and that life-sustaining treatments would only prolong dying. They also confirm that the patient is in a persistent vegetative state.	• Act allows withdrawing or withholding artificial nutrition and hydration. • Documents not valid for non-hospital emergencies. • Analgesic or palliative procedures can't be withheld or suspended.
Terminal condition declaration: The attending doctor must confirm that the condition is incurable and irreversible and would cause death shortly without life-sustaining treatments and that the patient is unable to make his own medical decisions. Permanently unconscious declaration: The attending doctor must confirm a lasting, unchanging condition in which thought, feeling, sensation, and awareness of self and the environment are absent.	• Act includes two forms: the terminal condition declaration and the permanently unconscious declaration. • Act authorizes withholding or withdrawal of tube feeding. • A pregnant patient's declaration will not be honored if the fetus would be viable with the continued application of life-sustaining treatment. • Not valid for non-hospital emergencies.

Living will laws continued

STATE LIVING WILL DOCUMENT	TESTATOR REQUIREMENTS	WITNESS REQUIREMENTS
• California Declaration • California Durable Power of Attorney for Health Care	Age 18 or older and of sound mind	• Declaration requires two witnesses who personally know the patient, excluding relatives, the patient's doctor, and operators or employees of the facility where the patient is confined. A patient in a nursing home must have a patient advocate or ombudsman as one witness. • At least one witness must be a person not entitled to all or part of the estate. • Durable Power of Attorney must be signed by either a notary public or two qualified witnesses.
• Colorado Medical Durable Power of Attorney for Health Care • Colorado Declaration as to Medical or Surgical Treatment	Age 18 or older and of sound mind	• Witnesses to Durable Power of Attorney should not be an agent, heir, health care provider, or employee of patient's health care provider, or a patient in the treating facility. They must sign to show that they personally know the patient and believe him to be of sound mind and free of duress. • Declaration requires two witnesses, age 18 or older, excluding the patient's heirs, any doctor, employees of the patient's doctor or the facility where the patient is confined, a claimant against the patient, and a patient in the same facility.
Connecticut Advance Directive	Adult of sound mind and able to understand the nature and consequences of health care decisions	• Advance directive must be notarized. • The agent cannot be a witness. • If the patient is in a facility for mental health or mental retardation, one witness must not be affliated with the facility, and one must be a doctor or clinical psychologist.
Delaware Declaration	Adult of sound mind	• Declaration requires two witnesses, age 18 or older, excluding relatives by blood or marriage, heirs, claimants against the patient's estate, those financially responsible for the patient's medical care, and employees of the hospital where the patient is confined.

MEDICAL REQUIREMENTS	ADDITIONAL INFORMATION
Two doctors must certify that the patient is terminally ill and that life-sustaining treatments would only artificially prolong dying. In addition, the patient's doctor must determine that death is imminent, whether or not life-sustaining treatments are undertaken.	• Includes withholding artificially administered nutrition and hydration. • Is void during pregnancy. • Not effective for out-of-hospital emergencies.
Attending doctor and one other doctor must certify that the patient has a terminal condition and has been unable to communicate medical decisions for at least 1 week.	• Act authorizes withholding or withdrawal of artificial nourishment. • Living Will must be notarized. • Durable Power of Attorney agent can be family member or close friend. An alternate agent can also be appointed. • Void if patient is pregnant and if the doctor believes the fetus is viable and could develop to live birth with continued application of life-sustaining procedures. • Not effective in non-hospital emergency.
The doctor must determine if the patient is in a terminal condition or permanently unconscious state and can no longer make his own medical decisions. If the patient is in a permanently unconscious state, a neurologist must examine him and confirm the doctor's opinion.	• Includes withholding or withdrawing artificial means of providing nutrition and hydration. • Act includes designating a conservator and making an anatomical gift (optional). • Advance directive is not effective until attending doctor receives a copy of it. • Not effective in an out-of-hospital emergency. • A pregnant patient's directive will not be honored. • Attorney-in-fact can make all medical decisions except to withhold or withdraw life support. Agent can make decisions to withhold or withdraw life support. One person can be named as agent and attorney-in-fact.
Two doctors must confirm, in writing, the patient's terminal condition, which is defined as any disease or illness from which recovery can't reasonably be expected and from which death would likely ensue despite the use or discontinuation of life support.	• Act doesn't mention withdrawal of tube feedings, but the patient can add personal instructions to the section titled "Other directions." • A pregnant patient's directive will not be honored.

Living will laws continued

STATE LIVING WILL DOCUMENT	TESTATOR REQUIREMENTS	WITNESS REQUIREMENTS
● District of Columbia Power of Attorney for Health Care ● District of Columbia Declaration	Adult of sound mind	● Power of Attorney must be signed in the presence of two witnesses who know the patient and believe him to be of sound mind and not under duress. Witness cannot be the attorney-in-fact or the doctor or his employee. At least one witness must not be related or an heir. ● Declaration requires two witnesses age 18 or older, excluding relatives, heirs, those financially responsible for the patient's medical care, the doctor, or health care employees. A nursing home resident must have a patient advocate or ombudsman as one witness.
● Florida Living Will ● Florida Designation of Health Care Surrogate	Adult of sound mind	● Two witnesses who know the patient, excluding the spouse and blood relatives, must sign the Living Will document. ● Two witnesses, excluding the surrogate, alternate, spouse, and blood relatives, must sign the Designation of Health Care Surrogate document.
● Georgia Durable Power of Attoney for Health Care ● Georgia Living Will	Age 18 or older and of sound mind	● Durable Power of Attorney must be signed in the presence of two witnesses age 18 or older; if in a facility, a doctor must be present. ● Living Will requires two witnesses age 18 or older, excluding blood relatives, spouse, heirs, those financially responsible for the patient's medical care, the doctor, and health care employees. If the will is signed in the hospital, the chief of the medical staff or an uninvolved staff doctor must act as a third witness; if signed in a skilled nursing facility, the medical director or an uninvolved staff doctor must act as a third witness.
● Hawaii Declaration ● Hawaii Durable Power of Attorney for Health Care Decisions	Adult of sound mind	● Declaration requires notarized signature of two witnesses age 18 or older who personally know the patient, excluding relatives by blood, marriage, or adoption; the patient's doctor; and employees of the doctor or health care facility. ● Durable Power of Attorney for health care decisions must be witnessed in the same manner as the declaration.

MEDICAL REQUIREMENTS	ADDITIONAL INFORMATION
Attending doctor and one other doctor must examine the patient and confirm in writing that his condition is terminal, whether or not life-sustaining treatments are used, and that these treatments serve only to artificially prolong dying.	• Before Power of Attorney can go into effect, two doctors, including one psychiatrist, must certify that the patient is unable to make health care decisions. • The act doesn't mention tube feeding. • Patient may appoint an attorney-in-fact to make health care decisions.
Attending doctor and one other doctor must determine that the patient is terminally ill, that life-sustaining treatments would only artificially prolong dying, and that death is imminent.	• If patient is physically unable to sign the Living Will, one witness may sign for him. • Designation of Health Care Surrogate Act allows an appointed relative or friend to make decisions. • Is void during pregnancy unless a person adds specific instructions authorizing the withholding and withdrawal of life-sustaining treatment. • A surrogate can be appointed in the Living Will to make decisions on the patient's behalf. Unlike the health care surrogate, the Living Will surrogate may act only when the patient is unable to make treatment decisions *and* is in a terminal condition. Appointing the same person in both documents will help avoid confusion.
Two doctors must examine the patient and then certify in writing that the patient has no reasonable expectation of recovery and that death is imminent.	• Durable Power of Attorney allows appointment of a surrogate and a guardian (not for health care). • If the patient has a Georgia Living Will and Durable Power of Attorney for Health Care, the patient's designee takes precedence.
Attending doctor must certify in writing that the patient's condition is terminal, that he can't participate in medical decisions, that death will shortly ensue if life-sustaining treatments aren't used, and that treatments would only artificially prolong dying. To enact Durable Power of Attorney, a licensed doctor must determine that the person is incapacitated.	• Will not honor a pregnant patient's declaration. • Allows for authorization of withholding and withdrawing artificial nutrition and hydration. • Durable Power of Attorney allows a surrogate to make care decisions.

Living will laws continued

STATE LIVING WILL DOCUMENT	TESTATOR REQUIREMENTS	WITNESS REQUIREMENTS
• Idaho Durable Power of Attorney for Health Care • Idaho Living Will	Age 18 or older, or an emancipated minor of sound mind	• Durable Power of Attorney requires notarized signature or two witnesses, age 18 or older, who personally know or have evidence of person's identity, excluding the agent, the doctor or other health care provider, and employees. • Living Will requires two witnesses who personally know the patient and believe him to be of sound mind.
• Illinois Power of Attorney for Health Care • Illinois Declaration	Person of sound mind at age of maturity or an emancipated minor	• Illinois Power of Attorney should be signed in the presence of one adult witness, preferably not the agent. • Declaration requires two witnesses, age 18 or older, who personally know the patient and believe him to be of sound mind, excluding relatives, heirs, and those financially responsible for the patient's medical care.
• Indiana Power of Attorney for Health Care Decisions and Appointment of Representatives • Indiana Living Will Declaration (A) • Life-Prolonging Procedures Declaration (B)	Age 18 or older and of sound mind	• Power of Attorney for Health Care Decisions must be signed in the presence of a notary public. • Declaration A must be signed by two witnesses, age 18 or older, who personally know the patient, excluding parents, spouse, children, heirs, and those responsible for the patient's medical bills. • Declaration B must be signed in the presence of two adult witnesses, age 18 or older, who personally know the patient.
• Iowa Declaration • Iowa Durable Power of Attorney for Health Care	Adult age 18 or older	• Declaration requires two witnesses who know the patient, excluding the doctor or other health care provider, employees of the health care provider, or anyone under age 18. At least one witness must not be related. • Durable Power of Attorney for Health Care can be witnessed in the same manner as Declaration. Alternatively, a person can sign in the presence of a notary public.
• Kansas Declaration • Kansas Durable Power of Attorney for Health Care	Adult of sound mind	• Declaration requires notarized signature or two witnesses who personally know the patient, excluding relatives by blood or marriage, heirs, and those financially responsible for the patient's medical bills. • Kansas Durable Power of Attorney can be witnessed in the same manner as the Declaration. Additionally, the witness cannot be the person appointed as health care agent.

MEDICAL REQUIREMENTS	ADDITIONAL INFORMATION
Two doctors must certify that the patient's condition is terminal, that life-sustaining treatments would only artificially prolong dying, and that death would be imminent whether or not treatments are used. Alternatively, the doctors must certify that the patient is in a persistent vegetative state.	• Act authorizes the withholding or withdrawal of tube feeding and hydration. • A proxy can be appointed through the Living Will to act on the patient's behalf when he is unable to make treatment decisions *and* is in a terminal condition. To avoid confusion, appoint the same person in all documents. • Under Durable Power of Attorney for Health Care, the patient's appointed agent makes decisions when he's incapacitated. • The Living Will doesn't apply during pregnancy.
Doctor must determine that patient has an incurable and irreversible injury, disease, or illness judged to be terminal. He must certify that death is imminent except for death-delaying procedures, which would only prolong the dying process.	• Power of Attorney gives agent authority to withdraw or withhold artificial nutrition or hydration on patient's behalf. • Not effective for non-hospital emergencies.
Attending doctor certifies in writing that the patient's condition is terminal, that death will occur shortly, and that life-sustaining treatments would only artificially prolong dying.	• Power of Attorney can even be granted to an emancipated minor (age 14, not dependent on parents, married, in the military, or authorized by another statute). This law provides for anatomical gifts and withdrawing or withholding artificial nutrition and hydration. • Living Will (A) allows a person to refuse life-prolonging procedures if he is terminally ill and can no longer make his own medical decisions. • Life-Prolonging Procedures Declaration (B) allows a person to request all life-prolonging procedures.
Attending doctor and one other doctor must confirm that the patient's condition is terminal.	• A pregnant patient's declaration will not be honored if the fetus is determined to be viable. • Iowa Durable Power of Attorney allows a person to name an agent to make medical decisions for him in the event that he is no longer able to make his own decisions.
The attending doctor and one other doctor must certify that the patient's condition is terminal, that death will ensue whether or not life-sustaining treatments are used, and that these treatments would only prolong dying.	• A pregnant patient's declaration will not be honored. • Durable Power of Attorney authorizes organ donation.

Living will laws continued

STATE LIVING WILL DOCUMENT	TESTATOR REQUIREMENTS	WITNESS REQUIREMENTS
Kentucky Advance Directive	Age 18 or older and of sound mind	● Advance Directive requires two adult witnesses, excluding heirs, blood relatives who would be the patient's beneficiary, the attending doctor, employees of the facility where the patient is confined, and those financially responsible for the patient's medical bills. Alternately, the signature may be witnessed by a notary.
Louisiana Declaration	Adult of sound mind age 18 or older	● Declaration requires two adult witnesses who personally know the patient, excluding anyone entitled to part of the patient's estate and relatives by blood or marriage.
● Maine Durable Power of Attorney for Health Care ● Maine Declaration to Physicians	Competent adult (age 18 or older)	● Durable Power of Attorney must be signed by two witnesses who also sign to show that the patient signed the document voluntarily. It also must be notarized. ● Declaration requires two witnesses who also sign to show that the patient signed the document voluntarily.
● Maryland Appointment of Health Care Agent (Part A) ● Maryland Advance Medical Directive Health Care Instructions (Part B)	Age 18 or older, or married or a parent	● Part A requires two witnesses, excluding the agent. At least one witness must not be an heir or claimant against the patient's estate. ● Part B requires two witnesses, at least one of whom is not an heir or claimant against the patient's estate.
Massachusetts Health Care Proxy	Competent adult (age 18 or older)	● Proxy must be signed in the presence of two adult witnesses who believe the patient to be at least age 18 and of sound mind.
Michigan Designation of Patient Advocate for Health Care	Competent adult (age 18 or older)	● Act requires two witnesses (excluding those related by blood or marriage, heirs, the doctor, employees of the patient's life or health insurance provider, or employees of the treatment or care facility) who show that the patient voluntarily signed the document.

MEDICAL REQUIREMENTS	ADDITIONAL INFORMATION
Attending doctor must determine that the patient has an incurable and irreversible condition, that death will shortly ensue, and that life-sustaining treatments would only prolong dying artificially. The doctor will determine if the patient can no longer make decisions.	● A person appointed as surrogate cannot be an employee, owner, director, or officer of a health care facility in which the patient is a resident, unless related by blood or marriage. ● The act allows withdrawal of tube feedings. ● The Living Will doesn't apply during pregnancy.
Attending doctor and one other doctor must certify in writing that the patient has a terminal condition or is in a profound coma without reasonable chance of recovery and that life-sustaining treatments would only artificially prolong dying.	● Act doesn't mention tube feeding. ● Secretary of State is required to establish a declaration registry, where the patient may choose to file his declaration. ● Declaration does not apply if patient has an irreversible condition that would not be considered terminal.
Attending doctor must certify in writing that the patient has an incurable, irreversible condition that would cause death shortly if life-sustaining treatments weren't used.	● Act authorizes the withholding or withdrawal of tube feeding. ● If the patient elects not to have fluids and nutrients artificially administered, he must indicate his wishes in writing.
Attending doctor and one other doctor must examine the patient and then confirm that his condition is terminal, that death is imminent with or without use of life-sustaining treatments, or that the patient is in a permanent vegetative state. The doctor must determine that the patient is incapable of making an informed decision.	● Appointed health care agent cannot be an owner, operator, or employee of the treating facility unless he is a relative, spouse, or close friend. ● Patient can list specific instructions in the event of pregnancy. ● Not effective for non-hospital emergencies. ● Act allows for withdrawing or withholding artificial nutrition and hydration.
Patient must be terminally ill, permanently unconscious, or minimally conscious due to brain damage, as determined by a doctor. For Health Care Proxy to be effective, doctor must determine in writing that the patient is unable to make or communicate health care decisions.	● Act allows patient to write his wishes regarding artificial nutrition and hydration.
Patient's doctor and one other doctor or licensed psychologist must certify in writing that the patient is unable to make medical treatment decisions. Living Will becomes effective if doctor certifies that the patient is terminally ill, permanently unconscious, or minimally conscious due to brain damage.	● A pregnant patient's advocate cannot authorize withholding treatment. ● Patient advocate must date and sign an acceptance of the designation before he can make decisions on the patient's behalf. ● The patient can refuse examination by a doctor because of religious convictions.

Living will laws continued

STATE LIVING WILL DOCUMENT	TESTATOR REQUIREMENTS	WITNESS REQUIREMENTS
● Minnesota Health Care Living Will ● Minnesota Durable Power of Attorney for Health Care	Adult of sound mind or emancipated minor	● Living Will requires two adult witnesses or a notary public; neither witness may be the patient's proxy or an heir. ● Durable Power of Attorney requires two witnesses at least age 18, excluding any agent and the doctor or his employee. Alternately, the document may be signed in the presence of a notary public who is not the patient's agent.
● Mississippi Durable Power of Attorney for Health Care ● Mississippi Declaration	Adult of sound mind	● Durable Power of Attorney requires two witnesses who know the patient, excluding the attorney-in-fact, the doctor, and his employees. At least one witness must not be a relative or heir. ● Declaration requires two witnesses who personally know the patient, excluding relatives by blood or marriage, heirs, claimants to the patient's estate, and the patient's doctor or one of his employees.
● Missouri Durable Power of Attorney for Health Care ● Missouri Declaration	Age 18 or older and of sound mind	● Durable Power of Attorney for Health Care must be signed in the presence of an attorney. ● Declaration requires two witnesses age 18 or older who personally know the patient.
● Montana Appointment of Agent ● Montana Declaration	Competent adult (age 18 or older)	● Appointment of Agent requires two witnesses at least age 18 (should not be the appointed agent). ● Declaration requires two witnesses at least age 18.
● Nebraska Power of Attorney for Health Care ● Nebraska Declaration	Competent adult (age 19 or older) or someone who is or has been married	● Power of Attorney requires notarization or two witnesses who know the patient, excluding the doctor, relatives by blood or marriage, the attorney-in-fact, and employees of the wife or health insurer. ● Declaration requires notarized signature or two witnesses, neither of whom is an employee of the patient's life or health insurer. At least one witness must not be an administrator or employee of the treating facility.

MEDICAL REQUIREMENTS	ADDITIONAL INFORMATION
Diagnosis of a terminal condition and the patient's inability to participate in medical decisions are required.	• The Living Will encourages personalization, including written wishes about artificial administration of fluids and nutrients. • A proxy can be named in the Living Will but can act only if the patient is terminally ill and unable to make treatment decisions. To avoid confusion, name the same person as proxy and agent. • A pregnant patient's Living Will is not honored if the fetus is deemed to be viable.
Attending doctor and two other doctors must agree that they do not expect the patient to recover consciousness or a meaningful (to the patient) state of health and that death would be immediate without use of life-sustaining treatments. They must also obtain a certified copy of the patient's declaration as proof that no revocation has been filed.	• Act doesn't specifically mention tube feeding. • To be legally valid, the Living Will must be filed with the Mississippi State Department of Health, Division of Public Health Statistics. • The Living Will is void during pregnancy.
Attending doctor certifies in writing that the patient's condition is terminal and that death will occur shortly, with or without life-sustaining treatments. Durable Power of Attorney becomes effective when patient's doctor and one other doctor certify that the patient is incapacitated and will remain so while treatment decisions are required.	• Agent cannot be the doctor or his employee, or the owner, operator, or employee of the treating health care facility unless the patient is related or both are bound by vows to a religious life. • Attorney-in-fact can refuse artificial nutrition and hydration on patient's behalf *only* if the patient specifically grants such authority. • Declaration is void during pregnancy. • Declaration does not cover conditions such as permanent unconsciousness.
Attending doctor must determine that the patient has a terminal condition and death would occur without the use of life-sustaining medical care.	• Appointed agent must be at least age 18. • Declaration will not be honored if patient is pregnant. • Montana documents are not valid for non-hospital emergencies.
Power of Attorney takes effect when the patient's doctor and another doctor certify in writing that the patient is incapable of making health care decisions. Declaration becomes effective when the attending doctor determines that the patient is incapable of making decisions about the use of life-sustaining treatment and is either terminally ill or in a persistent vegetative state.	• Pregnant patient's document will not be honored if the fetus is believed to be viable. • The attorney-in-fact cannot be the doctor or his employee; an owner, operator, or employee of the treating facility (unless related to patient); or anyone who is currently serving as attorney-in-fact for 10 or more people.

Living will laws continued

STATE LIVING WILL DOCUMENT	TESTATOR REQUIREMENTS	WITNESS REQUIREMENTS
• Nevada Durable Power of Attorney for Health Care • Nevada Declaration	Adult of sound mind	• Durable Power of Attorney requires two witnesses who personally know the patient, excluding the attorney-in-fact, doctor or his employees, or operator or employees of the health care facility. • Two witnesses required to sign the declaration.
• New Hampshire Durable Power of Attorney for Health Care • New Hampshire Declaration	Age 18 or older of sound mind and under no constraints or undue influence	• Durable Power of Attorney requires notarization and two witnesses, excluding the appointed agent, spouse, heir, and claimants against the patient's estate. • Declaration requires notarization and two witnesses, excluding the patient's spouse, heirs, doctor or his employees, and claimants against the patient's estate.
• New Jersey Appointment of a Health Care Representative • New Jersey Instruction Directive	Age 18 or older and legally competent	• Both documents require two witnesses, excluding the patient's health care representative (the proxy under patient's durable power of attorney), or a notarized signature.
• New Mexico Durable Power of Attorney for Health Care Decisions • New Mexico Declaration	Adult of sound mind and under no constraints or undue influences	• Durable Power of Attorney for Health Care Decisions must be notarized. • Declaration requires two witnesses.
• New York Health Care Proxy • New York Living Will	Competent adult (age 18 or older)	• Proxy requires two witnesses, excluding the agent. Special requirements for residents of a mental health or mental retardation facility. • No specific witnessing requirements for the Living Will.
• North Carolina Health Care Power of Attorney • North Carolina Declaration of a Desire for a Natural Death	Adult of sound mind	• Both documents require two witnesses, excluding relatives by blood or marriage, heirs, the attending doctor or any of his employees, and employees of the facility where the patient resides.

MEDICAL REQUIREMENTS	ADDITIONAL INFORMATION
Doctor will determine that the patient has an incurable and irreversible condition that, without life-sustaining treatment, will cause death shortly.	● Attorney-in-fact can't be the doctor or his employee, or the care facility operator or employee, unless one of these is a relative. ● Patient can authorize, in writing, the removal or withdrawal of artificial nutrition and hydration. ● The patient's directive is void during pregnancy.
Attending doctor and one other doctor must confirm, in writing, that the patient is permanently unconscious or in a terminal condition and that death is imminent, with or without life-sustaining procedures.	● The agent cannot be the doctor or his employee, or any care provider, unless one of these is a relative. ● Act is void during pregnancy if the fetus is considered viable. ● Allows for refusing artificial nutrition and hydration.
Act specifies four categories that allow refusal of treatment: imminent death; permanent unconsciousness (including a persistent vegetative state); terminal illness; or serious, irreversible illness in which the risks and burdens of intervention outweigh the benefits. Attending doctor and one other doctor must confirm the patient's condition.	● The health care representative cannot be the attending doctor or an operator, administrator, or employee of the treating facility unless the person is related. ● Act makes provisions for definition of death based on religious beliefs. ● Patient can refuse tube feedings and ventilator.
Attending doctor and one other doctor must certify in writing that the patient has a terminal condition or an irreversible loss of consciousness.	● No specific restrictions on who can be appointed attorney-in-fact. ● It is unclear whether the law gives the attorney-in-fact the power to make decisions to withhold or withdraw artificial nutrition and hydration.
Doctor determines that the patient is terminally ill or permanently unconscious or minimally conscious due to brain damage and will never regain the ability to make decisions.	● Proxy cannot be the attending doctor, an operator or employee of the treating facility, or anyone acting for 10 or more people. Relatives are exceptions. ● Proxy can order withholding or withdrawing of artificial nutrition or hydration only with written direction.
Attending doctor and one other doctor must certify in writing that the patient has a terminal, incurable condition.	● Agent must be at least age 18 and not a paid care provider. ● Patient can name in a notarized document the doctor who will determine his incapacity. ● Act allows for withholding or withdrawing artificial nutrition or hydration. ● Act provides good faith immunity from legal liability for agent and health care providers.

Living will laws continued

STATE LIVING WILL DOCUMENT	TESTATOR REQUIREMENTS	WITNESS REQUIREMENTS
● North Dakota Durable Power of Attorney for Health Care ● North Dakota Declaration	Age 18 or older and of sound mind	● Durable Power of Attorney requires two witnesses, excluding the agent, doctor or his employee, spouse, relative, heir, claimant against the estate, or operator or employee of a long-term facility. ● Declaration requires two witnesses who personally know the patient, excluding blood relatives or spouse, heirs, claimants against his estate, the doctor, and those financially responsible for the patient's medical care. If the patient is in a long-term care facility, one witness must be a regional long-term care ombudsman, attorney, or clergyperson.
● Ohio Durable Power of Attorney for Health Care ● Ohio Living Will Declaration	Competent adult (age 18 or older)	● Durable Power of Attorney can be witnessed in the same manner as the Living Will. ● Have Living Will signature witnessed by a notary or two adults who show that the patient signed in their presence and appears to be of sound mind. Witnesses cannot be relatives, the doctor, or administrator of patient's nursing home.

● Oklahoma Advance Directive for Health Care
  Living Will (Sec. I)
  Appointment of Health Care Proxy (Sec. II)
	Age 18 or older	● Document requires two witnesses, age 18 or older, excluding heirs.

● Oregon Advance Directive
  Appointment of Health Care Representative (Part B)
  Health Care Instructions (Part C)
	Adult of sound mind, an emancipated or married minor	● Document requires two witnesses who personally know the patient and can attest to soundness of mind and freedom from duress, excluding blood relatives or spouse, heirs, claimants against the estate, the doctor or his employees, and employees of the care facility. If the patient is in a long-term facility, one witness must be designated by the state's Department of Human Resources.

Pennsylvania Declaration	Age 18 or older of sound mind, or a minor who is married or a high school graduate	● Declaration requires two witnesses who also sign to show that the patient knowingly and voluntarily signed the document.

MEDICAL REQUIREMENTS	ADDITIONAL INFORMATION
Attending doctor and one other doctor must determine that the patient has a terminal condition and that death is imminent without life-sustaining medical care.	• Act authorizes withholding or withdrawal of tube feedings. • Agent cannot be the doctor or other health care provider or their employees. • A pregnant patient's declaration will not be honored.
Attending doctor and one other doctor must determine that the patient is terminally ill or permanently unconscious and that death would occur without life-sustaining medical care. They must also find no reasonable possibility that the patient will regain his capabilities.	• Agent cannot be the doctor or his employee or an operator or employee of the treating facility. Relatives or fellow members of a religious order are exceptions. • Agent can consent to withholding or withdrawing artificial nutrition and hydration.
Two doctors must certify that the patient is persistently unconscious or has a terminal condition.	• Document will not be honored during pregnancy. • Document allows patient to sign a request to withdraw or withhold artificial nutrition or hydration.
Attending doctor and one other doctor must certify that the patient has an incurable, terminal condition and that death is imminent whether or not life-sustaining procedures are used.	• Agent cannot be the attending doctor or his employee or an operator or employee of the care facility. • If the spouse is the agent, document is automatically revoked in the event of a divorce. • Act authorizes withholding or withdrawing of tube feedings.
Doctor determines that patient is incompetent and terminally ill or in a state of permanent unconsciousness.	• Declaration encourages personal instructions because Pennsylvania law is unclear on the definition of "terminal." • Pregnant patient's declaration will not be honored if the fetus is deemed viable.

Living will laws continued

STATE LIVING WILL DOCUMENT	TESTATOR REQUIREMENTS	WITNESS REQUIREMENTS
• Rhode Island Durable Power of Attorney for Health Care • Rhode Island Declaration	Competent adult (age 18 or older)	• Durable Power of Attorney requires two witnesses who know the patient and believe him to be of sound mind, excluding the agent, the doctor or his employees, and the operator or employees of the health care facility. At least one witness cannot be related or an heir. • Declaration requires two witnesses who know the patient and are not related to sign that he voluntarily signed the document.
• South Carolina Health Care Power of Attorney • South Carolina Declaration of a Desire for a Natural Death	Age 18 or older	• Health Care Power of Attorney must be signed in the presence of two witnesses, excluding the agent or alternate, relatives, doctor or his employees, those financially responsible for the patient's care, heirs, insurance beneficiaries, or claimants against the estate. • Declaration requires two witnesses who personally know the patient and believe him to be of sound mind, excluding blood relatives or spouse, heirs, insurance beneficiaries, claimants against the patient's estate, those financially responsible for the patient's medical care, and the doctor or his employees. No more than one witness can be an employee of the health care facility.
• South Dakota Durable Power of Attorney for Health Care • South Dakota Living Will	Competent adult	• Durable Power of Attorney can be witnessed by a notary or signed in the presence of two adult witnesses, who sign that they know the patient and believe him to be of sound mind. • Living Will must be signed in the presence of two witnesses.
• Tennessee Durable Power of Attorney for Health Care • Tennessee Living Will	Adult of sound mind	• Durable Power of Attorney requires notarized signatures of two witnesses who know the patient and believe him to be of sound mind. Witnesses can't be the attorney-in-fact, the doctor or his employees, or the operator or employees of the treating facility. • Living Will requires notarization and two witnesses who know the patient and believe him to be of sound mind.
• Texas Durable Power of Attorney for Health Care • Texas Directive to Physicians	Competent adult or emancipated minor	• Durable Power of Attorney requires two witnesses who know the patient and believe him to be of sound mind, excluding the agent, the doctor or his employees, heirs, or claimants against the estate. • Directive requires two witnesses, excluding blood relatives or spouse, heirs, claimants against estate, the doctor or any of his employees, and any health care employee who cares for the patient or is involved in the facility's finances.

MEDICAL REQUIREMENTS	ADDITIONAL INFORMATION
Doctor must determine that the patient has an incurable and irreversible condition and can no longer make his own medical decisions. It should be his opinion that death would occur without life-sustaining medical care.	● Agent cannot be the doctor or his employee or an operator or employee of a care facility. Relatives are the exception. ● A pregnant patient's declaration is void. ● Not effective for non-hospital emergencies.
Two doctors must examine the patient and then certify that the patient is terminally ill, that death will occur shortly without use of life-sustaining treatments, and that such treatments only artificially prolong dying.	● Act allows withholding or withdrawing artificial nutrition or hydration. ● Patient may appoint an agent in the declaration who is empowered only to enforce or revoke the declaration and cannot make medical decisions. ● Documents will not be honored during pregnancy. ● Documents must be notarized.
Attending doctor and one other doctor must confirm after an examination that the patient's condition is terminal and that life-sustaining treatments would only prolong dying.	● State law restricts the attorney-in-fact's power to withhold or withdraw artificial nutrition and hydration, even with the patient's written direction, if it is determined necessary to relieve pain.
Attending doctor must determine that the patient is terminally ill or in a coma or persistent vegetative state, that death is imminent, and that the use of life-sustaining treatments would only artificially prolong dying.	● Act allows withholding or withdrawing of tube feedings and organ donation. ● Agent can't be the doctor or his employee or an operator or employee of a care facility. Relatives and conservator are exceptions. ● Living Will detail is encouraged because the law is unclear as to when the patient is considered terminal.
Two doctors must certify in writing that the patient has an incurable and irreversible condition, that death is imminent, and that use of life-sustaining treatments would only artificially prolong dying.	● Appointed agent cannot be the doctor or his employee or an operator or employee of the residential care facility unless such person is related. ● Patient should add personal instructions to directive because Texas law is unclear in defining "terminal." ● Act doesn't mention tube feedings. ● Living Will is void during pregnancy.

Living will laws continued

STATE LIVING WILL DOCUMENT	TESTATOR REQUIREMENTS	WITNESS REQUIREMENTS
• Utah Directive to Physicians and Providers of Medical Services • Utah Special Power of Attorney	Adult of sound mind	• Directive requires two witnesses age 18 or older who know the patient, excluding blood relatives or spouse, heirs, those financially responsible for the patient's medical care, any employee of the patient's health care facility, or the person who signed the Directive at the patient's direction. • Special Power of Attorney must be signed in the presence of a notary.
• Vermont Durable Power of Attorney for Health Care • Vermont Terminal Care Document	Age 18 or older and of sound mind	• Durable Power of Attorney must be signed in the presence of two witnesses who know the patient and believe that he is of sound mind and understands the nature of the document, excluding the agent, the doctor or his employees, spouse, heirs, or claimants to the estate. • If the patient is in a nursing home or hospital, an ombudsman must sign the Durable Power of Attorney. • Terminal Care Document requires two witnesses, excluding the spouse, heirs, claimants against the patient's estate, and the patient's doctor or anyone under his direction.
Virginia Advance Medical Directive	Competent adult age 18 or older	• Directive requires two witnesses who know the patient, excluding relatives by blood or marriage.
• Washington Durable Power of Attorney for Health Care • Washington Health Care Directive	Adult of sound mind age 18 or older	• Two adult witnesses sign the Durable Power of Attorney. • Directive requires two witnesses who personally know the patient, excluding relatives by blood or marriage, heirs, claimants against the patient's estate, the doctor or any of his employees, and any employee of the patient's health care facility.
• West Virginia Living Will • West Virginia Medical Power of Attorney	Age 18 or older and of sound mind	• Living Will must be notarized and requires two witnesses age 18 or older, excluding relatives by blood or marriage, heirs, those financially responsible for the patient's medical care, the patient's doctor or any of his employees, any employee of the health care facility where the patient resides, and the person who signed the document on the patient's behalf. • Medical Power of Attorney witness requirements are the same as for the Living Will.

MEDICAL REQUIREMENTS	ADDITIONAL INFORMATION
Two doctors must examine the patient and then certify in writing that his injury, illness, or disease is terminal or that he is in a persistent vegetative state, and that use of life-sustaining treatments would only artificially prolong dying. Doctor must certify incapacitation.	● Act allows withdrawing or withholding tube feedings. ● The Directive is to be completed only after injury or illness. The patient does not have to be terminally or in a persistent vegetative state. ● Any Directive for medical services that the agent completes takes precedence over a Directive that the patient completed.
Patient must be in a terminal state with no reasonable expectation of recovery.	● The Act allows for withholding or withdrawing artificial nutrition or hydration. ● Agent can't be the doctor or his employee or any care provider. Relatives are the exception.
Attending doctor and one other doctor must certify that the patient's condition is terminal, that death is imminent, and that use of life-sustaining treatments would only artificially prolong dying.	● Court decisions have permitted withholding or withdrawing of tube feedings. ● Additional instructions are encouraged because the law is unclear about meaning of "terminal."
Attending doctor and one other must determine that the patient has developed a terminal condition and can no longer make his own medical decisions; this also applies to permanent unconsciousness and persistent vegetative state.	● Agent can't be the doctor or his employee or an operator or employee of the care facility. Relatives are the exception. ● A pregnant patient's directive is void. ● Act allows withholding or withdrawing of artificial nutrition and hydration.
Attending doctor and one other doctor must confirm in writing that the patient's condition is terminal or that he's in a persistent vegetative state.	● Agent can't be the doctor or his employee or an operator or employee of the involved facility. Relatives are the exception. ● Medical Power of Attorney requires written directions regarding artificial nutrition and hydration.

Living will laws continued

STATE LIVING WILL DOCUMENT	TESTATOR REQUIREMENTS	WITNESS REQUIREMENTS
• Wisconsin Power of Attorney for Health Care • Wisconsin Declaration to Physicians	Age 18 or older and of sound mind	• Power of Attorney for Health Care witness requirements are the same as those for the Declaration. • Declaration to Physician requires two witnesses, excluding relatives, heirs, the patient's doctor, any employee of the treating facility, claimants against the estate, and persons financially responsible for the medical care.
• Wyoming Durable Power of Attorney for Health Care • Wyoming Declaration	Adult of sound mind	• Durable Power of Attorney requires notarization or two witnesses who know the patient and believe him to be of sound mind, excluding the attorney-in-fact, the doctor or his employees, and the operator or employees of a community care or residential care facility. One witness must not be related to an heir. • Declaration requires two adult witnesses who know the patient, excluding relatives by blood or marriage, heirs, those financially responsible for the patient's medical care, or the person who signed the document on the patient's behalf.

to be reviewed periodically to keep pace with changes in technology. Some living wills are very detailed, multipage documents; some are a simple paragraph.

Immunity

If doctors, nurses, and other health care providers follow the wishes expressed in a living will authorized by law, they're generally immune from civil and criminal liability. No matter which state you work in, check your hospital's policy and procedures manual and seek advice from your hospital's legal department as needed.

Children and living wills

Although minors can't make valid *testamentary wills,* and adults can't make such wills for them, living wills are another matter. In a few states, adults

are authorized to make living wills for their minor children.

Most parents are unlikely to make a living will before a child's terminal illness is diagnosed. Even then, a living will is usually legally unnecessary. If the parents and the child agree that no extraordinary means should be used to prolong life, or if the child is too young to understand, the parents have the legal right to act for the child. They can require that the health care team not use extraordinary means to prolong his life. That principle applies in reverse: If the child wants to die but the parents want him treated, the parents' wishes prevail.

If a terminally ill adolescent doesn't want extraordinary treatment but his parents do, and the adolescent has written a living will, a doctor or hospital may use the will to petition a court in his behalf. Even though the will itself is legally invalid because it was written

MEDICAL REQUIREMENTS	ADDITIONAL INFORMATION
Attending doctor and one other doctor must determine if the patient has developed a terminal condition and can no longer make his own medical decisions or if he is in a persistent vegetative state.	• Act authorizes withholding or withdrawing of tube feedings. • Agent cannot be the doctor or his employee, an employee of the involved facility, or the spouse of these people. Patient's relatives are excepted. • A pregnant patient's declaration is void.
Attending doctor and one other doctor must certify that the patient's incurable injury, disease, or other illness is terminal and that death will occur whether or not life-sustaining treatments are used.	• Attorney-in-fact for Durable Power of Attorney cannot be the doctor or the operator or employee of the involved care facility. • Proxy in declaration may be enforced only when the patient is unable to make treatment decisions and is in a terminal condition. The patient should appoint the same person as proxy and attorney-in-fact.

by a minor, its very existence may prompt the court to consult the adolescent and, in its ruling, grant the patient his wishes.

Living will from another state or country

U.S. law applies to foreign citizens who are treated in the United States. That means a foreign citizen may execute a living will while in the United States, and it must be honored.

What about a patient who executes a living will in one state and later finds himself terminally ill in another? The law of the state where the living will decision will be carried out prevails. Therefore, if a patient has an out-of-state living will, you should determine whether it matches the criteria required by the laws of the state you're in. When dealing with an out-of-state living will, consult your hospital attorney.

What if a patient produces a living will executed in a foreign country? In general, the foreign country's law applies (regardless of whether the patient is a citizen of that country) and determines the extent to which a living will will be honored. Consult your hospital attorney.

When a living will becomes invalid

A living will needn't be honored if it has been revoked or is out of date. State law may mandate that a living will is valid only for a limited number of years. If the patient's family and attending medical personnel find that the patient made the living will many years ago and his life circumstances have changed substantially since then, they may have legal justification for disregarding the will. For this reason, publishers of living will forms suggest reviewing the will yearly, revising it if needed, and redating and re-signing it.

If the patient asks that the will be disregarded or tells his doctor to proceed with treatment that contradicts the will, such action effectively revokes the will.

When the family's wishes contradict the will

The patient's family can't contradict a patient's living will unless they can prove the will is invalid. Some states provide penalties for concealing a patient's living will or for falsely reporting that it has been revoked.

Drafting a living will

Like all legal documents, a living will must be written, signed, and witnessed. State laws specify the execution requirements. (To obtain forms, refer the patient to Choice in Dying — The National Council for the Right to Die, 200 Varick St., 10th Fl., New York, NY 10014-4810; (phone 1-800-989-WILL). If the patient asks for help drafting a living will, refer him to the hospital's legal department or to a local legal aid agency.

Although it's not required, a patient should be encouraged to file copies of his living will with his doctor and with family members who would attend him in the event of a terminal illness.

You may be asked to witness a living will. Check to see if your state law allows this. If it doesn't, ask your nursing supervisor what procedure you should follow.

If the patient drafts a living will while under your care, document this in your nurses' notes, describing factually the circumstances under which the will was drawn up and signed.

Oral statements

Patients most often make oral statements expressing their wishes about further medical treatment before or during a terminal illness.

Before terminal illness

When a patient has made his treatment wishes known to his family and doctor in advance, they will usually respect his wishes even if he later becomes comatose or otherwise incompetent. But if the doctor and the family disagree about what is best for the terminally ill, incompetent patient, they may have to settle the dispute in court.

During terminal illness

Every competent adult has the right to refuse medical treatment for himself, including the use of extraordinary efforts. If a competent terminally ill patient tells a doctor or nurse to discontinue extraordinary efforts, his wishes are binding.

If a patient tells you his wishes about dying, first write what he says in your nurses' notes, using his exact words as much as possible. Next, describe the context of the discussion — for example, was the patient in pain, or had he just been informed of a terminal illness? Be sure to also tell the patient's doctor about the discussion.

If the patient becomes incompetent, ensuring that orally-stated wishes are respected may be difficult. Oral statements *should* be respected, however, as guidelines for how the patient feels about his treatment.

Dealing with living wills

Federal legislation, the Patient Self-Determination Act of 1990, requires hospitals, *nursing homes, health maintenance organizations, hospices,* and home health care agencies that participate in Medicare and *Medicaid* to provide patients with written information about their rights under state law regarding living wills and **durable power of attorney** (together called **advance directives**) as well as about the hospital's procedure for implementing them. The law also requires the institution to document whether or not the patient has a living will or durable power of attorney.

If your patient has a living will, review your nursing or hospital manual for directions on what steps to take. For instance, you may need to inform the patient's doctor about it. Or you may need to ask your nursing supervisor to inform the hospital administration and the legal affairs department. With the patient's permission, make sure that his family knows about the will; if they don't, show them a copy.

If the patient is able to talk, discuss the will with him, especially if it contains terms that need further definition. As always, objectively document your actions and findings in the patient's record.

Beyond these actions, your responsibilities for a patient's living will will be determined by the circumstances involved — including the family's and doctor's responses to the will. If you feel strongly about the patient's right to have his wishes followed, work with family members and colleagues to come up with a unified plan of care.

Personal conflicts over a living will

If implementing a living will conflicts with your personal ethics or beliefs, you may wish to discuss the matter with a **clinical nurse specialist,** your nursing supervisor, a nursing administrator, the hospital chaplain, a hospital administrator, or a hospital ethics committee member. Then, after talking over your feelings with one of them, if you're still unable to accept the idea, you can ask for reassignment to another patient. Chances are your request will be honored and no disciplinary action will be taken against you.

Selected references

1995 Comprehensive Accreditation Manual for Hospitals. Oakbrook Terrace, Ill.: Joint Commission on Accreditation of Healthcare Organizations, 1994.

Feutz-Harter, S. "Nursing Case Law Update," *Journal of Nursing Law* 1(1):23-29, Autumn 1993.

Fiesta, J. "Legal Update, 1994, Part 1," *Nursing Management* 26(1):30, January 1995.

Fiesta, J. "Legal Update, 1994, Part 2," *Nursing Management* 26(3):10-11, March 1995.

Fiesta, J. "Staffing Implications: A Legal Update," *Nursing Management* 25(6):34-35, June 1994.

Grane, N. "Witnessing Informed Consent," *Nursing94* 24(5):17, May 1994.

Grant, A.B. *The Professional Nurse: Issues and Actions.* Springhouse, Pa.: Springhouse Corp., 1994.

Hyde-Robertson, B., et al. "A Strategy Against Elderly Mistreatment," *Caring* 13(11):40-44, November 1994.

King, B. "Working with a New Staff Mix," *RN* 58(6):38-41, June 1995.

Mulholland, D.K. "Privacy and Confidentiality of Patient Information: Challenges for Nursing," *Journal of Nursing Administration* 24(2):19-24, February 1994.

Rich, J. "13 Ways to Protect Your Practice," *Nursing93* 23(2):60-61, February 1993.

Salvatore, N.G. "Restraints: A Sampling of Current Practice," *Journal of Emergency Nursing* 19(5):417-21, October 1993.

Sherry, D. "Coping with Staffing Shortages: Strategies for Survival," *Home Healthcare Nurse* 12(1):38-42, January/February 1994.

Simonowitz, J. "Violence in the Workplace: You're Entitled to Protection," *RN* 57(11):61-63, November 1994.

Sullivan, G. "When Assignments Don't Match Skills," *RN* 58(4):57-60, April 1995.

Sullivan, M.P. *Nursing Leadership and Management,* 2nd ed. Springhouse, Pa.: Springhouse Corp., 1995.

4

Legal risks while off duty

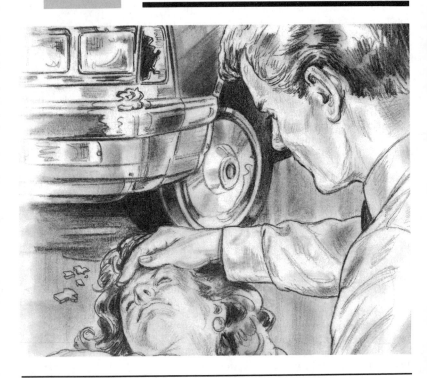

When you're on duty, numerous guidelines define the legal limits of your practice and your legal risks. They include hospital *policies, standards* issued by nursing organizations, and state or provincial *nurse practice acts. Statutory law* and *common law* provide additional direction. When you're off duty, however, you have few specific guidelines. Your legal responsibilities aren't as clear-cut.

For example, you probably wouldn't hesitate to perform the Heimlich maneuver to save a choking victim. But what if you panic, make a mistake, and injure the patient? Can you be sued by the victim or his estate? Can your nursing license be suspended or revoked? Does the law protect you because of your good intentions?

Fortunately, thus far, lawsuits resulting from off-duty nursing actions have been extremely rare. However, whether you frequently provide off-duty care or whether you just give free advice occasionally to your neighbor, it's important to act on sound legal footing.

Legal issues

This chapter discusses legal issues related to off-duty nursing. You'll find information on:

• *acting as a Good Samaritan* — your *liability* when you give emergency care at an accident scene or in a disaster

• *giving free health care advice* — legal ramifications of giving advice to family members and friends

• *donating nursing services* — protecting yourself legally when you volunteer your nursing skills

• *acting during disasters* — legal aspects of providing nursing services during emergencies and declared *disasters.*

You'll learn to distinguish between what the law requires and what the law allows. You'll also find out how your nurse practice act and other state laws apply to off-duty actions. (Incidentally, you may discover that except for *Good Samaritan acts,* the law has relatively little to say about off-duty nursing.)

Legal protection for Good Samaritans

Imagine yourself driving in heavy traffic. Not far ahead, you see an automobile accident and a bloodied motorist gesturing for help. Nearby, another victim lies sprawled at curbside. What should you do? Your conscience and compassion prompt you to help the victim in any health care emergency. Your common sense prompts you to ask if helping out means courting legal trouble.

Your options

You have three options. You can:
• help the accident victim at the scene
• leave the scene, stop at the nearest phone, and call for an ambulance or other rescue service
• pass the scene and make no attempt to call for help.

In almost every state, you have the legal right to choose any of these options. In most cases, off-duty nurses in the United States and Canada have no legal duty to rescue anyone.

Obligation to rescue

In general, the only people with a legal duty to rescue others are individuals who perform rescues as part of their jobs — fire fighters, police officers, emergency medical technicians, and a few others, such as public transportation workers. In a few states, such as Vermont, Minnesota, and Wisconsin, *"duty to rescue" laws* may apply to nurses. Unless you're covered by a duty-to-rescue law, your decision to help remains voluntary and personal.

Common and statutory law

If you choose to help the accident victim, two kinds of law protect you: common law and statutory law, specifically the Good Samaritan acts.

Common law is the cumulative result of court decisions over the years. These decisions may provide guidelines for acting in an accident situation.

Good Samaritan acts grew out of *health care professionals'* concerns that common law didn't sufficiently protect their actions. For one thing, common law doesn't prevent a victim from pursuing a lengthy and costly court battle. In response, health care professionals lobbied for stronger protection. And most states obliged with Good Samaritan acts. (See *State Good Samaritan acts,* pages 182 to 186.)

(Text continues on page 187.)

State Good Samaritan acts

	Alabama	Alaska	Arizona	Arkansas	California	Colorado	Connecticut	Delaware	Dist. Columbia
Statute	6-5-332	9.65.090	32-1471	17-93-101	2727.5	13-21-108	52-557b	16 §6802	2-1344
Covers in-state nurses	●				●		●		
Covers in-state and out-of-state nurses			●				●	●	
Covers "any person"		●	●	●		●			●
Separate Good Samaritan act for nurses								●	
Covers only gratuitous services	●		●	●		●	●		●
Covers emergencies occurring in health care facilities		●				●			
Specifically protects against failure to provide or arrange for further medical treatment	●		●						
Specifically covers transportation from the scene of the emergency to a destination for further medical treatment								●	
Specifically mentions that acts of gross negligence or willful or wanton misconduct are not covered (1,2,3)		●	●	●	●	●	●	●	●
Includes "duty to rescue" statute (4)									

(1) Arizona: applies only to MDs. (2) Florida: in hospitals only. (3) Georgia: with restrictions.
(4) Hawaii: at scene of crime.

Use this chart to familiarize yourself with your state's Good Samaritan act. You may want to check with your board of nursing to make sure your state hasn't passed any amendments that would affect how this law pertains to your practice.

Florida	Georgia	Hawaii	Idaho	Illinois	Indiana	Iowa	Kansas	Kentucky	Louisiana	Maine	Maryland
45 §768.13	51-1-29	663-1.5	§5-330	111 P3505.1	34-4-12-1	613.17	65-2891	411.148	9:2793	14§164	CJ5-309
								•			
				•		•					
•	•	•	•		•	•			•	•	•
•	•	•		•	•	•		•	•	•	•
•						•					
•	•				•				•		
			•			•			•		•
•	•	•	•	•	•	•	•	•	•	•	•
		•									

(continued)

State Good Samaritan acts continued

	Massachusetts	Michigan	Minnesota	Mississippi	Missouri	Montana	Nebraska	Nevada	New Hampshire
Statute	112:12B	14.563	604A.01	73-25-37	537.037	27-1-714	25-21,186	41.505	326-B:18
Covers in-state nurses		●							
Covers in-state and out-of-state nurses	●				●			●	●
Covers "any person"			●	●		●	●		
Separate Good Samaritan act for nurses (5)			●	●					●
Covers only gratuitous services	●		●		●	●	●	●	●
Covers emergencies occurring in health care facilities			●						
Specifically protects against failure to provide or arrange for further medical treatment							●	●	
Specifically covers transportation from the scene of the emergency to a destination for further medical treatment			●	●					
Specifically mentions that acts of gross negligence or willful or wanton misconduct are not covered		●	●	●	●	●		●	
Includes "duty to rescue" statute			●						

(5) Mississippi: covers nurse practitioners.

New Jersey	New Mexico	New York	North Carolina	North Dakota	Ohio	Oklahoma	Oregon	Pennsylvania	Rhode Island	South Carolina	South Dakota
2A:62A-1	24-10-3	8§6909	90-21.14	39-08-04.1	2305.23	76§5	30.800 to 30.807	42-§8331	5-34-34	15-1-310	20-9-3
		●					●	●	●		●
●	●		●	●	●	●				●	
		●				●			●		
	●	●	●	●	●	●	●		●	●	
										●	
●					●		●				
	●	●	●	●	●	●	●	●	●	●	

(continued)

State Good Samaritan acts continued

	Tennessee	Texas	Utah	Vermont	Virginia	Washington	West Virginia	Wisconsin	Wyoming
Statute	63-6-218	Title 4 74.001	26-8-11	12§519	8.01-225	4.24.300	55-7-15	895.48	1-1-120
Covers in-state nurses									
Covers in-state and out-of-state nurses			●						
Covers "any person"	●	●		●	●	●	●	●	●
Separate Good Samaritan act for nurses									
Covers only gratuitous services	●	●		●	●	●	●	●	●
Covers emergencies occurring in health care facilities		●							
Specifically protects against failure to provide or arrange for further medical treatment									
Specifically covers transportation from the scene of the emergency to a destination for further medical treatment	●				●	●			
Specifically mentions that acts of gross negligence or willful or wanton misconduct are not covered	●	●	●	●	●	●			
Includes "duty to rescue" statute				●					

Proving malpractice

To bring a *malpractice* suit to a jury trial, the patient must establish the following:
• you owed a *duty,* based on a nurse-patient relationship
• you breached that duty in some way
• the patient was harmed
• your *breach of duty* caused the harm.
Consider these points as they apply to the auto accident.

Your legal duty

As long as you pass the accident scene—whether or not you stop down the road to call for help—you owe the victim no legal duty. He's not your patient, and he has no legal claim to your professional services. (Remember, ethical questions aren't at issue here.)

But just by stopping your car at the scene, you incur a legal duty. From now on, you can't leave the victim until he's being cared for by another health care professional with at least as much training as you have or until the police order you from the scene.

When you stop your car at the scene, you give the appearance to other potential rescuers that you'll take care of the victim. At that point, you establish a nurse-patient relationship for that particular emergency. And you owe the victim the normal duty you owe any patient—treatment that meets the *standard of care* of a *reasonably prudent nurse* in a similar situation.

Breach of duty

Once you've stopped to help, you can avoid breaching your duty by using the same good judgment that you use every day on the job. But what if you do breach your duty in this unusual situation?

If your performance falls below standard, the court will decide whether your act worsened the victim's condition. If your act didn't make the victim measurably worse, the court may find that the harm committed doesn't warrant damages. Your act must cause measurable harm for the court to consider you legally responsible.

How the courts measure harm

The victim must prove that the probability is better than 50% that your error (whether an act of commission or omission) caused his injuries. Historically, the courts have recognized the 50% figure as the standard. Because the typical victim has already suffered injuries from the accident, he's likely to have a hard time proving that your error caused or worsened his injuries.

In making it hard for the accident victim to prove you negligent, the courts balance the victim's right to justice against society's need to encourage trained professionals to assist in emergencies.

Good Samaritan laws

Good Samaritan acts limit your liability for any service you render at an accident or emergency scene. To win a malpractice suit against you under Good Samaritan law, a patient must prove that you intentionally caused his injury or were grossly negligent in your care. In effect, the Good Samaritan acts offer you *immunity from lawsuits* as long as you don't intentionally or recklessly cause the accident victim harm.

Determining gross negligence

No law can protect you if you commit an act of *gross negligence*—an extremely careless act or omission that seriously violates the applicable standard of care.

In court, jury members decide whether your error constitutes "ordinary" negligence or "gross" negligence. To make this distinction, they measure your error against the local standard of care, which may vary from

Care tips for Good Samaritans

When you stop at a motor vehicle accident or similar emergency to offer your assistance, always observe professional standards of nursing care, regardless of the setting. To reduce your malpractice risk, follow these guidelines:
- Care for the victim in the vehicle if you can do so safely.
- Assess the possibility of fractures.
- Move the victim only if he's in danger and if conditions permit. Avoid moving him needlessly, and don't try to straighten his arms and legs.
- Let him lie or sit quietly. Don't carry him or force him to walk.
- Keep his airway open.
- Stop his bleeding.
- Keep the victim warm.
- Determine his level of consciousness.
- Ask the victim where he feels pain.
- Avoid speculating about who or what caused the accident.
- Allow only skilled personnel to attend or treat the victim.
- Stay at the accident site until skilled personnel arrive to assume care of the victim.
- Guard the injured person's personal property. Release it only to the police or members of his family.

place to place. For example, what may qualify as ordinary negligence in rural Georgia may be gross negligence in metropolitan New York. However, as more nurses take certification exams that are national in scope, members of the profession will be held increasingly accountable to a national standard, just as doctors are.

Additionally, the court considers your training and experience to decide whether you've breached the standard of care and, if so, to what degree. This means that the court holds *RNs* — even as Good Samaritans — to a higher standard than it holds *LPNs* or *LVNs*. (See *Care tips for Good Samaritans*.)

Legal discrepancies
Good Samaritan protection varies. Some acts specifically include nurses, whereas other acts — those in Florida and Alaska, for example — protect any person who offers help to a victim. Some acts protect out-of-state nurses only if they are trained in cardiopulmonary resuscitation. In some jurisdictions, Good Samaritan acts include only "practitioners of the healing arts." The courts usually interpret this to mean doctors and dentists. (See *Understanding Good Samaritan acts*.)

Compensated care
Keep in mind that most Good Samaritan acts apply only to uncompensated rescues. If you charge or accept money for your services, the law usually says that you forfeit the special protections afforded by such acts.

Invoking Good Samaritan law

Regardless of the kind of Good Samaritan act your state or province has, remember that accident victims rarely sue Good Samaritans. In fact, nurses have never invoked a Good Samaritan act as a defense. And so far, the common law has served as a deterrent.

Ironically, though, auto accident victims sometimes claim that a Good Samaritan act requires a nurse or doctor to respond at an accident scene. To date, the courts have rejected this argument.

In some states, doctors have invoked a Good Samaritan act as a defense against malpractice suits, claiming that

Understanding Good Samaritan acts

Am I covered by a Good Samaritan act if I respond to an emergency outside the hospital while I am officially on duty?
That depends on two things: the wording of the act in your state and court decisions, if any, that interpret that act. All Good Samaritan laws cover aid at the scene of an emergency, accident, or disaster. If an emergency occurs just outside the hospital, and you provide care while on duty, most likely this would be considered providing care in an emergency setting and, therefore, would be covered under Good Samaritan law. Note that some states' Good Samaritan statutes specifically cover emergencies outside of the hospital, doctor's office, and other places that have medical equipment.

I live and work in Kansas. Every year, I go skiing in a different state. What if I help an accident victim while I'm vacationing? Does the Good Samaritan act of the state I'm in apply to me?
It does if that state's act says it applies to "any person." It may not, however, if the act specifically states that it applies only to "nurses." The designation "nurse" in a law or act may mean an RN, LPN, or LVN licensed in that state.

Does the Good Samaritan act apply if I accept money from the person I've helped?
Not usually. By accepting money in such a situation, you establish a professional relationship with the person you've helped.

For how long am I responsible to the person I've helped?
Statutory law doesn't address this subject, but common law does. The courts say your responsibility ends:
• when the emergency ends (when you're certain that the victim is no longer in danger)
• when an authorized rescue or other qualified medical service takes over for you
• when the victim is pronounced dead.

If a doctor and I respond to the same emergency, does the Good Samaritan act cover us equally?
Not necessarily. In some states, the Good Samaritan act for nurses differs completely from the Good Samaritan act for doctors. Contact your state nursing board to find out what's true for your state.

the act protects them from liability for emergency services they provided in a hospital. In Illinois, a doctor responded to an in-hospital emergency where both patients (mother and fetus) later died, and the estate brought suit. The doctor successfully invoked, as part of his defense, the Illinois Good Samaritan Act. The Appellate Court found that the Act protected the doctor from liability for a true hospital emergency where the service was provided in good faith and without fee. Using this argument in California, doctors have met with mixed results. The same argument will not hold for nurses in California because the Good Samaritan act covers nurses only during emergencies "outside both the place and course" of employment.

Duty to rescue

Four states and most Canadian provinces (and most European countries)

Minimizing legal risks when giving advice

Here are some steps to take to minimize your risk when giving health care advice to friends or family members.

What to do

• Be sure that your advice reflects accepted professional and community nursing standards.

• Check whether your professional liability insurance (or your employer's) covers such off-the-job nursing activities as giving advice.

• Know what – if anything – your state's nurse practice act says about giving advice to friends.

• Give advice only within the confines of your nurse practice act, education, and experience.

• Make sure that the advice you give is up-to-date. You'll be judged on current nursing standards if your advice results in a lawsuit.

What not to do

• Don't charge a fee or accept money for your advice.

• Avoid speculating about your friends' illnesses or ailments.

• Never suggest that friends change or ignore their doctors' orders.

• Steer clear of offering advice about medical care.

• Avoid giving any directions that, if wrong or misinterpreted, could result in serious or permanent injury.

posed to grave physical harm. The Vermont law requires anyone (Vermont resident or not) who can help a victim to do so, provided he won't be endangering himself or interfering with important duties he owes to others. Minnesota has a similar law, as do Wisconsin (which has a "duty to rescue crime victims" law) and Wyoming (where the duty-to-rescue law applies only to doctors).

The Vermont statute provides for criminal penalties for failure to render assistance as required under the law. By contrast, the Quebec statute provides no penalties for violation of its mandate to render assistance. Minnesota makes the failure to render "reasonable assistance at the scene of an emergency" a petty *misdemeanor.*

How a duty-to-rescue law would apply to nurses remains uncertain. For example, if you pass an accident scene on the way to your dentist, the duty-to-rescue law requires you to stop and try to help. But what if you're on your way to work? Would your nursing job be considered an important duty owed to others? The answer to this question will eventually come from the courts.

Giving free health care advice

Most likely, friends and family members rely on you for advice on health matters. Respond cautiously, even though this may seem unnatural when speaking with individuals you know well. Keep in mind that you can be sued for giving inappropriate advice. And if you decide not to give advice at all, be reassured: The law doesn't require it.

If you choose to offer advice, be aware of positions on the issue taken by your nurse practice act, the common law, and professional organizations. (See *Minimizing legal risks when giving advice.*)

have taken the Good Samaritan principle a step further by requiring potential rescuers to help a victim. Vermont's law, the first of its type in the United States, defines *rescuer* as any person who knows that another is ex-

Free advice and the law

In a hospital setting, giving health care advice may be construed to be a part of patient teaching, a recognized nursing function. Outside of the hospital setting, giving advice may subject you to liability if, in providing the advice, you do not act as a reasonably prudent nurse.

The person suing you for harm caused by inappropriate advice must prove that you owed him a specific duty, that you breached that duty, that he was harmed, and that the harm was a result of the breach of duty.

Establishing breach of duty

For a duty to exist, you must have a nurse-patient relationship with the person asking for your advice. This rarely occurs in everyday, short-lived conversations with other people. Suppose, for example, that you're a guest at a cocktail party. Another guest finds out that you're a nurse and bombards you with questions about his health. If you decide to answer, you have a duty to answer as correctly as any reasonably prudent nurse would, but you have no duty to follow up after the party is over and no duty to monitor the outcome of your advice. The person who's asking your advice hasn't established, or indicated that he intends to establish, an ongoing nurse-patient relationship with you.

Establishing probable reliance

The situation may be different if you decide to give advice to a neighbor. For instance, imagine that your neighbor calls across the yard and asks you about her child's fretfulness. You observe honestly that the child's activity doesn't appear to warrant a call to the doctor. A day later, you see the mother and child together outdoors, and the child appears particularly listless. If you discover that the child has a fever

or other signs and symptoms of illness, you are legally and professionally responsible for telling the mother to take the child to a doctor as soon as possible. This holds true no matter what your original advice was.

You must respond to the mother's probable reliance on you for further advice, even though your original intention was not to form a nurse-patient relationship with her and her child.

Again, if you realize that your neighbor now relies on you for further advice, you have an obligation—a legal and professional duty—to keep your advice current as the situation changes. Or you may opt to take formal steps to break off the relationship by telling the mother to look elsewhere for help.

Keep in mind that the principles that apply to your on-duty work also apply to off-duty advice. The help and advice you give your patient Monday morning may have to be changed by Tuesday afternoon. What's more, if a patient's questions reveal that his problem may be beyond the scope of nursing practice, you have a clear duty to call in the doctor (see *Neighborly advice: Some legal safeguards*, page 192).

Professional standards

Whenever you establish a professional relationship with an individual seeking advice, you must give an answer as good as any reasonably prudent nurse would give in similar circumstances.

Do this by applying the same standards that you're expected to apply in your regular work. If you feel confident that you know the answer—and your education and experience support you—you're legally free to give it. Naturally, you must be sure that your answer is correct and that giving it falls within your scope of nursing practice.

To protect yourself, you might say something like, "I think your problem sounds like arthritis, but it could be

Neighborly advice: Some legal safeguards

My best friend Sara and I have babies the same age. Sara isn't a nurse, and I know she relies on my judgment a lot. How should I answer her when she asks questions? For instance, yesterday she asked, "If your Richie had a rash like Tommy's, would you take him to the doctor?"

If you answer yes, no harm will result from your advice, and you'll be on safe legal ground. If you answer no, and if following your advice results in harm to the child, you may be liable. In such a situation—best friend or not—conservative advice is legally safer, especially if you have any doubts.

I seem to be the neighborhood ear-piercer. Of course, with children I require a parent's permission, and I warn everyone about the risks of infection and how to reduce them. Still, I'm worried: If someone got an infection and sued me, would this verbal warning protect me from malpractice liability?

Some states have legislation or regulations governing ear piercing, so check with your state licensing board. If your state doesn't have regulations on ear

piercing, your warnings about possible infection protect you only if infection results from piercing done according to accepted standards. The warning doesn't protect you if the infection results from your negligence.

One of my neighbors comes to see me whenever one of her family members gets sick or enters the hospital. She's a good friend and I'm glad to help, but I think she's making a habit of asking my advice. I feel especially uncomfortable when she asks me to explain everything the doctor tells her. Once she said, "The doctor says my husband might have adhesions from a previous operation. What does that mean? Is that common?" How can I answer her questions and protect myself too? Should I say, "I can only tell you what I know from my own experience"?

You'd be better off saying, "I can tell you what those terms usually mean, but not what they mean in your husband's case." You can best serve your neighbor, though, by encouraging her to ask the doctor to explain anything she doesn't understand.

something more serious, and I'm not sure. You should ask a doctor."

Remember, you're always legally protected if you refer the questioner to his doctor. However, the law doesn't require you to make that suggestion if you're honestly convinced that it isn't necessary and that a reasonably prudent nurse wouldn't make it either.

Guard against the temptation to say "Don't worry" when family members or friends ask for advice. Reassure them only if you're certain that nothing is seriously wrong. The law requires you

to apply this standard: If I were at work and one of my patients asked the same question, what would I tell him? Try to imagine that an inquiring family member or friend is a complete stranger. Then give your best professionally considered answer.

Medical advice

Giving health care advice can lead to legal problems if the advice can be interpreted as medical advice. Then you may be at risk for *practicing medicine without a license.*

Donating nursing services

Many health care professionals, including nurses, donate their professional services to community organizations or activities.

Usually, when you volunteer your nursing services, no pay is involved. At times, you may "volunteer" services for pay by providing nursing care outside of your usual paid work. In such situations, you're volunteering your personal time while being paid for your nursing services.

You might donate your nursing services to family members, friends, or such community organizations and activities as the following:
• a community ambulance service
• a bloodmobile or hypertension outreach program
• a home and school association panel discussion on child health issues.

As a licensed nurse, whether RN, LPN, or LVN, your responsibilities to patients don't change when you donate your services. However, your legal status does. It becomes less defined than when you're paid. In most states, nurse practice acts specify only the legal limits of paid nursing practice.

Donated services and the law

Being exempt from your state's nurse practice act if you donate nursing services doesn't mean you'll be exempt from a lawsuit. In such a situation, the court can use the provisions of your state nurse practice act — together with *expert witness* testimony and applicable standards of nursing care — to determine if you acted as a prudent nurse would have acted in similar patient care circumstances. If the court finds that your care didn't conform to the requirements of your state's nurse practice act,

Minimizing legal risks when volunteering

When offering your time and skills for free, observe the same standards of care that you observe in your paid job. Consider these guidelines:

Have necessary orders
Obtain a doctor's order or a standing order before giving any treatment or medication that requires such an order.

Document your actions
Document your donated care as carefully as you document the care you give on the job. Keep a copy of your nurses' notes so you have a permanent record of your actions should a question ever arise.

Check your coverage
Check your professional liability insurance coverage and its limitations from every angle before agreeing to donate your services to any organization. Also check the coverage provided by the organization that receives your volunteer services. Does your or the organization's coverage include the volunteer nursing duty that you're considering? Is the coverage adequate in light of the potential damages and legal fees that you might pay if sued?

you may be facing a malpractice suit. (See *Minimizing legal risks when volunteering*.)

Even if no lawsuit results, you may be subject to discipline by your state nursing board if the board finds that your services fall below the accepted standard of care. In such a situation, the board may suspend or even revoke your license.

Volunteering out of state

If you travel to a state in which you're not licensed to practice, you're not prohibited from donating your nursing services as long as that state's nurse practice act covers only paid nursing care. But if you're sued, the court will probably evaluate your actions and their consequences against whatever standard of nursing care would apply in that situation.

Good Samaritan acts

Good Samaritan laws won't cover you in day-to-day situations in which you donate nursing services. These acts apply only to accidents or other emergency situations. In addition, not all state Good Samaritan acts extend coverage to all nurses.

Acting during a disaster

A tornado levels a part of your community. Spring floods take life and property at the south end of town. A freight train derails, blanketing the community with toxic vapor. The brakes fail on an airplane carrying 137 passengers; the craft careens off the runway. Any of these disastrous events can overload local medical and nursing resources. In situations such as these, nurses have special responsibilities and legal rights.

Contract duties

When you give nursing care during a disaster, professional, ethical, and legal concerns figure heavily in every decision you make. In general, with the exception of *declared emergencies,* a nurse's responsibilities in a disaster don't differ legally from her everyday responsibilities. You may have specific duties to perform in specific kinds of disasters, and you may be legally bound to perform those duties, but that is likely to be based on your employment contract and not on laws or precedent-setting legal cases.

If you work in a city hospital, for example, your employment contract may contain a provision that you can be called to work whenever a government official declares a *state of emergency.* If you refuse to come in, you can be disciplined, suspended, or fired. This rule applies even if the work you're assigned to do isn't normally part of your job description.

If you're already on the job when a disaster occurs, the same contractual provisions may be invoked to keep you from going home at the end of your shift. And the same penalties apply if you refuse to cooperate.

Similarly, if you're an unpaid volunteer for a community service, such as the *Red Cross* or an ambulance unit, you may be expected to report for duty in any local disaster as long as your reporting doesn't conflict with your regular employment. If you refuse, the service can drop you from its roster; if you're a paid, part-time worker for such an organization, you can be dismissed. These duties apply even if your work arrangements are unwritten but are part of an oral agreement.

Contract defenses

Because reporting for work in an emergency, including a disaster, is usually a contract matter, specific *contract defenses* apply if you're disciplined for failing to fulfill your duties. One such contract defense is that of *impossibility.* If reporting is impossible for you, and you can prove it—even if you're contractually required to do so and would be paid for the work—you can't be disciplined or prosecuted. For example, if a blizzard absolutely prohibits travel from your home to the hospital, or disastrous flooding causes the governor to ban all travel in your area, what your contract says doesn't matter much. And if you're disciplined, you have a legal defense. But watch for exceptions to travel bans — for example, a ban may be announced for all but "required personnel" or "persons with medical or nursing training." In those situations, obviously you must report for duty.

Volunteering during a disaster

No law prevents you from voluntarily donating your services, and specific statutory or common laws may provide protection. If you want to volunteer your help in a disaster, do it, whether or not anyone in authority has asked you. (See *Minimizing legal risks during a disaster*.)

Suppose you're working in a hospital that doesn't have a policy mandating that health care personnel report to work when a disaster occurs. You can still volunteer to stay for extra shifts or to perform services outside your normal scope of employment. The hospital will almost certainly accept your offer, if they have not already asked for help. That is especially likely if emergency conditions prevent other staff nurses from reporting to work.

You can't necessarily expect your pay to reflect the extra work performed during a disaster. Most institutions will try to pay for the overtime, but some may not. If you're curious, find out what your institution's policy is before a disaster occurs. The policy may depend on union *rules* or, if you work in a city or state hospital, on city ordinances or state regulations.

Volunteering in another state

Nurse practice acts don't legally restrict you from volunteering during a disaster in an out-of-state location. For

---

Minimizing legal risks during a disaster

By taking a few precautions, you can help assure protection from liability when working under disaster conditions.

Be prepared

Don't wait for a disaster to happen before you ask your charge nurse what you'll be required to do during a disaster. Keep any equipment you're likely to need available and in working condition.

Follow instructions

In any disaster, public officials and other authorities — such as medical personnel, public health workers, or municipal staff — will probably issue orders. Even if these people aren't normally your superiors, follow their directions as much as possible. Offer advice only when you think necessary.

Know your limits

Don't work beyond the point of effectiveness. If you're so tired that you can't make correct decisions, no one will benefit from your care. Describe your fatigue to the person in charge, and ask for a rest break.

---

instance, suppose you're licensed in California and while you're on vacation in Oregon, a disaster occurs. You can give your nursing services during the disaster without concern that you're breaching California's or Oregon's nurse practice act. That's because most nurse practice acts have a special exemption for care given in emergencies that usually includes disasters.

Right to refuse

If you don't want to volunteer, and your hospital policy or contract doesn't require it — or, as happens rarely, if you don't have a contract — in most states you have the right to refuse. Most nurse practice acts don't require you to provide emergency care in disasters, any more than they require you to perform any care. They only permit such care. Similarly, Good Samaritan acts provide some legal immunity for giving emergency care but don't require you to provide that care — except in states with duty to rescue laws.

Civil defense laws, also known as disaster relief laws, do not apply in most states to nurses who aren't already involved in civil defense work — although in a declared national emergency, nurses (like anyone else) can be drafted. Alternatively, martial law may be imposed, which makes all citizens subject to public authority. Many civil defense laws authorize state or federal governing bodies to enforce special regulations dealing with the duties of medical and nursing personnel in a declared emergency. Some states already have such plans ready for use in a sufficiently serious disaster.

Deciding whether to volunteer

When deciding whether to help out in a disaster, assess your actual ability to help. Caring for the disaster victims may require particular skills — for example, knowledge of a special area such as toxicology. Alternatively, the skill required may be as simple as rowing a boat in a flood.

Also consider whether you can get to the disaster site or to the place where care will be provided. If an airliner crashes, for example, and emergency departments throughout the city are treating victims, your ability to get to your hospital or another hospital quickly may figure in whether you decide to volunteer. What if, for example, the disaster involves a riot occurring during a total blackout in your city, and the mayor decrees, "Don't travel to work unless you're within walking distance"? If you try to drive into the city from your suburban home, you'll only complicate driving conditions — and you probably won't get to your hospital in time to be helpful.

You may also consider whether volunteering in the disaster will keep you from working and earning your regular salary. Find out, too, whether your *professional liability insurance* covers off-the-job activities.

Working outside your scope of practice

In a disaster, you may find yourself performing duties outside your usual *scope of practice.* If you're an LPN or LVN, you may be asked to perform duties that ordinarily would be restricted to RNs, and nurses' aides may be asked to do work you usually do. If you're an RN, you may find yourself doing tasks usually reserved for medical residents. And either you or a resident may be asked to do work a nurses' aide would normally do. Provided you have the knowledge and skill to meet minimum safety requirements, you're permitted to give such substitute care in disasters based on the same exemption in nurse practice acts that lets an out-of-state nurse volunteer her services in a disaster. This exemption may be construed as letting you expand the scope of your practice in a disaster. Even if it can't be construed this way, statutory or common laws usually permit regulatory authorities to place the public welfare above strict enforcement of the letter of the law.

Selected references

Curtin, L.L. *Nursing into the 21st Century.* Springhouse, Pa.: Springhouse Corp., 1996.

Fiesta, J. *Twenty Legal Pitfalls for Nurses to Avoid.* Albany, N.Y.: Delmar Pubs., 1994.

Helminski, F. "Ghost from Samaria: Good Samaritan Laws in the Hospital," *Mayo Clinic Proceedings* 68(4):400-01, April 1993.

Page, J. "Go and Do Thou Likewise...Read the Story of the Good Samaritan," *Journal of Emergency Medical Services* 19(12):7-8, December 1994.

Sullivan, G.H. "Good Samaritan Laws Don't Provide Blanket Protection," *RN* 58(3):51, March 1995.

"Trade Center Bombing Puts New York RNs to the Test," *AJN* 93(4):101-02, April 1993.

Ufema J. "Oklahoma City Bombing: Touched by a Distant Catastrophe," *Nursing95* 25(8):30, August 1995.

5

Malpractice liability

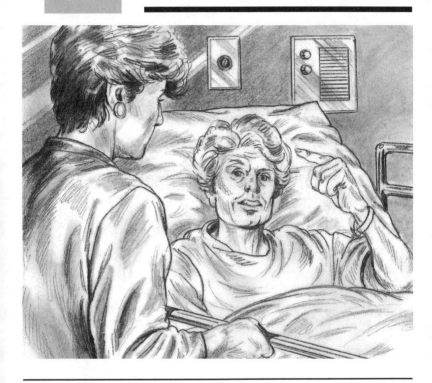

No legal issue sparks as much anxiety among nurses as *malpractice* liability. That's because malpractice litigation can be emotionally harrowing and financially devastating. Unfortunately, more and more nurses are being named in lawsuits, and this trend shows no sign of changing. Several reasons exist for this phenomenon:

• Patients are becoming increasingly knowledgeable about health care, and their expectations are higher.

• The health care system is becoming increasingly reliant on nurses and pro-viders other than doctors to help contain costs.

• Nurses are becoming increasingly autonomous in their practice.

• The courts are expanding the definition of *liability,* holding all types of professionals to higher and higher standards of accountability.

Losing a malpractice lawsuit can jeopardize your career. Prospective employers and insurance companies will want to know if you've ever lost a nursing malpractice lawsuit, or if you've ever been a *defendant* in one. If you have, you may find job hunting more difficult. (See *National Practitioner Data Bank,* pages 200 and 201.) You'll also pay a higher premium for *professional liability insurance,* and some insurance companies may simply refuse to cover you.

What's more, a judgment against you may involve a large amount of money. According to the *American Nurses' Association* (ANA), the average award in a claim against a nurse is $145,000. In contrast, the highest award against a nurse was $5 million. It occurred after a nurse failed to read a medication label and administered 10 times the ordered dose of lidocaine.

Fortunately, you can limit your vulnerability to malpractice litigation. The most important strategy is to give your patients the best possible nursing care, according to the highest professional *standards.* Standards of care consist of the limitations stated in every state's nurse practice act, policies and procedures established by the health care institution where you work, standards adopted by the ANA, and standards of clinical specialty nursing organizations. Every nurse should be familiar with the nurse practice act of her state and other standards applicable to her practice.

You can further protect yourself by becoming familiar with malpractice *law.* This chapter describes malpractice issues, defines key legal terms, and explains legal doctrines that may be used as a defense during a malpractice lawsuit. You'll find extensive information on steps to take to avoid malpractice suits and advice on how to shop for professional liability insurance.

Even if you are meticulous in your practice and carefully avoid unnecessary legal risks, you can't completely escape the risk of being named in a lawsuit. To prepare you for this reality, you'll find guidelines in this chapter for

facing a court appearance with a minimum of anxiety.

Understanding malpractice law

Our legal system's view of malpractice has evolved from the premise, basic to all law, that everyone is responsible, or *liable,* for the consequences of his own actions. Malpractice law deals with a professional's liability for improper or immoral conduct. (See *Understanding tort law,* pages 202 and 203.)

Nursing liability

As late as the 1930s, nurses were expected to follow every doctor's order almost without question. Nursing responsibilities under the law were minimal. In *Byrd v. Marion General Hospital* (1932), the Supreme Court of North Carolina stated: "The great weight of authority...establishes the principle that nurses, in the discharge of their duties, must obey and diligently execute the orders of the doctor or surgeon in charge of the patient unless, of course, such order was so obviously negligent as to lead any reasonable person to anticipate that substantial injury would result to the patient from the execution of such order or performance of such direction. Certainly, if a doctor or surgeon should order a nurse to stick fire to a patient, no nurse would be protected from liability."

After World War II, however, the educational and licensing requirements for nurses increased. Tasks became more complex and the nursing profession more specialized. These changes meant that nurses had to make independent judgments. Although this increased responsibility provides a more

National Practitioner Data Bank

In 1990, the National Practitioner Data Bank began operation. As a result, doctors, dentists, nurses, and other health care practitioners who are forced to pay malpractice judgments are going to have a much harder time concealing their professional histories from potential employers. The data bank, which will store malpractice data on an unprecedented nationwide scale, was created under the Health Care Quality Improvement Act of 1986 and the Medicare and Medicaid Patient and Program Protection Act of 1987.

Reporting requirements

The National Practitioner Data Bank collects information about practitioners who may endanger the public welfare and puts this information at an employer's fingertips. All hospitals and health care institutions, professional health care societies, state licensure boards, and insurance companies are now required to report the following information about nurses to the data bank:

• malpractice payments made by a nurse (including judgments, arbitration decisions, and out-of-court settlements)
• actions taken against a nurse's clinical privileges
• adverse licensure actions, including revocations, suspensions, reprimands, censure, or probation.

Failure to report a nurses' malpractice payment of any amount—no matter how small—carries a $10,000 fine. However, the fact that a suit has been filed is not, by itself, reportable; only the making of a payment is. Adverse clinical privilege actions against nurses may be reported at the discretion of the reviewing health care agency.

Federal agencies

Under the law, federal agencies aren't required to report to the National Practitioner Data Bank. However, the Department of Defense, the Drug Enforcement Administration, and the Department of Health and Human Services have voluntarily agreed to observe the regulations.

Availability of information

The information in the data bank isn't available to the general public. State licensing boards, hospitals, professional societies, plaintiff's attorneys, and health care institutions involved in peer review may access the data bank. Individual nurses have access to records that pertain to themselves.

All hospitals must check the data bank when a nurse applies for clinical privileges. The hospital must request information on the nurse again every 2 years. The courts will presume that the hospital is aware of any information the data bank contains on any nurse or other practitioner in its employ. If the information contained in the data bank, if known, would have resulted in a denial of clinical privileges, the hospital could be held liable for negligence in a malpractice lawsuit.

Information in the data bank

Reports made to the data bank will include the following information:

• the nurse's full name, home address, date of birth, professional schools attended and graduation dates, place of employment, Social Security number, and license number and state
• name, title, and phone number of the official submitting the report

National Practitioner Data Bank continued

- relationship of reporting person to practitioner
- dates of judgment or settlement and amount paid
- description of judgment, settlement, or action.

Disputing a report

If a report about you is submitted to the data bank, you'll receive a copy for your review. If you believe that the report is in error, ask the official submitting the report to correct it. Any corrections must be submitted to the data bank by the official making the report.

If you fail to get satisfaction from the reporting official, you'll have to follow a detailed procedure for disputing the report. This must be done within 60 days of the initial processing of the report. Ultimately, you may request review from the Secretary of Health and Human Services.

---

rewarding working environment, it also makes nurses more liable for errors and increases their likelihood of being sued.

Causes of lawsuits against nurses

Patient falls and medication errors are the two most common causes of lawsuits against nurses. Other problems that can prompt lawsuits include:
- operating room errors, such as sponges or instruments being left inside the patient (unperformed or inaccurate needle and sponge counts)
- mix-ups during patient transfers, either between departments or units within a hospital or from one hospital to another
- communication breakdowns between nurses and doctors or between one nursing shift and the next
- inadequate observation of patients leading to misdiagnoses or injuries.

In addition, nurses who work in special practice areas may be especially vulnerable to lawsuits. (See *Liability in special practice settings*, pages 204 to 206.)

Negligence vs. malpractice

The court's view of nursing liability has changed significantly. At one time, nurses were only charged with *negligence.* But now courts in several states,

including Wyoming, Louisiana, and Rhode Island, have recognized nursing negligence as a form of malpractice.

Negligence is the failure to exercise the degree of care that a person of ordinary prudence would exercise under the same circumstances. A claim of negligence requires that there be a *duty* owed by one person to another, that the duty be breached, and that injury results. Malpractice is a more restricted, specialized kind of negligence, defined as a violation of professional duty to act with reasonable care and in good faith.

The distinction shows that the courts are beginning to recognize nursing as a legitimate profession. This emerging professional status may affect the *statute of limitations* applicable in a particular case. These statutes define the time period in which a suit may be filed. Many states have statutes of limitations for medical malpractice claims that are shorter than those for ordinary negligence actions.

Criminal negligence

Whereas negligence is generally a civil matter — concerned with the rights and duties of persons in contracts and *torts* — trying to conceal it can be a criminal offense. In *State of New Jersey v. Laura Winter* (1984), a nurse was

Understanding tort law

Most lawsuits against nurses fall into the tort category. If you're ever a defendant in a lawsuit, understanding the distinctions in this broad category may prove especially important.

A tort is a civil wrong or injury resulting from a breach of a legal duty that exists by virtue of society's expectations regarding interpersonal conduct (as opposed to a legal duty that exists by virtue of a contractual relationship). More generally, you may define a tort as "any action or omission that harms somebody." Malpractice refers to a tort committed by a professional acting in his professional capacity.

Unintentional vs. intentional torts

The law broadly divides torts into two categories—unintentional and intentional. An *unintentional tort* is a civil wrong from the defendant's negligence. If someone sues you for negligence, he must prove four things in order to win:
• that you owed him a specific duty (in nursing malpractice cases, this duty is equivalent to the standard of care)
• that you breached this duty
• that the plaintiff was harmed physically, mentally, emotionally, or financially
• that your breach of duty caused the harm.

An *intentional tort* is a direct invasion of someone's legal right. In a malpractice case involving an intentional tort, the plaintiff doesn't need to prove that you owed him a duty. The duty at issue (for example, not to touch people without their permission) is defined by law, and you're presumed to owe him this duty. The plaintiff must still prove that you breached this duty and that this breach caused him harm. These lawsuits are usually based on a theory of lack of informed consent.

When lawyers use the word "intentional" in a noncriminal case they don't mean that the defendant meant to do harm. Intentional here indicates that the defendant "meant to perform the complained-of action," whether or not she meant that action to hurt the patient.

TORT CLAIM	ACTIONS THAT LEAD TO CLAIM
Unintentional tort	
Negligence	• Leaving foreign objects inside a patient after surgery • Failing to observe a patient in the intensive care unit as the doctor ordered • Failing to obtain informed consent before a treatment or procedure • Failing to report a change in a patient's vital signs or status • Failing to report a staff member's negligence that you witnessed • Failing to provide for a patient's safety • Failing to provide the patient with appropriate teaching before discharge

Understanding tort law continued

TORT CLAIM	ACTIONS THAT LEAD TO CLAIM
Intentional torts	
Assault	• Threatening a patient
Battery	• Assisting in nonemergency surgery without the consent of the patient • Forcing a patient to ambulate against his wishes • Forcing a patient to submit to injections • Striking a patient
False imprison-ment	• Confining a patient in a psychiatric unit without a doctor's order • Refusing to let a patient return home
Invasion of privacy	• Releasing private information about a patient to third parties • Allowing unauthorized persons to read a patient's medical records • Allowing unauthorized persons to observe a procedure • Taking pictures of the patient without his consent
Slander	• Making false statements about a patient to a third person, which causes damage to another's reputation

charged with administering blood of an incompatible type to a patient undergoing surgery. The state alleged that when she discovered her error, she attempted to cover up her negligence. In the prosecution that resulted, the jury found her actions "reckless and wanton negligence...showing an utter disregard for the safety of others under circumstances likely to cause death." The jury found that the nurse's negligence constituted manslaughter, and the trial court sentenced her to 5 years in prison.

Malpractice defenses

Over the years, the law has developed special doctrines, or theories, to apply to cases involving subordinate-superior relationships. These doctrines may be used in a nurse's defense during a lawsuit. Exactly how much protection they offer, however, depends on the circumstances of the case and the development of the law in the nurse's state or province.

Respondeat superior

One of the most important malpractice defenses is the doctrine of **respondeat superior** (Latin for "let the master answer"), also called the theory of vicarious liability.

This doctrine holds that when an employee is found negligent, the employer must accept responsibility if the employee was acting within the scope of his employment. The doctrine applies to all occupations, not just health care — a utility company, for instance, is liable for injuries that result if one of its on-duty truck drivers negligently hits a pedestrian.

To the extent that a nurse is working as the hospital's functionary, she can claim some protection under this theory. This doctrine is attractive to

(Text continues on page 206.)

Liability in special practice settings

Although errors can be made in virtually any practice setting, nurses who work in certain practice settings are more vulnerable to malpractice charges because their errors usually prove more costly for patients. In addition, the courts may expect a higher standard of practice from a nurse who practices in a specialty area.

Critical care nursing

Compared to nurses in other units, critical care nurses spend proportionately more of their time in direct contact with their patients, thus increasing the opportunity for error and the number of potential lawsuits. Because of the many invasive and potentially harmful procedures performed in this setting, critical care nurses are especially vulnerable to charges of negligence or battery. If they perform expanded-role duties and procedures, nurses working in this area may be accused of practicing medicine without a license.

Additional tort claims that may be leveled against critical care nurses include:
● abandonment – the unilateral severance of a professional relationship with a patient without adequate notice and while the patient still needs attention. A critical care nurse who fails in her duty to observe the patient closely for any subtle changes in condition is vulnerable to this charge.
● invasion of privacy, intentional infliction of emotional distress, or battery – such cases usually involve a patient who was placed on or removed from a life-support system
● failure to obtain informed consent – this is more likely to occur in a critical care setting because of the inherent pressure and urgency for immediate treatment.

Critical care nurses who deny a competent patient the right to refuse treatment – even if lack of treatment results in the patient's death – expose themselves to charges of various intentional torts.

Emergency department nursing

Many of the day-to-day practices of emergency department nurses fall into a legal gray area because the law's definition of a *true emergency* is open to interpretation; for instance, health care workers who treat a patient for what they regard as a true emergency may be liable for battery or failure to obtain informed consent if the court ultimately concludes that the situation was not a true emergency.

One of the most common charges filed against emergency department nurses is failure to assess and report a patient's condition. Inadequate triage may be considered negligence.

All too often, the use of high-tech equipment combined with a hectic daily pace increases the potential for lawsuits.

Other tort claims made against emergency department nurses may involve:
● failure to instruct a patient adequately before discharge
● discounting complaints of pain from a patient who is mentally impaired by alcohol, medication, or injury
● failure to obtain informed consent, which gives rise to claims of battery, false imprisonment, and invasion of privacy.

Psychiatric nursing

Malpractice cases dealing with psychiatric care usually involve failure to obtain informed consent. A nurse may wrongly assume she does not need informed con-

Liability in special practice settings continued

sent, especially if the patient's condition interferes with his awareness or understanding of the proposed treatment or procedure. Violation of a patient's right to refuse treatment may stem from the mistaken belief that all mentally ill patients are incompetent. (The right to refuse treatment is not absolute, however, and can be abrogated if medications or treatments are required to prevent serious harm to the patient or others.)

A nurse who reveals personal information about a patient to someone not directly involved in the patient's care is vulnerable to malpractice charges. Violation of a patient's right to privacy and confidentiality is a common complaint in lawsuits against psychiatric health care workers, probably because of the stigma still associated with seeking care for mental illness.

Malpractice allegations may also stem from failing to protect a patient from inflicting foreseeable harm to himself or others. If a nurse fails to report information given by the patient, even in confidence, that could have prevented the harm, she may be held liable for violating her duty to assess and report his condition.

Obstetric nursing

Cases involving obstetric errors have at least two plaintiffs: the mother and the infant. (Because the courts recognize a legal duty owed to the unborn, an obstetric nurse may also be charged with violating the rights of a fetus.) Monetary damages tend to be large because of the permanent or long-term injuries that can occur to newborns.

An obstetric nurse may be held liable for:
• negligence through participation in transfusion of incompatible blood, especially in relation to Rh factor incompatibility
• failure to attend to or monitor the mother or the fetus during labor and delivery
• failure to recognize labor symptoms and to provide adequate support and care
• failure to monitor contractions and fetal heart rate, particularly in obstetric units that have internal monitoring capabilities
• failure to recognize high-risk labor patients who show signs of preeclampsia or other labor complications
• failure to warn parents of the risks of diagnostic tests – or the consequences of refusing such tests – if the failure contributes to maternal or fetal injury
• abandonment of a patient in active labor
• failure to exercise independent judgment, such as knowingly carrying out medical orders that will harm the patient
• failure to ensure that a patient has given informed consent for various procedures or treatments, including physical examinations, administration of a potent medication, type of delivery method, sterilization, and postdelivery surgical procedures.

Other common sources of malpractice suits filed against obstetric nurses include failure to attend to the infant in distress, failure to monitor equipment, use of defective equipment, failure to monitor oxygen levels, and failure to recognize and report newborn jaundice during the immediate postnatal period.

Parents can file a *wrongful birth* lawsuit if a nurse failed to advise them of contraceptive methods or the methods' potential for failure, possible genetic defects, the availability of amniocentesis to detect

(continued)

Liability in special practice settings continued

defects, or the option of abortion to prevent birth of a defective child. A child with a genetic defect can file a *wrongful life* lawsuit if a nurse failed to inform the parents about amniocentesis and the option of abortion.

Failure to provide adequate genetic counseling and prenatal testing when the mother has a history of Down's syndrome can also result in a wrongful birth or wrongful life lawsuit.

---

plaintiffs as well as employees, because hospitals usually have much more money available to pay claims than nurses do (a reality that's facetiously known as the "deep pocket" doctrine).

Consider, for example, *Nelson v. Trinity Medical Center* (1988). In this case, a nurse delayed placing a woman in labor on a continuous fetal heart rate monitor, despite **standing orders** to do so. The child was born severely brain-damaged, a condition that might have been prevented if the monitor had been operating to alert the doctor, and if a cesarean section had been performed. But it was the hospital, not the nurse, who was found liable for the actions of its employee. (The doctor settled out of court before the trial.) The parents were awarded $5.5 million.

In another case, *Crowe v. Provost* (1963), a mother returned with her child to her pediatrician's office one afternoon after having been there earlier that morning. She said her child was convulsing. The doctor was at lunch, so the office nurse briefly examined the child. She then called the doctor, told him that she didn't feel the child's condition had changed since he had examined her, and advised that he needn't rush back. After the nurse left the office, the child vomited violently, stopped breathing, and died before the receptionist could contact the doctor.

The mother filed negligence charges against the nurse. At the trial, the court found the nurse's negligence was indeed the **proximate cause** of the child's death. However, the doctor was also liable, according to the doctrine of *respondeat superior*, because the nurse was working as the doctor's employee.

Borrowed servant

A concept closely related to *respondeat superior* is the **borrowed servant** or **captain of the ship** doctrine. It is still applied in malpractice lawsuits, but not as often as in the past. The borrowed servant doctrine might apply when you, as a hospital employee, commit a negligent act while under the direction or control of someone other than your supervisor, such as a doctor in the operating room. Because the doctor is an **independent contractor** and you're responsible to him during surgery, you're considered his borrowed servant at the time. If you're sued for malpractice, his liability is vicarious, meaning that even though the doctor didn't direct you negligently, he's responsible because he was in control.

Many states haved moved away from strict application of the borrowed servant theory. One reason for this shift is that operating room procedures are becoming so complex that they're beyond the direct control of any one person, thus making it too difficult for courts to determine responsibility under the borrowed servant doctrine.

Res ipsa loquitur

The Latin phrase *res ipsa loquitur* literally means, "The thing speaks for itself." *Res ipsa loquitur* is a rule of evidence designed to equalize the plaintiff's and the defendant's positions in court, when otherwise the plaintiff could be at a disadvantage in proving his case — a disadvantage not of his own making. (*Res ipsa loquitur* doesn't apply when a plaintiff simply fails to prove his case.) Essentially, the rule of *res ipsa loquitur* allows a plaintiff to prove negligence with **circumstantial evidence,** when the defendant has the primary, and sometimes the only, knowledge of what happened to cause the plaintiff's injury.

Res ipsa loquitur derives from a 19th-century English case, *Byrne v. Boadle* (1863). In this case, the injured person had been struck by a flour barrel that fell from a second-floor window of a warehouse. In the ensuing lawsuit, the plaintiff wasn't able to show which warehouse employee had been negligent in allowing the barrel to fall. The court applied the concept of *res ipsa loquitur* to the warehouse owners, who were found liable in the absence of proof that the employees weren't responsible for the plaintiff's injury.

Applying *res ipsa loquitur*

In most medical malpractice cases, the plaintiff has the responsibility for proving every element of his case against the defendant; until he does, the court presumes that the defendant met the applicable **standard of care.** However, when a court applies the *res ipsa loquitur* rule, the burden of proof shifts from the plaintiff to the defendant. The defendant must prove that the injury was caused by something other than his negligence.

For the *res ipsa loquitur* rule to apply, three circumstances must be met:

- The act that caused the plaintiff's injury was exclusively in the nurse's control.
- The injury wouldn't have happened in the absence of the defendant's negligence.
- No negligence on the plaintiff's part contributed to his injury.

Court case

For example, this rule was invoked in *Sanchez v. Bay General Hospital* (1981). In this case, Mrs. Sanchez entered Bay General Hospital for a laminectomy. After the surgery, the surgeon implanted an arterial catheter to minimize the chance that an air embolism would form in her heart.

When Mrs. Sanchez was transferred to the postoperative ward, her condition began to deteriorate. She was still unconscious and unable to contribute to her injury in any manner. The nurses in the postoperative ward who were responsible for her care made several initial errors:

- They didn't examine the patient's chart, so they weren't aware that the catheter had been put in place.
- They neglected to check the patient's neurologic status.
- They didn't report her deteriorating vital signs to a doctor.

Mrs. Sanchez went into cardiac arrest, and an emergency department doctor ordered immediate administration of medication. The nurses administered the medication through the arterial catheter, mistaking it for an I.V. line. The medication went directly to Mrs. Sanchez's heart, causing **brain death** a few hours later. The children of Mrs. Sanchez later sued the hospital for the wrongful death of their mother.

The court, invoking the *res ipsa loquitur* rule, granted a **directed verdict** to the children of Mrs. Sanchez. The court indicated that the hospital had the burden of proving that Mrs. Sanchez's death was caused by something other than the *staff's* negligence — or, alternatively, that she died even though the staff had given due care to prevent her death. The hospital was unable to refute the court's presumption of negligence. The hospital appealed the directed verdict, but the *appellate court* sustained the trial court's judgment in favor of Mrs. Sanchez's children.

Courts also apply the *res ipsa loquitur* rule in cases in which the defendant is the only one in a position to know what caused the injury. Courts won't apply the rule if the evidence offered by the defendant satisfactorily explains the facts that appeared to constitute blatant negligence.

Incidents associated with *res ipsa loquitur*

Perhaps the most common incident associated with the *res ipsa loquitur* rule is the foreign-object case, in which a sponge, a needle, pin, or other object is left inside the patient after surgery. Courts have also been willing to invoke the rule because of injuries to plaintiffs involving body parts completely unrelated to the plaintiffs' surgery.

Consider the Wisconsin malpractice case, *Beaudoin v. Watertown Memorial Hospital* (1966). A patient suffered second-degree burns on the buttocks during vaginal surgery. She brought suit, claiming negligence. The court applied the *res ipsa loquitur* rule on the basis that injury to an area unrelated to surgery automatically results from failure to exercise due care.

For and against *res ipsa loquitur*

Critics of this rule call it "the rule of sympathy" and believe the courts have been too lenient in allowing plaintiffs to use it. *Health care professionals* usually contend that the rule puts them at an unfair disadvantage during a malpractice defense. They feel that, by assigning them the burden of proof, the court singles them out for more negligence liability than other types of defendants. Also, invoking the rule usually eliminates the plaintiff's responsibility to introduce expert testimony.

Supporters of the rule feel that it draws attention to the fact that a plaintiff's unusual or rare injury is, in itself, sufficient to cause suspicion that the defendant was negligent.

State interpretations

In some states, courts cannot apply the *res ipsa loquitur* rule. Most states, however, do allow courts to apply some form of it. For example, neither Michigan nor South Carolina uses the rule by name, but both permit circumstantial evidence of negligence, which is, in effect, the same concept. (See also *Challenging a malpractice suit.*)

Canadian cases

In *Holt v. Nesbitt* (1953) and again in *Cardin v. City of Montreal* (1961), the Supreme Court of Canada clearly stated that the rule of *res ipsa loquitur* applied in malpractice cases. In *Holt v. Nesbitt*, the plaintiff was a patient of the defendant, an oral surgeon. While the plaintiff was under general anesthesia, a sponge lodged in his windpipe, causing death by suffocation. The court decided that failure to apply the *res ipsa loquitur* rule would give the health care practitioner unfair — and therefore unwarranted — protection in a malpractice lawsuit. In effect, the court put the patient's protection from bad medical practice above the health care practitioner's protection from a difficult malpractice lawsuit.

The Canadian courts progress slowly in mediating malpractice lawsuits. That's because differences in expert opinion are the rule, not the exception, and because many lawsuits present issues not previously resolved. The Canadian courts do, however, seem to want to ensure that the rule doesn't

Challenging a malpractice suit

If your attorney can establish one of the following malpractice defenses, the court will either dismiss the allegations against you or reduce the damages for which you're liable.

DEFENSE	RATIONALE
False allegations	Does the plaintiff have legally sufficient proof that your actions caused his injuries? If he doesn't, the court may rule that the allegations against you are false and dismiss the case.
Contributory negligence	Did the plaintiff, through carelessness, contribute to his injury? If he did, some states permit the court to charge the plaintiff with failing to meet the standards of a reasonably prudent patient. Such a ruling may prevent the plaintiff from recovering any damages. A few states permit the court to apportion liability, which prevents the plaintiff from recovering some, but not all, of the damages he claims.
Comparative negligence	Has more than one defendant been named in the lawsuit? In some states, the court may apportion liability according to the negligence of the defendants involved, with the total damages divided up among them in proportion to the fault of each.
Assumption of risk	Did the plaintiff understand the risk involved in the treatment, procedure, or action that allegedly caused his injury? Did he give proper informed consent and so voluntarily expose himself to that risk? If so, the court may rule that the plaintiff assumed the risk, knowingly disregarded the danger, and so relieved you of liability.

place too heavy a burden on the defendant.

Understanding the statute of limitations

A statute of limitations specifies a particular number of years within which one person can sue another. For malpractice lawsuits, the statute of limitations is specified in each state's medical malpractice law. These limits vary widely from state to state, and it's important to know the limits in your state. Contact the attorney, lobbyist, or legislative committee members of your state nurses' association for information about the statutes of limitations in your state. (For a list of state nurses' associations, see pages 5 to 9.) Stat-

utes of limitations also vary widely from province to province in Canada, and even within a province.

Purpose of statutes of limitations

Statutes of limitations are useful because as time passes, evidence vanishes, witnesses' memories fail, and witnesses die. A time limit for bringing a lawsuit ensures that enough relevant evidence exists for a judge or jury to decide a case fairly.

Statutes of limitations for general negligence usually give a person 3 years to sue another for damages. Plaintiffs may invoke these limits in general personal-injury lawsuits. But in response to pressure from medical and insurance groups, states established shorter statutes of limitations for professions that require independent judgments and frequent risks. The statutes of limitations of medical malpractice laws, for example, usually give the patient 2 years or less to sue for damages.

Determining which statute applies

In many states, only doctors and dentists are expressly subject to medical malpractice statutes of limitations. These states view the nurse as someone carrying out orders and not making independent, risk-taking judgments.

If a nurse alleges a patient's claim is invalid because he didn't file suit until after the statute of limitations had expired, the court must determine which applies: the statute of limitations for state medical malpractice law or the statute of limitations for general personal-injury lawsuits. (The malpractice law's statute of limitations is usually shorter.) The court bases its decision on the two following considerations:

• *how much statute of limitations protection the court believes the defendant-nurse's job warrants.* If her job forces her to make many independent patient care judgments, the court may apply a strict, or short, statute of limitations. A short time limit offers more protection for the nurse, because the patient has less time to seek damages.

• *the type of negligent act the plaintiff-patient claims the nurse committed.* An injured patient may sue a nurse for any one or for several of the charges that constitute negligence or malpractice. The patient's attorney determines which charge has the best chance of winning the most damages for his client, and structures his case accordingly. Then, if a statute of limitations is used as part of the nurse's defense, the court will decide which statute of limitations to apply in relation to the patient's charges.

Court case

In a Michigan case, *Kambas v. St. Joseph's Mercy Hospital of Detroit* (1973), a myocardial infarction patient lost full use of his arms after receiving anticoagulant drug injections. Because the patient brought the suit over 2 years after the incident, the defendant-nurse's attorneys tried to invoke Michigan's 2-year medical malpractice statute of limitations. The plaintiff-patient's attorney argued that the state's 3-year general negligence statute should apply. The state supreme court ruled for the patient, concluding that because nurses don't exercise independent judgment, as doctors do, they aren't entitled to the protection of the medical malpractice statute of limitations.

Applying the statute of limitations

Suppose a patient files suit long after the statute of limitations has expired. Don't think your worries are over. Remember, the patient's attorney knows about the statute of limitations, and he's filing suit anyway. That means he believes the court may set aside the statute of limitations.

Normally, the statute begins to run on the date the plaintiff's injury occurred. But what if the plaintiff doesn't know he was injured or doesn't find out he has grounds for a suit until after the normal limitations period expires? Determining when the applicable statute actually begins to run has become the pivotal question whenever a defense attorney invokes the statute of limitations.

Legislatures and the courts — which are continually struggling with this question — have devised a series of rules to help decide, in individual malpractice cases, when a statute should properly begin to run. A court can apply these rules, when a plaintiff-patient's attorney requests that it do so, to extend the applicable statute of limitations beyond the limit written in the law. That means that the defendant-nurse's use of a statute of limitations as a defense is invalidated, and the plaintiff-patient's right to sue is affirmed.

Occurrence rule

This rule allows the statute of limitations to begin to run on the day a patient's injury occurs. The occurrence rule generally leads to the shortest time limit. In several states, the courts have interpreted the occurrence rule strictly, so that even badly injured patients have been prevented from bringing suit after the applicable statute of limitations had expired.

Termination-of-treatment rule

The courts may apply this rule when a patient's injury results from a series of treatments extended over time, rather than from a single treatment. The termination-of-treatment rule says that a statute of limitations begins on the date of the last treatment. In devising this rule, the courts reasoned that for the patient, a series of treatments could obscure just how and when the injury occurred.

The Supreme Court of Virginia applied this rule in *Justice v. Natvig* (1989). In this case, a patient filed a lawsuit 8 years after an allegedly negligent operation. The patient had continued to receive treatment during this interval. The defendant doctors argued that the statute of limitations had elapsed. The court ruled, however, that the statute didn't begin to run until the treatment had ended, so the patient's lawsuit was valid.

Constructive continuing treatment rule

This rule is essentially the same as the termination-of-treatment rule, but it applies even after the patient leaves a nurse's or a doctor's care. For example, suppose a patient you cared for is injured later, in someone else's care, and sues. Under the constructive continuing treatment rule, if the subsequent health care providers relied on decisions you made earlier in caring for the patient, the court may extend the statute of limitations in malpractice cases.

Discovery rule

Under this rule, the statute of limitations properly begins to run when a patient discovers the injury. This may take place many years after the injury occurred and after the applicable statute of limitations has formally run out. The discovery rule considerably extends the time a patient has to file a malpractice lawsuit.

Two types of cases in which the discovery rule is usually applied are foreign object and sterilization cases. When a nurse or a surgeon leaves a scalpel, sponge, or clamp inside a patient, the patient might not discover the error until long after his surgery. Under the discovery rule, the applicable statute of limitations wouldn't begin to run until the patient found out about the error.

A court's decision to apply the discovery rule depends on whether it believes that the patient could have discovered the error earlier. If evidence indicates the patient should have recognized that something was wrong (for example, if he had chronic pain for months after the surgery but didn't take legal action until long afterward), the court could apply the termination-of-treatment rule instead.

Time limits for applying the discovery rule in foreign-object cases vary from state to state. Missouri allows the longest period, up to 10 years after discovery of injury. California has the shortest period, 1 year from discovery of injury.

COURT CASE

Extending the statute of limitations

If a plaintiff-patient can prove that a nurse or doctor willfully deceived him, the court may lengthen the statute of limitations for filing a lawsuit.

Painful overtreatment

Consider the case of *Lopez v. Swyer* (1971). Mary Lopez, age 32, underwent a radical mastectomy after discovering a lump in her breast. Several doctors prescribed postsurgical radiation treatments, which were performed by a radiologist.

These treatments occurred six times a week for more than a month, and left painful radiation burns over most of her body. When Mrs. Lopez asked why the complications were so severe, her doctors assured her that the burns weren't unusual. They never suggested that the treatments could have been too numerous or too strong.

Mrs. Lopez's condition worsened. Over the next several years, she was hospitalized 15 times, including twice for reconstructive surgery made necessary by the radiation treatment. But she didn't file a malpractice lawsuit until she heard a consulting doctor tell other doctors, gathered near her hospital bed, that she was a victim of negligence.

Extra time for the plaintiff

A lower court dismissed the suit because the 2-year statute of limitations for malpractice had expired. But an appeals court ruled that the statute of limitations didn't begin until Mrs. Lopez learned that her doctors had concealed the truth from her. This effectively lengthened the statute of limitations by nearly 10 years. The appeals court ruling allowed Mrs. Lopez to bring the facts of her case before a jury.

In lawsuits involving tubal ligations or vasectomies, the courts have sometimes allowed the discovery rule to apply when a subsequent pregnancy occurs. In these cases, the courts' reasoning is that a patient can't discover the negligence until the procedure proves unsuccessful, no matter how long after the surgery this proof occurs.

Because the discovery rule is so generous to plaintiffs, some states, notably Texas, have restricted its application. A number of states have adopted separate statutes of limitations, one for readily detected injuries and one for injuries discovered later. Other states permit statute of limitations extensions only in foreign-object cases.

Proof of fraud

Courts, in most states, will extend the limitation period indefinitely if a plaintiff-patient can prove that a nurse or doctor used *fraud* or falsehood to conceal from the patient information about his injury or its cause. In most cases, the law says that the concealment must be an overt act, not just the omission of an act. The most flagrant frauds involve concealing facts to prevent an inquiry, elude an investigation, or mislead a patient. (See *Extending the statute of limitations*.)

Consider, for example, *Garcia v. Presbyterian Hospital Center* (1979). In this case, a patient who sued was operated on for cancer of the prostate gland twice in 1972 and once again in 1973. He'd repeatedly asked his doctor and attending nurses why the third operation was needed, but he hadn't received any explanation. Some time later, he learned that the third operation had resulted from retention of a catheter in his body during the second operation. The court held that the applicable statute of limitations did not prevent the patient from bringing suit.

Minor or mentally incompetent patients

In most states, laws give special consideration to *minors* and *mentally incompetent* patients because they lack the legal capacity to sue. Some states postpone applying the statute of limitations to an injured minor until he reaches the *age of majority* — age 18 or 21, depending on the state. And some states have specific rules about how statutes of limitations apply to minors.

Cases involving mentally incompetent patients who file after statutes of limitations have expired usually follow the *discovery rule* or a special law. Most of these special laws say that a statute of limitations doesn't begin until the patient recovers from his mental incompetence.

Using the statute-of-limitations defense

When a defendant-nurse and her attorney use a statute of limitations as a defense, they're making, in legal jargon, an *affirmative defense*. The defendant must prove that the statute of limitations has run out. If the court decides the statutory time limit has expired, the plaintiff-patient's case is rendered invalid.

Retaining medical records

Because a patient may file a malpractice suit years after he claims his injury occurred, accurate *medical records* should be kept on file for years. The complexity of malpractice cases re-

quires you to recall specific clinical facts and procedures. Complete *documentation* of your care is usually found only in the records. These records provide your best defense. Without them, you're legally vulnerable.

Few states have laws setting precise time periods, but many legal experts urge hospitals and other health care facilities to maintain medical record files long after patients are discharged. New Jersey, for example, requires hospitals to keep medical records for 7 years.

Some states have adopted the Uniform Business Records Act, which calls for keeping records for no less than 3 years. Some states allow microfilm copies of medical records to be admitted as evidence in malpractice cases, but other states insist that only the original records can be used in court.

Avoiding malpractice liability

You can take steps to avoid tort liability by using caution and common sense and maintaining heightened awareness of your legal responsibilities. Follow the guidelines described below. (See *Everyday situations that can trigger lawsuits*, pages 214 and 215.)

Know your own strengths and weaknesses

Don't accept responsibilities for which you're not prepared. For example, if you haven't worked in pediatrics for 10 years, accepting an assignment to a pediatric unit without orientation only increases your chances of making an error. If you do make an error, claiming you weren't familiar with the unit's procedures won't protect you against liability.

As a professional, you shouldn't accept a position if you can't perform as

Everyday situations that can trigger lawsuits

Everyday nursing situations present many legal hazards. The following examples of nursing liability, based on actual court decisions, show how deviating from accepted standards can harm a patient and result in lawsuits. By being aware of how certain common situations can cause you legal entanglements, you can avoid making similar mistakes.

Failing to perform a proper assessment

When a man traveling between cities began having chest pain and numbness in his left shoulder and arm, he and his companion stopped at a small hospital for help. The nurse on duty in the emergency department (ED) advised him to continue on to a bigger hospital 24 miles away. She failed to perform a physical assessment or obtain a formal history. On his way to the other hospital, the man had a massive myocardial infarction and died.

Clearly, the nurse failed to assess her patient accurately. Her mistake may have cost the patient his life and resulted in a landmark decision that established a nurse's independent relationship with her patient.

The court held the nurse responsible and accountable for her omissions, stating that she had failed to meet her duty to protect the patient from harm.

Failing to take appropriate precautions

An elderly senile patient with a history of falling down was left in bed with the side rails down. She fell out of bed and hurt herself.

Another patient, an alert 28-year-old, was instructed by a nurse to call for help

before getting out of bed. After the nurse left the room, the patient got herself out of bed and fell.

In the first case, the nurse was found liable for failing to raise the side rails. When a patient is at clear risk for injury, the nurse must take extra measures to protect her.

In the second case, the nurse was not held liable for the patient's injuries. Her patient, a competent adult, had received appropriate instructions and chose to ignore them. In such circumstances, a court will hold the patient responsible for her own actions.

Neglecting to document and communicate information

A mother took her two sons to an ED with head and chest rashes and high fevers. The mother gave the nurse an accurate history, which included the recent removal of two ticks from one of the boys.

The nurse didn't tell the doctor about the ticks or record the information in the chart. The doctor diagnosed measles in both boys and sent them home.

Two days later, one of the boys died of Rocky Mountain spotted fever, which is transmitted by ticks.

Neither the hospital nor the doctor was held responsible for the boy's death. But the nurse's omission was found to be a contributing cause of death.

Performing nursing procedures incorrectly

A nurse administered an intramuscular injection in the wrong quadrant of a patient's buttocks. He later developed footdrop from sciatic nerve damage.

In this case, both the nurse and the hospital were found negligent. The law

Everyday situations that can trigger lawsuits continued

expects a nurse to administer drugs and treatments without injuring patients by following set standards of care. (Drug-related errors are one of the most common sources of negligence claims against nurses.)

The hospital's liability was established under the legal doctrine *respondeat superior,* which holds an employer responsible for an employee's errors.

Failing to report another's mistakes

While delivering a patient's baby, an obstetrician made an incision in the patient's cervix to relieve a constrictive band of muscle. After delivery, he failed to suture the incision.

The patient was sent to the postpartum unit for care and observation. The patient's nurse, noticing that the patient was bleeding heavily, called the obstetrician three times. He assured the nurse that the bleeding was normal. Within 2 hours, the patient went into shock and died.

Even though the nurse contacted the patient's doctor, the court held the nurse negligent for failing to intervene further. The courts expect nurses to exercise professional, *independent* judgment and to object when a doctor's orders are inappropriate. In this case, the nurse should have reported the facts to her manager or the unit's medical director, insisting that the patient receive proper care.

Being involved in a surgical team's error

During a cholecystectomy, the surgical team accidentally left a sponge in the patient's body. When the sponge was discovered later, the patient needed another operation to remove it.

When the court awarded damages, both the surgeon and the nurse paid. At one time, the surgeon would have been fully responsible under the "captain of the ship" doctrine. Today, all members of the surgical team are responsible for their actions.

---

a *reasonably prudent nurse* would in that setting. Courts may, however, be more lenient when dealing with nurses who work in emergency settings, such as a fire or flood. But simply being told "We need you here today" doesn't constitute an emergency.

Evaluate your assignment

You may be assigned to help out on a specialized unit, which is reasonable as long as you're assigned duties you can perform competently and as long as the experienced nurse on the unit assumes responsibility for the specialized duties. Assigning you to perform total patient care on the unit is unsafe because you don't have the skills to plan and deliver that care.

For example, if you're assigned to coronary care, you could monitor the I.V. lines, take vital signs, and report your observations to the coronary care nurse. She'll check the monitors, administer the medications, and make decisions. This arrangement fragments the patient's care, however, so it's not appropriate as a permanent solution to a staffing problem.

Delegate carefully

Exercise great care as a supervisor when delegating duties because you may be held responsible for subordinates. Inspect all equipment and machinery regularly, and make sure that subordinates use them competently and safely. Report incompetent health care personnel to superiors through the institutional chain of command.

Carry out orders cautiously

Never treat any patient without orders from his doctor, except in an emergency. And don't prescribe or *dispense* any medication without authorization. In most cases, only doctors and pharmacists may legally perform these functions.

Don't carry out any order from a doctor if you have any doubt about its accuracy or appropriateness. Follow your hospital's policy for clarifying ambiguous orders. Document your efforts to clarify the order and whether or not the order was carried out.

If, after you carry out an order, the treatment is adversely affecting the patient, discontinue it. Report all unfavorable signs and symptoms to the patient's doctor. Resume treatment only after you've discussed the situation with the doctor and clarified orders. Document your actions.

Keep in mind that a doctor can change his orders at any time, including while you're off duty. A patient may know something about his prescribed care that no one has told you. If a patient protests a procedure, medication dosage, or medication route—saying that it's different from "the usual," or that it's been changed—give him the benefit of the doubt. Question the doctor's orders, following your hospital's policy.

If you're an inexperienced nurse, you should take steps to clarify all standing orders. Contact the prescribing doctor for guidance. Or tell your supervisor that you're uncertain about following the order, and let her decide what to do.

Administer medications carefully

Medication errors are the most common and potentially most dangerous of nursing errors. Mistakes in dosage, pa-

tient identification, or drug selection by nurses have led to vision loss, brain damage, cardiac arrest, and death. In *Norton v. Argonaut Insurance Co.* (1962), an infant died after a nurse administered injectable digoxin at a dosage level appropriate for elixir of Lanoxin, an oral drug. The nurse was unaware that digoxin was available in an oral form. The nurse questioned two doctors who were not treating the infant about the order but failed to mention to them that the order was written for elixir of Lanoxin and failed to clarify the order with the doctor who wrote it.

The nurse, the doctor who originally ordered the medication, and the hospital were found liable.

Maintain rapport with the patient

Trial attorneys have a saying: "If you don't want to be sued, don't be rude." Failing to communicate with patients is the cause of many legal problems.

Always remain calm when a patient or his family becomes difficult. Tell patients the truth about adverse outcomes, but always do so discreetly and sensitively. (See *Who's looking for litigation?*)

Do not offer opinions

Avoid offering your opinion when a patient asks you what you think is the matter with him. If you do, you could be accused of making a medical diagnosis, which is *practicing medicine without a license.* Don't volunteer information about possible treatments for the patient's condition or possible choices of doctors, either.

Avoid making any statement that could be perceived by the patient as an admission of fault or error. Don't criticize other nurses or health care practitioners, or the care they provide, if the patient can hear you. Don't discuss with the patient or visitors which members of the health care team are covered by malpractice insurance.

Who's looking for litigation?

Patients who are more likely to file lawsuits against nurses share certain personality traits and behaviors. What's more, nurses who are more likely to be named as defendants also have certain characteristics in common.

Beware of these patients

Although not all persons displaying the behaviors listed below will file a lawsuit, a little extra caution in your dealings with them won't hurt. Providing professional and competent care to such patients will lessen their tendency to sue.

A patient who is likely to file a lawsuit may:
- persistently criticize all aspects of the nursing care provided
- purposefully not follow the plan of care
- overreact to any perceived slight or negative comment, real or imagined
- unjustifiably depend on nurses for all aspects of care and refuse to accept any responsibility for his own care
- openly express hostility to nurses and other health care personnel
- project his anxiety, fear, or anger onto the nursing staff, attributing blame for all negative events to health care providers
- have filed lawsuits previously.

Nurses at risk

Nurses who are more likely to be named as defendants in a lawsuit display certain characteristic behaviors. If you recognize any of these attributes within yourself, changing your behavior will reduce your risk of liability.

A nurse who is likely to be a defendant in a lawsuit may:
- be insensitive to the patient's complaints or fail to take them seriously
- fail to identify and meet the patient's emotional and physical needs
- refuse to recognize the limits of her nursing skills and personal competency
- lack sufficient education for the tasks and responsibilities associated with a specific practice setting
- display an authoritarian and inflexible attitude when providing care
- inappropriately delegate responsibilities to subordinates.

Be careful not to discuss a patient's care or personal business with anyone except when doing so is consistent with proper nursing care.

Read before you sign

Never sign your name as a *witness* without fully understanding what you're signing as well as the legal significance of your signature.

Document care accurately

From a legal standpoint, documented care is as important as the actual care. If a procedure wasn't documented, the courts assume it wasn't performed. Documentation of observations, decisions, and actions is considered much more solid evidence than oral testimony.

The patient's chart, when taken into the jury room, is a nurse's "best evidence" of the care given. The chart should follow the "FACT" rule: Be factual, accurate, complete, and timely.

Use *incident reports* to identify and report any accidents, errors, or injuries to a patient. Instead of placing incident reports in the patient's chart, give them directly to the institution's *risk manager.* A long period may elapse between an incident and subsequent court proceedings and this documentation may be the only proof of what happened.

Don't ever correct or revise a patient's medical record after he has filed a lawsuit. The case of *Carr v. St. Paul Fire and Marine Insurance Co.* (1974) illustrates the liability a hospital may incur when nurses or other employees alter or destroy patient records. In this case, the patient came to the hospital emergency department (ED) suffering severe pain. One of the nurses on duty refused to call a doctor for the patient, so he returned home and died a short time later. The nurses on duty in the ED that night testified that they'd taken the patient's vital signs, but this couldn't be proved or disproved because the patient's records had been destroyed. In instructing the jury, the judge indicated that they could find the hospital negligent.

The case of *Sweet v. Providence Hospital* (1995) held that a rebuttable presumption of negligence arises if a health care facility's records are unavailable to a plaintiff and the plaintiff can demonstrate that the missing records are necessary to prove his negligence claim.

Exercise caution when assisting in procedures

Don't assist with a surgical procedure unless you're satisfied that the patient has given proper *informed consent.* Never force a patient to accept treatment that he has expressly refused. Don't use equipment you're not familiar with, not trained to use, or that seems to be functioning improperly. And, if you're an operating room nurse, always check and double-check that no surgical equipment, such as sponges or instruments, are unaccounted for after an operation is completed.

Document the use of restraints

Restraints need to be applied correctly and checked according to hospital or health facility policy and procedure. Documentation must be exact about the reason for, amount, and kind of restraint used and the status of the restrained patient. An omission or failure to monitor a restrained patient may result in a malpractice claim.

Take steps to prevent patient falls

Patient falls are a very common area of nursing liability. Patients who are elderly, infirm, sedated, or mentally incapacitated are the most likely to fall. The case of *Stevenson v. Alta Bates* (1937) involved a patient who'd had a stroke and was learning to walk again. As two nurses, each holding one of the patient's arms, assisted her into the hospital's sunroom, one of the nurses let go of the patient and stepped forward to get a chair for her. The patient fell and sustained a fracture. The nurse was found negligent: The court said she should have anticipated the patient's need for a chair and made the appropriate arrangements before bringing the patient into the sunroom.

Comply with laws about advance directives

The Patient Self-Determination Act, a federal law, requires that every patient who is admitted to a hospital be given information concerning living wills and durable power of attorney. Follow the health care facility's policy and procedure for providing the required information. (Do not, as one of the patient's health care providers, witness a living will or a durable power of attorney.) You should also be aware of state laws concerning living wills and advance directives.

Follow hospital policies and procedures

You have a responsibility to be familiar with the policies and procedures of the hospital where you work. If the policies and procedures are sound and you follow them carefully, they can protect you against a malpractice claim. The court in *Roach v. Springfield Clinic* (1992) held that "hospital policies are admissible as standards of care for the treatment of patients within that hospital."

The medication procedure may involve checking all medication cards against a central Kardex. If you do this and the Kardex is in error, you may not be liable for a resulting medication error because you followed all appropriate procedures and acted responsibly.

The person who made the original error, however, would be liable. But if you didn't follow the procedure, you might also be liable because you didn't do your part to prevent the error.

Inexperienced nurses are high liability risks. The RN must be able to recognize her limitations and admit to them, if the safety of the patient is at issue. If the nurse doesn't know how to perform a nursing function or doesn't understand the reason for a particular treatment, it's her duty to obtain assistance that is timely and appropriate.

Keep policies and procedures up to date

As nursing changes, so should the hospital's policies and procedures. As a professional, you're responsible for maintaining up-to-date procedures.

For instance, does your facility have written policies on dealing with emergency situations? "We've always done it this way" isn't an adequate substitute for a clearly written, officially accepted policy.

If *administrators* are reluctant to make policy changes based on one nurse's suggestion, join with colleagues to present the legal implications.

Provide a safe environment

When providing care, you should not use faulty equipment. If the equipment isn't working properly, clearly mark it as defective and not usable. Even after repairs are done, don't use the equipment until technicians demonstrate that it's operating properly. Document steps you took to handle problems with faulty equipment to show that you followed the facility's policy and procedure.

Liability insurance

Your expanded health care role makes having *professional liability* coverage crucial. In any work setting, you are at risk for malpractice suits. The risk increases if you work in a specialized setting, such as the *intensive care unit.*

Some nurses believe that purchasing professional liability insurance makes them a more attractive target for *compensation* claims and increases their chances of being sued. They also believe that, as hospital employees, they are protected by *respondeat superior* and the hospital's insurance policy. That's dangerous thinking: Given the legal risks you face on the job, you simply can't afford to be without insurance.

Understanding insurance coverage

When you buy professional liability insurance, you get protection under contract for a designated period from the financial consequences of certain professional errors. The type of insurance policy you buy defines the amount that the insurance company will pay if the judgment goes against you in a lawsuit.

You may purchase a policy designated with "single limits" or "double limits." In a single-limits policy, you buy protection in set dollar increments, for example, $100,000, $300,000, or $1,000,000. The stipulated amount will shield you if a judgment, arising out of a single nursing malpractice occurrence, goes against you.

In the double-limits policy, you buy protection in a combination package, such as $100,000/$300,000, $300,000/$500,000, or $1,000,000/$3,000,000. The smaller sum is what your insurance company will make available to protect you from any one injury arising out of a single nursing malpractice occurrence. The larger sum is the maximum amount that will be paid for all claims under that policy in a given year. Although the single-limits policy will also protect you against injuries to more than one patient, the double-limits policy makes considerably more money available to protect you if you're involved in multiple lawsuits.

Occurrence and claims-made policies

Professional liability insurance may cover either the time the malpractice occurred (*occurrence policy*) or when a lawsuit is filed (*claims-made policy*).

An occurrence policy protects you against any incidents occurring during a policy period, regardless of when the patient files a claim against you — even after the policy ends.

The claims-made policy protects you only against claims made against you during the policy period. A claims-made policy is less expensive than an occurrence policy because the insurance company is at risk only for the duration of the policy. However, you can purchase an extended-reporting endorsement, or tail coverage, which in effect turns your claims-made policy into an occurrence policy.

Excess judgment

You are personally responsible for any excess judgment — a judgment that exceeds the policy limits. Depending on the laws in your state, almost everything you own, except for a limited portion of your equity in your home and the clothes on your back, can be taken to satisfy the uninsured portion of a judgment.

Insurance costs

Fortunately, premiums for insurance coverage of $1 million aren't much greater than they are for smaller limits. That's because a substantial part of the premium pays for the insurance company's assumption of risk; higher limits don't increase the premium disproportionately.

General duty RNs usually pay less for coverage than critical care nurses, operating room nurses, emergency room nurses, and post-anesthesia care nurses. In recent years, nurses specializing in obstetrics usually have paid the highest rates, in part because of the large number of lawsuits filed against obstetricians.

Insurance companies offer a wide variety of liability insurance policies. (See *Choosing liability insurance.*) If possible, choose an agent who is experienced in professional liability insurance. Organizations such as the ANA or your state nurses' association offer group plans at attractive premiums. You'll still want to review the extent of coverage with your agent to make sure it's adequate for your needs.

Insurer's role in a lawsuit

Professional liability insurance supplies you with more than just financial protection. The insurance company also provides defense counsel to represent you for the entire course of litigation. Insurance companies aren't in business to lose money; they will retain highly experienced attorneys with considerable experience in defending malpractice lawsuits.

When preparing your defense, attorneys will investigate the subject of the lawsuit; obtain *expert witnesses;* handle motions throughout the case; and

Choosing liability insurance

To find the professional liability coverage that fits your needs, compare the features of a number of policies. Understanding insurance policy basics will enable you to shop more aggressively and intelligently for the coverage you need. You should work with an insurance agent who's experienced in this type of insurance. If you already have professional liability insurance, the information below may help you better evaluate your coverage.

Type of coverage

Ask your insurance agent if the policy covers only claims made before the policy expires (claims-made coverage) or if it covers any negligent act committed during the policy period (occurrence coverage). Keep in mind that an occurrence policy provides more coverage than a claims-made policy.

Coverage limits

All malpractice insurance policies cover professional liability. Some also cover personal liability, medical payments, assault-related bodily injury, and all property damage.

The amount of coverage varies, as does your premium. Remember that professional liability coverage is limited to acts and practice settings specified in the policy. Make sure your policy covers your nursing role, whether you're a student, a graduate nurse, or a working nurse with advanced education and specialized skills.

Options

Check whether the policy would provide coverage for the following incidents:
- negligence on the part of nurses under your supervision

- misuse of equipment
- errors in reporting or recording care
- failure to properly teach patients
- errors in administering medication
- mistakes made while providing care in an emergency outside your employment setting.

Also ask if the policy provides protection if your employer (the hospital) sues you.

Definition of terms

Definition of terms can vary from policy to policy. If your policy includes any restrictive definitions, you won't be covered for any actions outside those guidelines. So for the best protection, seek the broadest definitions possible and ask the agent for examples of actions the company hasn't covered.

Duration of coverage

Insurance is an annual contract that can be renewed or canceled each year. The policy usually specifies how it can be canceled – in writing by either you or the insurance company. Some contracts require 30 days' notice for cancellation. If the company is canceling the policy, you'll probably be given at least 10 days' notice.

Exclusions

Ask your agent about exclusions – areas not covered by the insurance policy – for example, "this policy does not apply to injury arising out of performance of the insured of a criminal act" or "this policy does not apply to nurse anesthetists."

Other insurance clauses

All professional liability insurance policies contain "other insurance" clauses that address payment obligations when a

Choosing liability insurance continued

nurse is covered by more than one insurance policy, such as the institution's policy and the nurse's personal liability policy:

• The *pro rata* clause states that two or more policies in effect at the same time will pay any claims in accordance with a proportion established in the individual policies.

• The *in excess* clause states that the primary policy will pay all fees and damages up to its limits, at which point the second policy will pay any additional fees or damages up to its limits.

• The *escape clause* relieves an insurance company of all liability for fees or damages if another insurance policy is in effect at the same time; in effect, the clause states that the other company is responsible for all liability.

If you are covered by more than one policy, be alert for "other insurance" clauses and avoid purchasing a policy with an escape clause for liability.

Additional tips

Here is some additional information that will guide you in the purchase of professional liability insurance:

• The insurance application is a legal document. If you provide any false information it may void the policy.

• If you are involved in nursing administration, education, research, or advanced or nontraditional nursing practice, be especially careful in selecting a policy because routine policies may not cover these activities.

• After selecting a policy that ensures adequate coverage, stay with the same policy and insurer, if possible, to avoid potential lapses in coverage that could occur when changing insurers.

• No insurance policy will cover you for acts outside of your scope of practice or licensure. Nor will insurance cover you for intentional torts if intent to do harm is proved.

• Be prepared to uphold all obligations specified in the policy; failure to do so may void the policy and cause personal liability for any damages. Remember that any act of willful wrongdoing on your part renders the policy null and void and may lead to a breach of contract lawsuit.

• Check out the insurance company by calling your state's insurance commission or regulatory office to inquire about the company's financial condition.

---

prepare medical models, transparencies, photographs, and other court exhibits, if necessary. The cost incurred in preparing a defense will be covered by your insurance.

Out-of-court settlements

During litigation—and indeed even before a lawsuit is actually filed in court—your insurance company will seek an out-of-court *settlement* from the patient's attorneys. Although this saves time and money, it may not be in

your best professional interests. In the United States, if you believe your professional reputation is at stake, you may be able to refuse to agree to an out-of-court settlement. If your policy contains a threshold limit, your insurer can't settle a case out of court for an amount greater than the threshold limit without your permission. Without a threshold limit, your insurer has total control over out-of-court settlements.

If the lawsuit against you goes to court, the insurer has the right to control how the defense is conducted. The insurer's attorney makes all the decisions regarding the case's legal tactics and strategy.

You have a right to be kept advised of every step of the case. Most insurers will keep you informed. After all, the insurer knows that a successful defense depends in part on the defendant's cooperation. Also, you can sue the insurance agency if it fails to provide a competent defense.

If you lose a malpractice lawsuit, the insurance company will cover you for jury-awarded general and special damages. In the United States, juries award *general damages* to compensate for:
• pain and suffering
• worsening change in life-style.

Juries award *special damages* to relieve:
• present and future medical expenses
• past and future loss of earnings
• decreased earning capacity.

Punitive damages

The court may award *punitive damages* to punish actions that involve malice or reckless disregard for another. Historically, insurance companies haven't had to pay punitive damages. But recently, courts have been forcing insurers to pay punitive damages if the policy states that the company will pay "all sums which the insured shall become legally obligated to pay as damages." The courts have also directed insurers to expressly exclude punitive damages from coverage when writing the policy, if that is the insurer's intent.

Multiple insurers

You may have more than one insurance policy that covers a patient's claim against you. For example, you might have malpractice coverage through the hospital where you work, through membership in a professional organization, and through your own insurance policy.

All three insurance companies might become involved in settling a lawsuit. Determining who pays is complex. Be sure to promptly notify every company you have a policy with that you're the target of a malpractice lawsuit. That will prevent any company from using the *policy defense* of lack of notice or late notice. Such defenses frequently enable the insurance company to avoid responsibility for providing coverage.

Indemnification suits

If several insurance companies are representing different parties in a malpractice lawsuit, they'll typically file counteractions against the other parties, seeking compensation, or *indemnification,* for all or part of any damages the jury awards.

Many states now permit damages to be apportioned among multiple defendants, the extent of liability depending on the jury's determination of each defendant's relative contribution to the harm done. This is called *comparative negligence.* The jury "compares" the negligence of various defendants and apportions it accordingly. For example, suppose you were the nurse responsible for the instrument count during surgery in a foreign-object case, and the court found you to be 75% responsible. Your insurance company would pay 75% of the total award. The other insurance companies would be held liable for the remaining 25%, in proportion to the percentage of harm attributed to each remaining defendant. However, if one of the codefendants, such as the surgeon, decided that he'd been judged negligent only because of your negligence, he could instruct his insurance attorneys to file a separate new lawsuit in his name against you.

Indemnification suits are becoming increasingly common. This is another reason for carrying liability insurance.

Controlling liability costs

Many states are taking steps to decrease malpractice litigation. In addition to establishing special statutes of limitations, some states have imposed a maximum limit on how much a jury can award in general damages. That restriction, however, has been challenged as being unconstitutional.

Medical associations and insurance companies are also trying to limit malpractice awards in other ways: by forcing malpractice claims into *arbitration* — thus removing them from the province of *lay juries* — and by requiring that they be screened by a medical malpractice screening panel. A few states, such as Ohio, provide for submission to nonbinding arbitration panels if all parties agree to it. State laws may also provide for binding arbitration if specified by a written contract between a patient and the doctor or hospital.

If a malpractice screening panel decides the plaintiff's claim isn't valid, the plaintiff can't file suit unless he posts a bond to cover his defense costs in advance. More than half the states have set up screening panels, although the panels have been criticized by consumer groups and plaintiffs' attorneys and challenged in court as being unconstitutional.

Your employer's insurance

Virtually all health care institutions carry insurance to protect against their liability for an employee's mistakes. Without professional liability insurance, the insititution would have to pay damages awarded in a lawsuit out of its own funds, which could lead to bankruptcy.

You should make a point of finding out the degree of professional and financial protection you're entitled to under your employer's liability insurance. This information will help you to more wisely assess your own professional liability insurance needs.

Consider obtaining a copy of the hospital insurance policy from your employer and letting your professional liability insurance agent review it. Your agent, usually without a fee, should be willing to determine the extent, limits, and exclusions of your employer's insurance coverage.

Coverage limits

Each health care institution's professional liability insurance policy has a maximum dollar coverage limit. Your employer can purchase coverage that exceeds the basic limit; many hospitals do so for extra protection.

Deductible limit

Most hospitals also have a deductible provision that makes them responsible for damages under a certain figure. The higher the deductible limit, the lower the premium charged by the insurer. You should pay careful attention to the deductible limit because your employer can settle a claim against you under that figure without ever consulting you or the insurer. Because you won't have a chance to defend yourself and because many people interpret a settlement as an admission of guilt, such an action could tarnish your professional reputation. A tarnished reputation in turn could jeopardize your ability to get your own professional liability insurance or to get a new job. Therefore, in the event of a lawsuit, you should maintain close contact with your employer's legal staff, and insist on being informed about each step in the case.

Threshold limit

Most health care institutions demand control over when an insurer can settle a case. To gain this control, the employer normally sets a threshold limit, usually $3,000. The insurer can settle a case below the threshold without the employer's permission. But to settle a case above the threshold, the insurer must get the employer's permission. The employer wants the threshold to protect its reputation for safety and quality care — the same reason you have for not wanting your insurance provider to settle a lawsuit against you without informing you. If an insurer were allowed to settle cases behind an employer's back, the employer could become more prone to malpractice lawsuits as its reputation deteriorated.

Provisions for your defense

If you're sued and your employer's insurance covers you, the insurer has a duty to provide a complete defense, including assigning an attorney to handle the entire case. The insurer will pay the attorney fees as well as any investigation costs and expert witness fees.

The attorney will provide you with an opportunity to confer with him and give your side of the story. If your employer grants written consent to settle the case, the insurer may do so, or it may decide to try the case in court if its legal advisors overrule the employer. If the plaintiff wins the lawsuit, the insurer is obliged to pay damages awarded to the patient up to the insurance policy's coverage limit.

Stipulations for denying coverage

Insurance companies that provide professional liability coverage for hospitals and other health care institutions reduce the risk they assume under *respondeat superior* in several ways. One way is by stipulating a precise coverage period, typically 1 year. Another way is by defining the type of coverage they'll provide — whether, for example, it's an occurrence or claims-made policy.

A third way is by putting exclusions into malpractice policies. These exclusions vary considerably from policy to policy, but all list specific acts, situa-

tions, or personnel that the insurance doesn't cover.

Besides exclusions, insurers may deny coverage to you or your employer due to other circumstances, such as the following:

• The insurance policy lapses because your employer failed to pay the premiums.

• Your employer refuses to cooperate with the insurance company, for whatever reason.

• The insurer discovers that your employer made misstatements on the insurance application.

In some malpractice situations, an insurer could agree to provide you with a defense but refuse to pay damages awarded to a patient. The insurer agrees to defend you in this situation because he doesn't want to be accused of *breach of contract.* But he must notify you of his intention not to pay damages in a reservation-of-rights letter. This letter informs you and your employer that the insurer believes the case falls outside what's covered by the insurance policy. When your employer and the insurer disagree about whether insurance coverage exists, the dispute may have to be resolved through separate legal action. Similarly, you have the right to bring such action against your employer's insurance company if it refuses to cover you.

Special considerations

Keep in mind a few other concerns when reviewing your employer's policy. One is that the policy may only provide coverage for *incidents* that occur while you're on the job. You may be held liable for nursing actions off the job, unless your actions are covered under a *Good Samaritan act,* a state law which protects health care professionals who act in an emergency.

Second, many employers provide only a claims-made policy. If a suit is filed against you after you've stopped working there, for an incident that took place while you were still an employee, you probably won't be covered by your former employer's insurance plan.

Third, if you're an independent contractor, such as a private-duty nurse, you're not usually considered by the court to be under the hospital's direct supervision and control. Consequently, the hospital won't be considered responsible for your actions, and its insurance probably won't cover you.

Finally, intentional acts of harm — such as striking a patient — in most cases wouldn't impute liability to your employer. In such cases, you'd be responsible for any criminal or *civil penalties* levied against you.

Defending yourself in a lawsuit

Imagine you're at the nurses' station, catching up on paperwork, when a stranger approaches and asks for you. He thrusts some legal papers into your hands and starts to walk away. Baffled, you ask, "What's this all about?" He replies, "You've just been sued."

As you look over the papers, you recognize the name of a former patient listed as plaintiff, and you see your name listed as the defendant. You learn that you've been accused of "errors and omissions." A nagging worry for most nurses has just become reality: you've been sued for nursing malpractice.

Failing to respond to the complaint could result in a default judgment against you. You need to act immediately. Your next step depends on whether you have professional liability insurance. (See *Responding to a malpractice summons.*)

Contacting appropriate personnel

If you're covered by your employer's insurance, immediately contact your legal services administrators at work. They'll tell you how to proceed.

If you have your own professional liability insurance, consult your policy and read the section that tells you what to do when you're sued. Every policy describes whom you should notify and how much time you have to do it. Immediately telephone this representative and tell him you've been sued. Document the time, his name, and his instructions. Then, hand-deliver the lawsuit papers to him, if possible, and get a signed, dated receipt for them. Alternatively, send lawsuit papers by certified mail, return receipt requested, so you're assured of a signed receipt.

If you don't contact the appropriate representative within the specified time, the insurance company can refuse to cover you. So to protect yourself, act quickly, document your actions, and get a receipt.

In addition, contact the National Nurses Claims Data Bank established by the ANA. Provide a full report of the incident in question, including the date, time, and persons involved. This contact will give you access to national data that may support your case, and your data will, in turn, help other nurses who are involved in lawsuits. Your name and address will be kept confidential.

Insurance company considerations

When you notify your insurance company that you've been sued, it will first consider whether it must cover you at all. The insurer does this by checking for any policy violations you may have committed. For example, your insurance company will check whether you gave late notice of the lawsuit, gave

Responding to a malpractice summons

If you ever receive a summons notifying you that you're being sued, your response early on can have a significant effect on the outcome of the suit.

You should immediately cease communication with the plaintiff, his family, and his attorney. If you are insured, you should politely insist to your agent that your claim be handled by an attentive, experienced claims adjuster (the insurance company representative who investigates your claim and makes estimates for settlement) and a qualified attorney.

Be prepared to maintain your own separate file on the case. Ask for copies of all relevant documents and reports from the claims adjuster, your attorney, and the patient's attorney. Check the status of your case regularly.

Selecting a defense attorney

One of your first concerns will be finding a qualified attorney to represent you.

If the patient names your hospital in the lawsuit, the hospital's insurance company will supply an attorney to defend you as the hospital's employee. If you're sued alone, your insurance carrier will appoint a defense attorney to represent you. If you're uninsured, you'll have to find an attorney on your own.

If the dollar amount for which you're being sued exceeds your insurance coverage, consider hiring a private lawyer. This attorney will be working exclusively for you, not for your insurance carrier. He'll notify your primary defense attorney and your insurer that, should the judgment exceed your coverage, the carrier may be held liable.

Shop around

When seeking a qualified attorney, consider doing the following:

• consulting with your hospital's legal services department
• consulting with your state nurses' association or other appropriate professional organization
• asking friends or relatives with legal experience, whose judgments you can trust
• calling your local bar association, which is listed in the Yellow Pages.

When you meet with a prospective attorney, ask him about his experience with malpractice cases. If he has too little experience, or if too many of his cases were decided for the plaintiff, you have the right to ask your insurance carrier for another attorney.

Working with your attorney

Establishing a good working relationship with your attorney is crucial. It's your job to educate the attorney to the medical information he needs to defend you. Be prepared to spend many hours reviewing charts, licensing requirements, hospital procedures, journals, and texts, as well as your professional qualifications and the details of the case. Do the following:
• Provide your attorney and claims adjuster with all the information you can about the case, including anything relevant you remember that may not appear in the record.
• Supply your attorney with the nursing practice standards for your specialty.
• Discuss how you feel about settling out of court with your attorney.
• Develop a list of experts qualified to testify on the standards of care in your specialty and present it to your attorney. Avoid recommending friends, because the jury may believe them less objective.
• Review all available records, including those obtained by your attorney that are normally inaccessible to you, such as the records of the patient's private doctor.

false information on your insurance application, or failed to pay a premium on time. If the company is sure you've committed such a violation, it will use this violation as a *policy defense,* and it can simply refuse to cover you. If the company thinks you've committed such a violation but isn't sure it has evidence to support a policy defense, it will probably send you a letter by certified mail informing you that the company may not have to defend you, but that it will do so while reserving the right to deny coverage later, withdraw from the case, or take other actions. Meanwhile, the company will seek a declaration of its rights from the court. If the court decides the company doesn't have to defend you, the company will withdraw from the case.

Usually, however, an insurance company takes this action only after careful consideration. That's because denying coverage may provide you with grounds for suing the company. But if you receive such a letter, find your own attorney to defend you in the lawsuit and to advise you in your dealings with the insurance company. If your case against the insurance company is sound, he may suggest that you sue the insurer.

If your insurance company doesn't assert a policy defense, your company representative will select and retain an attorney or a law firm specializing in medical malpractice cases as your *attorney of record* in the lawsuit. Once so designated, this attorney is legally bound to do all that's necessary to defend you.

Your employer will almost certainly be named as a codefendant in the lawsuit. But even if that isn't the case, notify your employer that you're being sued. Your insurance company may try to involve your employer as a defendant.

Finding an attorney

If you don't have insurance, your own or your employer's, you'll have to find your own attorney. Don't even consider trying to defend yourself. You need an attorney who's experienced in medical malpractice, because the case will be complex and the opposition will be composed of experienced attorneys.

Make appointments with a few attorneys who seem qualified to defend you. In most cases, you won't be charged for this initial consultation. When you meet with each one, ask how long he thinks the lawsuit will take and how much money he will charge. Also, try to get a feeling for the attorney's understanding of the issues in your case. Then choose one as your attorney of record. Do this as soon as possible.

Preparing your defense

Your attorney will file the appropriate legal documents in response to the papers you were served. He'll ask you for help in preparing your defense. He should give you a chance to present your position in detail. Remember, all discussions between you and your attorney are *privileged communication,* meaning that your attorney can't disclose this information without your permission. Your attorney will also obtain complete copies of the pertinent medical records and any other documents he or you feel are important in your defense.

Interrogatories, depositions, and examinations

Your attorney will use *discovery devices* to uncover every pertinent detail about the case against you. Discovery devices are legal procedures for obtaining information. Discovery devices may include:

- *interrogatories* — questions written to the other party that require answers under oath
- *depositions* — oral cross-examination of the other party, under oath and before a court reporter
- *defense medical examination* — a medical examination of the injured party by a doctor selected by your attorney or insurance company.

The plaintiff-patient's attorney will also use discovery devices, so you may have to answer interrogatories and appear for a deposition as well. Your attorney will carefully prepare you for these procedures.

Neither the interrogatory nor the deposition should be taken lightly. Don't speculate in answering any question. Work closely with your attorney in preparing your written answers to the interrogatory.

That doesn't mean, however, that you must say or do anything he asks. If you feel your attorney is asking you to do or say things that aren't in your best interest, tell him so. You have the right to change attorneys at any time. If you believe an attorney selected by your insurance company is more interested in protecting the company than in protecting you, discuss the problem with a company representative. Then, if you still feel that he isn't defending you properly, hire your own attorney. You may have grounds for subsequently suing the insurance company and the company-appointed attorney.

Preparing for court

Plan on spending a fairly considerable amount of time preparing your case before you appear in the courtroom.

Don't talk about the case

Don't try to placate the person suing you by calling him and discussing the case. Your chances of talking him into dropping his lawsuit are very slim. And every word you say to him can be used against you in court. In fact, before the trial, don't discuss the lawsuit with anyone except your attorney. That will help prevent information leaks that could compromise your case. And to protect your professional reputation, don't even mention to your colleagues that you've been sued.

Study copies of the medical records

Your attorney will ask you to study relevant medical records as soon as possible. Examine the complete medical chart, including *nurses' notes,* laboratory reports, and doctors' orders. On a separate sheet of paper, make appropriate notes on key entries or omissions, but don't make any changes on the records. Such an action will hurt your case by undermining your credibility. Remember, you're not the only person with a copy of these records.

Create your own legal file

Ask your attorney to send you copies of all documents and correspondence pertaining to the case. Try to maintain a file that's as complete as your attorney's. Also, make sure you understand all the items in your file. If you receive a document that you don't understand, ask your attorney to explain it. Maintaining such a file should keep you current on the status of your case and prevent unpleasant surprises in court.

Take steps to protect your property

Many states have *homestead laws* that permit you to protect a substantial part of the equity in your house, as well as other property, from any judgment against you. Ask your attorney about the law in your state or province. Such protection is essential if you don't have insurance or if damages awarded to the plaintiff exceed your insurance coverage.

Events leading to trial

While your attorney prepares your defense, he'll also explore the desirability of reaching an out-of-court settlement. If he decides an out-of-court settlement is in your best interest, he'll try to achieve it before your trial date. (See *Settling out of court.*)

If your case does go to trial, your attorney will participate in selecting the jury. During this process, attorneys for both sides will question prospective jurors, and your attorney will ask your opinion on their suitability. Either attorney may reject a small number of prospective jurors without any reason (a *peremptory challenge*). You, the plaintiff, or either attorney may reject an unlimited number of jurors for specific reasons. For instance, you may reject someone who knows the plaintiff or someone who has a personal interest in the lawsuit (*challenge for cause*).

To help prepare you to testify, your attorney will ask you to review the complete medical record, your interrogatory answers, and your deposition. In addition, you should review the entire legal file you've been keeping, to make sure you understand all aspects of the case.

Deposition
Before the trial, you'll probably be called to testify at the deposition. (If you've been called to testify as an expert witness, you should be aware that some states don't permit expert witnesses to give pretrial depositions.) Where you give the deposition can vary. It can take place in an attorney's office or in a special room in the courthouse set aside for that purpose. The deposition takes place in a less formal atmosphere than a courtroom provides, but don't forget that a court reporter will be transcribing every word you and the attorneys say. In a way, it's a rehearsal of the actual trial. At the trial, the plaintiff's and the defendant's attorneys have the right to use your pretrial testimony to bolster their respective cases.

Trial

Be prepared for your trial to last several days — or even weeks. After all the witnesses have given their testimony, the jury, not the judge, will decide if you're liable. If the jury finds you liable, it will also assess damages against you. (See *The trial process: Step by step,* pages 232 and 233.) In some instances, an arbitration proceeding is used instead of a jury trial, but that is the exception.

Testifying in court
When you're called to testify in a malpractice lawsuit, as a defendant or an expert witness, you may be expected to respond quickly to a confusing presentation of claims, *counterclaims,* allegations, and contradictory evidence. You can use a number of techniques to help reduce stress and enhance the value of your testimony.

Courtroom demeanor
How you come across to the jury from the witness stand is very important. The jury may form its first, and sometimes lasting, impression of your credibility while you are testifying.

Your attorney will help prepare you to testify at the trial. He'll tell you how to dress — conservatively, as if you were going to an important job interview — and how to act. Your attorney may recommend, for example, that you sit with both feet on the floor with your hands folded in front of you and pay polite attention to other speakers. Keep in mind that the purpose of these instructions is to help win the case. Remember also that your failure to cooperate with an attorney provided by an insurance company can be used by the insurance company to deny coverage.

Settling out of court

Only 10% of malpractice lawsuits that are filed actually go to court, and of those that go to court, only 10% actually end with a final judgment. The rest, the vast majority of cases, are settled out of court.

Making a compromise

Settling your case out of court isn't an admission of wrongdoing. The law regards settlement as a compromise between two parties to end a lawsuit and to avoid further expense. You may choose to pay a settlement rather than incur the possibly greater expense, both financial and emotional, of defending your innocence at trial.

Determining your settlement rights

If you're covered by professional liability insurance, the terms of your policy will determine whether you and your attorney, or the insurance company, can control the settlement. Most policies do not permit the nurse to settle a case without the consent of the insurance company. In fact, many policies, especially those provided by employers, permit the insurance company to settle without the consent of the nurse involved.

Review your policy to determine your settlement rights. If the policy isn't clear on this point, call the insurance company representative and ask for clarification.

Evaluating a possible settlement

Offer your attorney and your insurance company's representative all the information you can about the case, so they can evaluate not only your liabilities, but also a possible settlement with the plaintiff. As an attending nurse, you may be in the best position to provide crucial observations concerning the patient's state of mind—in many cases, the basis of a successful settlement.

Malpractice lawsuits are notoriously slow-moving. Interruptions occur in the form of recesses, attorneys' lengthy arguments in judges' chambers, and the calling of witnesses out of turn. Be patient no matter what happens. And when you're asked to appear, be prompt. You may not score points by your punctuality, but you'll definitely lose a few if you aren't in court when you're called to testify.

When you testify, the jury doesn't expect you to be letter-perfect or to have instant or total recall. If you don't know the answer, say so. Listen closely to questions, and answer only what the questioner has asked. Always answer the questions simply and in lay terms, and never elaborate or volunteer information. If you're going to be describing a piece of equipment that's unfamiliar to a lay audience, get your attorney's approval to bring it to the courtroom and show it to the jury.

Above all, be honest. Especially when your testimony must be critical of a colleague or of your hospital's policies, you may be tempted to bend the truth a little. Don't.

During the trial, your professional reputation will be at stake. Project a positive attitude at all times, suggesting that you feel confident about the trial's outcome. Never disparage the plaintiff inside or outside the courtroom. Characterizing him as a gold digger, for instance, can only generate bad feelings that may interfere with the settlement. You won't want to speak to him

(Text continues on page 235.)

The trial process: Step by step

The chart below summarizes the basic trial process from complaint to execution of judgment. If you're ever involved in a lawsuit, your attorney will explain the specific procedures that your case requires.

Pretrial preparation

1 Complaint
Plaintiff files a complaint stating his charges against the defendant.

2 Summons
Court issues defendant a summons stating plaintiff's charges.

3 Answer or counterclaim
Defendant files an answer and may add a counterclaim to plaintiff's charges.

Trial

7 Opening statements
Plaintiff's and defendant's attorneys present facts as they apply to their cases.

8 Plaintiff presents case
Plaintiff's witnesses testify, explaining what they saw, heard, and know. Expert witnesses review any documentation and give their opinions about specific aspects of the case.

9 Cross-examination
Defendant's attorney questions plaintiff's witnesses.

13 Defendant closes case
Plaintiff's attorney may claim defendant hasn't presented an issue for the jury to decide.

14 Closing statements
Each attorney summarizes his case for the jury.

15 Jury instruction
Judge instructs the jury in points of law that apply in this particular case.

4 Discovery
Plaintiff's and defendant's attorneys develop their cases by gathering information by means of depositions and interrogatories and by reviewing documents and other evidence.

5 Pretrial hearing
Court hears statements from both parties and tries to narrow the issues.

6 Negotiation for settlement
Both parties meet to try to resolve the case outside the court.

10 Plaintiff closes case
Defendant's attorney may make a motion to dismiss the case, claiming plaintiff's evidence is insufficient.

11 Defendant presents case
Defendant's witnesses testify, explaining what they saw, heard, and know. Expert witnesses review any documentation and give their opinions about specific aspects of the case.

12 Cross-examination
Plaintiff's attorney questions defendant's witnesses.

16 Jury deliberation and verdict
Jury reviews facts and votes on verdict. Jury announces verdict before judge and both parties.

17 Appeal (optional)
Attorneys review transcripts. The party against whom the court ruled may appeal if he feels the judge didn't interpret the law properly, instruct the jury properly, or conduct the trial properly.

18 Execution of judgment
Appeals process is completed and the case is settled.

Courtroom controversy: Nurses as expert witnesses

Testimony by experts is an essential ingredient in malpractice cases for both plaintiff and defendant. But in lawsuits against nurses, the court's position on the use of expert witnesses is ambivalent.

Double standard?

Although most courts recognize nursing as a profession, they usually don't require expert testimony to establish whether a defendant-nurse breached the standard of care. Remember, however, that lawsuits against doctors don't always involve expert witness testimony. If a doctor slams his office door on the hand of a patient or closes an incision leaving a surgical sponge in the patient's abdomen, the court recognizes that no expert is needed to establish negligence.

In many cases, doctors have provided expert testimony on standards of nursing care. In other cases, nurses have provided expert testimony on such standards. To date, no uniform standard for expert testimony has been established for lawsuits involving nurses.

Qualifications of an expert

A nurse expert witness testifying for the plaintiff in a negligence case must be able to describe the relevant standard of care, show how the nurse deviated from the acceptable standard, and explain how failure to meet acceptable nursing standards caused or contributed to the patient's injury. Defense counsel will also provide a nurse expert who will testify to the standard and whether the defendant nurse met the standard.

An expert witness's credentials must match or exceed the defendant's. For example, a psychiatric nurse-defendant with 2 years' experience may insist that a pro-

spective expert witness have comparable experience. Some courts allow an RN to testify about the care an LPN or LVN provides, but not the reverse. Some courts won't allow an LPN or LVN to testify about nursing standards.

On occasion, a nurse may testify as an expert about a doctor's care—when the doctor performs a nursing function, such as drawing blood.

Case study

The case of *Wood v. Rowland* (1978) illustrates some of the questions that may arise when a nurse is called to give expert witness testimony. After Cecil Wood died, his wife charged that his nurses had been negligent. Mrs. Wood planned to base her case on the expert testimony of an RN, Mrs. Miller. Mrs. Miller reviewed the hospital records and was prepared to testify that the nurses who cared for Cecil Wood failed to meet a reasonable standard of care.

Mrs. Miller took the witness stand but was never able to testify. The defendant's attorney pointed out that Mrs. Miller had been employed by only one hospital.

Mrs. Miller had described her qualifications: She'd graduated from a diploma program in 1963 and then had worked at the same hospital for 3 years. For the next 2 years, she'd worked as an office nurse, after which she had not been employed for 5 years.

In May 1973—1 month after Cecil Wood's death—Mrs. Miller had started working again as a nurse in the same hospital where she'd worked before.

Mrs. Miller testified that her education and experience made her familiar with local nursing standards, even though she'd never worked in the hospital where Cecil

---

Courtroom controversy: Nurses as expert witnesses continued

Wood had been a patient. But the defendant's attorney asked if Mrs. Miller knew the standards of nursing care or procedures in other hospitals. She said no.

The defendant's attorney then said that policies may vary from hospital to hospital. He asked the judge to refuse to allow Mrs. Miller to testify as an expert witness and to enter a directed verdict in favor of the hospital. The judge agreed.

Mrs. Wood appealed. The appellate judge ruled that the trial judge's refusal to accept Mrs. Miller as an expert witness was an error. According to the appellate judge, Mr. Wood's care didn't concern hospital administrative standards, which would require an expert witness familiar with the standards adopted by various hospitals. Instead, the Wood case concerned professional nursing standards in general.

The courts define an expert as someone who has superior knowledge on a subject. Since Mrs. Miller's education and experience were not common to the average person, she met this test. That she worked in only one hospital might have affected the weight of her testimony, but it didn't disqualify her from giving it, the court ruled.

---

during the trial, but if you do, always be polite and dignified.

Cross-examination

During *cross-examination,* the opposing attorney will try to discredit your testimony. This may take the form of an attack on your credentials, experience, or education — especially if you're testifying as an expert witness. (See *Courtroom controversy: Nurses as expert witnesses.*)

Another way of discrediting expert testimony is by the "hired gun" insinuation. The cross-examining attorney may imply that because you accept payment for your testimony, you're being unethical. Just remember that as an expert witness you have the right to expect compensation for the time you spend on behalf of the case in and out of the courtroom. Say so if necessary.

Another ploy the opposing attorney can use to discredit your testimony is the "hedge." He may try to get you to change or qualify an answer you gave previously on *direct examination* or at the deposition. He may also try to confuse the issue by asking you a similar, but hypothetical, question with a slightly different — but significant — slant. Just remember that a simple but sincere "I don't know" often reinforces a jury's belief in your honesty and competence. Your best protection against cross-examination jitters is adequate preparation.

Selected references

Catalano, J.T. *Ethical and Legal Aspects of Nursing,* 2nd ed. Springhouse, Pa.: Springhouse Corp., 1995.

Feutz-Harter, S. "Nursing Case Law Update," *Journal of Nursing Law* 1(2):57-61, Winter 1994.

Feutz-Harter, S. "Nursing Case Law Update," *Journal of Nursing Law* 1(3):47-52, Spring 1994.

Feutz-Harter, S. "Nursing Case Law Update," *Journal of Nursing Law* 2(1):51-55, Autumn 1995.

Fiesta, J. "Law for the Nurse Manager: Assessment and Communication," *Nursing Management* 26(6):22, 24, June 1995.

"Following Hospital Policy: A Legal Risk?" *Nursing94* 24(5):26, May 1994.

George, J.E., et al. "Phone Consultations with the ED Physician: Is There Nursing Liability?" *Journal of Emergency Nursing* 21(2):163-64, April 1995.

Grant, A.B. *The Professional Nurse: Issues and Actions.* Springhouse, Pa.: Springhouse Corp., 1994.

Kelly, L.Y., and Joel, L.A. *Dimensions of Professional Nursing,* 7th ed. New York: McGraw-Hill Book Co., 1995.

Masoorli, S. "When I.V. Practice Spells Malpractice," *RN* 58(8):53-55, August 1995.

Moniz, D. "The Clock Stops Ticking on Potential Lawsuits — Eventually," *RN* 58(7):57, July 1995.

Moore, G.M. "Surviving a Malpractice Lawsuit: One Nurse's Story," *Nursing93* 23(10):54-57, October 1993.

Nurse's Problem Solver. Springhouse, Pa.: Springhouse Corp., 1995.

Pozgar, G.D. *Legal Aspects of Health Care Administration,* 5th ed., Gaithersburg, Md.: Aspen Pubs., Inc., 1993.

"Professional Liability Insurance: Taking Stock," *Nursing93* 23(10):81, October 1993.

Purnell, L. "What to Do If Called Upon to Testify," *Accident and Emergency Nursing* 3(1):19-21, January 1995.

Tammelleo, A.D. "Are You Responsible for the Doctor 'Covering' for You?" *Reagan Report on Medical Law* 28(6):4, June 1995.

6

Legal aspects of documentation

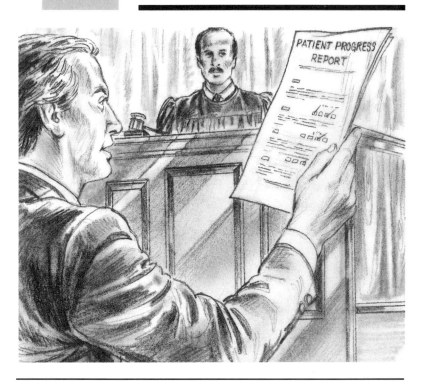

J ust how important is good nursing documentation?

Ask Lauren Ball, RN, a nurse at the Good Samaritan Hospital in West Islip, N.Y. In 1987, Ms. Ball failed to document in her **nurses' notes** that a patient, Gerolamo Kucich, reported seeing a bearded man in a white lab coat put "something" in his I.V. line. The bearded man, Richard Angelo, was subsequently convicted of assaulting Kucich and killing four others by injecting the drug Pavulon (pancuronium) to paralyze their breathing. Ms. Ball saved Kucich's life and was a key wit-

ness in the trial against Angelo. Nevertheless, in 1991, she was charged with **negligence** and professional misconduct and faced possible revocation of her license and a $10,000 fine *simply for failing to document the patient's observation.*

Thankfully, incidents like this are rare. Nevertheless, the fact that the state pressed charges against Ms. Ball underscores the seriousness of the nurse's responsibility to document in the eyes of the law. Nursing documentation has become increasingly scientific and complex. Its quality likewise has taken on greater legal significance.

In this chapter, you'll learn about the legal significance of the *medical record*—the principal tool used by the health care team to plan, coordinate, and document the care given to each patient. You'll also read about the importance of good nursing documentation, examine several court cases in which documentation quality affected the outcome, and review guidelines for avoiding errors. You'll find a discussion of computerized medical records and their legal implications. (See *Documentation tips.*) Finally, you'll learn about new documentation systems prompted by health care reform initiatives and the pressure to reduce costs.

Purpose and value of accurate documentation

The trend toward increasing specialization means that patients are being assessed, cared for, and treated by more health care professionals than ever before. Complete, accurate, and timely documentation is crucial to the continuity of each patient's care. The medical record is also a legal and business record with many uses. A well-documented medical record:
• reflects the patient care given
• demonstrates the results of treatment
• helps to plan and coordinate the care contributed by each professional
• allows interdisciplinary exchange of information about the patient
• provides evidence of the nurse's legal responsibilities toward the patient
• demonstrates adherence to standards, rules, regulations, and laws of nursing practice
• supplies information for analysis of cost-to-benefit reduction
• reflects professional and ethical conduct and responsibility

• furnishes data for a variety of uses—continuing education, risk management, diagnosis-related group (DRG) assignment and reimbursement, continuous quality improvement, case-management monitoring, and research.

Legal significance of the medical record

The medical record provides legal proof of the nature and quality of care the patient received. The weight it carries in legal proceedings cannot be overemphasized. The record may be the focus of inquiry in personal injury, professional *malpractice,* or product liability claims, as well as in *workers' compensation,* child custody, and employment disputes.

A factual, consistent, timely, and complete record defends you against allegations of negligence, improper treatment, and omissions in care. Health care professionals have a legal duty to maintain the medical record in sufficient detail, and inadequate documentation of care may result in *liability* or nonreimbursement by third-party payers.

In fact, documentation of care has become synonymous with care itself, and failure to document implies failure to provide care. Despite the recent introduction of charting by exception—a system that implies all standards have been met with a normal or expected response unless otherwise documented—the prevailing rule remains "If it isn't documented, it hasn't been done."

In *Collins v. Westlake Community Hospital* (1974), a boy was hospitalized with a fractured leg, which was put in a cast and placed in traction. The evening nurse recorded the condition of the boy's toes several times during her shift. The night nurse, however, didn't record the condition of his toes until 6

Documentation tips

If you're ever involved in a malpractice lawsuit, how you documented, what you documented, and what you didn't document will heavily influence the jury and the outcome of the trial. Following these tips can assure that your records don't tip the scales of justice against you.

How to document

• Use the appropriate form, and document in ink.
• Record the patient's name and identification number on every page of his chart.
• Record the complete date and time of each entry.
• Be specific. Avoid general terms and vague expressions.
• Use standard abbreviations only.
• Use a medical term only if you're sure of its meaning.
• Document symptoms by using the patient's own words.

What to document

• Document any nursing action you take in response to a patient's problem. For example: "8 p.m.—medicated for incision pain." Be sure to include the medication name, dose, route, and site.
• Document the patient's response to medications and other treatment.
• Document safeguards you use to protect the patient. For example: "raised side rails" or "applied safety belts."

• Document any incident in two places: in your progress notes and in an incident report. Don't mention the report in the patient's record, unless your institution or state requires it.
• Document each observation. Failure to document observations will produce gaps in the patient's records. These gaps will suggest that you neglected the patient.
• Document procedures after you perform them, never in advance.
• Write on every line. Don't insert notes between lines or leave empty spaces for someone else to insert a note.
• Sign every entry.
• Chart an omission as a new entry. Never backdate or add to previously written entries.
• Draw a thin line through an error and write "error" above it with the date and your initials. Never erase or obliterate an erroneous entry.
• Document only the care you provide. Never document for someone else.
• Understand and follow the documentation standards of your institution and your state or province. These standards are usually defined in state or provincial nurse practice acts (the statutes governing nursing practice) and in state or provincial administrative codes (the rules and regulations governing nursing practice).

---

a.m., when she noted that they were dusky and cold and that his doctor had been contacted. The leg required partial amputation, and the boy's family sued the hospital, claiming that the amputation was necessary because the night nurse had negligently failed to observe the condition of the toes in a timely fashion.

In her defense, the nurse testified that she had observed the toes periodically and that they were normal. Experts for the defense testified that only abnormal findings required documentation. But the jury disagreed, concluding that failure to document implied failure to observe, and held the nurse liable for malpractice.

Contents of the medical record

Federal regulations, such as those governing **Medicare** and **Medicaid** reimbursement, partially determine the form and content of the medical record. Although state laws vary in their stringency and specificity, all states require health care institutions to maintain the medical record in sufficient detail. (See *Documentation systems* and *Legal risks of charting by exception,* page 243.)

The following documents are usually included in the medical record:
• patient admission form and history
• doctor's order form and progress notes
• **nursing assessment** and **nursing diagnoses**
• patient's medication record
• nurses' notes and progress notes
• diagnostic and laboratory test results
• X-ray and other radiologic reports
• operative and other treatment reports
• flow sheets, checklists, and graphic sheets
• discharge summary
• referral summaries
• **consent forms,** such as **advance directives**, living wills, do-not-resuscitate orders, and the name of a health care proxy or legal guardian
• home care instruction sheet.
(See *Using flow sheets,* page 244, and *Documenting discharge planning,* page 245.)

Failure to properly maintain the medical record

As a general rule, the medical record is presumed to be accurate if there is no evidence of *fraud* or tampering. Evidence of tampering can cause the record to be ruled inadmissible as evidence in court. Medical records may be corrected if the portion in error remains legible; deleting or rendering the entry illegible can impose liability. Late entries are usually acceptable if they're clearly marked "late entry" when made.

Loss of the medical record raises a *rebuttable presumption* of negligence (which may be overcome by contrary evidence).

Nursing documentation

With a large number of health care professionals involved in each patient's care, nursing documentation must be complete, accurate, and timely to foster continuity of care. It should cover the following:
• initial assessment using the nursing process and applicable nursing diagnoses (*Note:* Nursing diagnoses have received judicial recognition [*Sermchief v. Gonzales,* 1983].)
• nursing actions, particularly reports to the doctor
• ongoing assessment, including the frequency of assessment
• variations from the assessment and plan
• accountability information, including forms signed by the patient, location of patient valuables, and patient education
• notation of care by other disciplines, including doctor visits, if practical
• health teaching, including content and response
• procedures and diagnostic tests
• patient response to therapy, particularly to nursing interventions, drugs, and diagnostic tests
• statements made by the patient
• patient comfort and safety measures.

Sources of documentation duties and standards

Factors that influence nursing documentation standards include:
• federal statutes and regulations
• state regulations and statutes, including licensing statutes and **nurse practice acts**

Documentation systems

Properly documented, the medical record provides legal evidence that can be used to protect the patient, the hospital, or the health care team. Two major record-keeping systems—source-oriented and problem-oriented—have evolved over the years to serve the needs of caregivers and patients. Another traditional system, the narrative record, is now usually combined with another system. Newer documentation approaches include focus charting, problem-intervention-evaluation charting, and charting by exception.

Source-oriented system

Hospitals have been using the source-oriented system since record keeping began. Under this system, each professional group keeps a separate record.

This system was widely practiced until recently, with doctors charting the progress notes and nurses charting the nurses' notes. A drawback is that you must consult several sources to get an accurate picture of the patient's condition. Also, failure to consult all the individual records carries potentially serious consequences for both the patient and staff. For example, in a case from Louisiana, *Villetto v. Weilbaecher* (1979), nurses observed that a patient had developed several blisters 8 days after knee surgery. They recorded their observation in the nurses' notes and reported the problem to the doctor. However, the doctor did not mention the blisters in his notes until 6 days after that. The patient sued and was awarded damages for pain and scarring; the doctor was found liable for failure to treat the blisters. (The nurses, however, were found not liable because the record showed that they had met their standard of care.)

Problem-oriented system

Many hospitals have adopted problem-oriented records, which give a comprehensive picture of the patient's clinical status and response to therapy. All members of the health care team combine their data into a format known by the acronym SOAP: **S**ubjective patient data; **O**bjective findings on observation, assessment, and examination; **A**ssessment of the subjective complaints and objective findings; **P**lan, both for present and future therapy.

For instance, the nurse may note a problem: pain on ambulation. Under the SOAP system, she would record:
S—The patient says, "My side hurts when I walk."
O—Favoring left side. Appendectomy performed 11/15/96. Approximately 2-cm erythematous area surrounding stitches.
A—Local inflammation of appendectomy stitches causing pain.
P—Report to doctor. Assist when walking.

Narrative record

In this approach, the nurse documents ongoing assessment data, nursing interventions, and patient responses in chronological order. This system has several drawbacks. Writing narrative notes is time consuming and repetitive. Also, tracking problems and trends can be difficult because the entire record must be read to identify the patient outcome. Today, this system, when used, is typically combined with the source-oriented system.

Newer charting methods

These include focus charting, PIE charting, and charting by exception.

Focus charting

This charting technique identifies patient care problems as foci of concern. A focus may be a nursing diagnosis, a sign or symptom, a patient behavior, a special need, or an acute change in the patient's

(continued)

Documentation systems continued

condition. The focus is identified by reviewing assessment data and then is documented precisely in a progress note.

Advantages and disadvantages
- Highlights patient concerns
- Provides structure for progress notes
- Enhances documentation of the nursing process
- Promotes analytical thinking
- Can be adapted to any clinical setting
- Must be monitored regularly to ensure compliance with response component
- May require in-depth training to use
- Involves many checklists and flow sheets
- May be difficult for some nurses to write accurate, logical notes using this system

PIE charting

In this system, information is grouped into one of three categories: Problem, Intervention, and Evaluation. PIE charting integrates the plan of care into the nurses' progress notes, omitting the need for a separate plan of care. The nurse keeps a daily patient assessment flow sheet and progress notes.

Advantages and disadvantages
- Encourages use of nursing diagnoses
- Simplifies charting by incorporating plan of care in progress notes
- Calls for evaluation of each identified problem at least once every shift
- Time-consuming; may lead to repetitive entries by requiring reevaluation of each problem every shift
- May require in-depth training to use
- Eliminates the planning step of nursing process
- Does not provide opportunity to document expected outcomes

- Eliminates the plan of care or protocol to guide care
- Not well suited to long-term care

Charting by exception

Gaining support in the current managed-care environment, **C**harting **B**y **E**xception (CBE) requires documentation of only abnormal or significant findings. It relies on written standards of practice that identify nurses' basic responsibilities to patients and protocols for interventions. The CBE format includes a standardized plan of care based on nursing diagnoses as well as several types of flow sheets, which allow easy tracking of trends.

Advantages and disadvantages
- Eliminates the need to document routine care through use of nursing standards
- Decreases charting time and report time
- Allows patient data to go directly to the permanent record
- Reduces the risk of transcribing errors
- Gives other caregivers access to most current patient data
- Standardizes assessments so that all caregivers evaluate and document findings consistently
- Makes trends in patient's care status obvious
- Markedly reduces chart size
- Requires large time commitment by hospital to develop clear guidelines and standards of care
- Requires major teaching effort for implementation
- Must be thoroughly understood and correctly used by all staff members to be effective
- Has questionable legal basis

Legal risks of charting by exception

Charting by exception (CBE) omits all charting related to routine nursing care. Instead, it relies on written standards of practice that identify the nurse's basic patient responsibilities.

Because this charting system requires the nurse to document only information that deviates from the expected, it can raise legal concerns. To ensure a legally sound patient record, well-defined guidelines and standards of care for using CBE must be understood by all nursing staff members.

When CBE violates the law

Lama v. Boras, a 1994 Puerto Rico case, illustrates what can go wrong when nurses don't follow accepted standards of care when using CBE. On May 15, 1985, Roberto Romero Lama had surgery for a herniated disk. Two days later, a nurse wrote in his chart that the bandage covering the surgical wound was "very bloody." An entry the next day indicated that the patient had pain at the incision site.

On May 19, a nurse documented the bandage as "soiled again." The next day, Mr. Romero began to complain of severe back discomfort; he spent that night screaming in pain. On May 21, the doctor diagnosed an infection in the space between the vertebral disks and ordered antibiotics. The patient was hospitalized for several months to treat the infection.

Mr. Romero sued the hospital and the doctors who treated him, alleging that they failed to prepare and monitor proper medical records. The hospital did not dispute the charge that nurses did not supply the required notes; instead, it pointed out that they followed the hospital's official CBE policy.

The court ruled against the hospital on the grounds that Puerto Rico law requires qualitative nurses' notes for each nursing shift and that violation of this regulation had caused Mr. Romero's injury. The court reasoned that a more complete picture of his evolving condition was unavailable because the hospital's CBE policy called for nurses to note qualitative observations only when needed to chronicle important clinical changes. Although objective aspects of the patient's care and condition (temperature, vital signs, and medications) were documented regularly, important details (the changing condition of the surgical site and the patient's reports of pain) were not.

Playing it safe

Although CBE complies with legal principles, the system may be questioned in court until it becomes more widely known. If you believe your institution's CBE policy is unsafe or ambiguous, confer with your colleagues and supervisors, and then approach an administrator about clarifying it.

- custom
- accrediting bodies
- standards of practice issued by professional organizations
- institutional *policies* and procedures.

Professional organizations and accrediting bodies have developed and refined recommendations and standards of practice for nursing documentation.

Sometimes these standards are more stringent than those required by state law.

The *American Nurses' Association* (ANA) has included documentation in its Standards of Nursing Practice. The ANA says documentation must be systematic, continuous, accessible, com-

Using flow sheets

Flow sheets are record-keeping forms used for tracking information about the repetitive tasks you perform throughout the day, such as giving medication or monitoring your patient's vital signs or fluid balance. Using a flow sheet enables you to keep all routine measurements in one place and to compare data quickly. Flow sheets come in a variety of styles, including blank-ruled paper, multi-columned paper, and graph paper, to suit various documenting needs.

Advantages

A flow sheet offers the following advantages:
● It displays a specific aspect of your patient's condition, such as his temperature, at a glance. You don't have to search through pages of notes to determine his temperature pattern over the past 48 hours.
● It saves you time. You can note the vital signs or medication given without having to write a full descriptive entry every time. You can use your nurses' notes to describe how the patient is responding to treatment.
● It documents that you're giving the patient continuous care.
● It provides a mechanism for nonlicensed personnel to record their care and observations. Because nonlicensed personnel usually aren't permitted to

chart in the nurses' notes, any information they have about patient care may be lost. Instead, you can ask them to describe their care and initial each entry on a flow sheet. Then, if you have a question about the status of your patient's skin, for example, you can check the flow sheet to identify the nurses' aide who administered that day's bed bath.

Common errors

Flow sheets can create a legal tangle if you don't avoid two common mistakes.

The first mistake is to treat flow sheets casually. For instance, some nurses will routinely check off whatever the previous shift checked off on the flow sheet, regardless of the care given, and then carefully chart the actual care in the nurses' notes. As part of the legal medical record, the flow sheet must accurately reflect the care provided.

The second mistake is to depend too heavily on flow sheets. Flow sheets can help you document, quickly and accurately, what care was given and who provided it. But don't neglect to record the patient's *response to care* in your nurses' notes. Like any other chart form, retain the flow sheet as part of the permanent chart so that you have a progressive picture of the patient's status and a record of your care.

municated, recorded, and available to all members of the health care team.

The *Joint Commission on Accreditation of Healthcare Organizations* (JCAHO) also sets standards. Current standards for documentation stress a change from source-oriented to a fully integrated, multidisciplinary approach.

Documentation should reflect the collaborative planning and provision of care and treatment. The JCAHO does

not specify a format for medical record documentation. Therefore, patient care, treatment, and rehabilitation may involve many forms — from preprinted forms to handwritten reports to electronic records — and may include decision algorithms, care paths, and care maps.

Many of the professional specialty societies, such as the American Association of Critical-Care Nurses, the

Documenting discharge planning

When planning a patient's discharge, be sure to document in his chart that he or his family is aware that treatment and care will be discontinued on a specific date. Also document the alternative resources and specific plans that must be organized to ensure continuity of care.

Writing a discharge summary

The final document in each patient's record, the discharge summary highlights the patient's condition, treatment, status at discharge, discharge nursing diagnoses, and all medications. It should also include a home care instruction sheet, the name of an escort, the patient's discharge address, and his transportation mode.

Taking it step-by-step

When preparing a discharge summary, take the following steps:
- First, review the patient's nursing diagnoses or problem list, care plan, flow sheets, and progress notes to develop an overall impression of his hospital stay.
- Follow your hospital's policies regarding the format and content of the summary.
- Include any exceptional details or unusual findings.
- Outline all patient teaching and provide written instructions in a language the patient understands.

Reviewing the summary

Make sure that your discharge summary:
- summarizes the patient's care
- provides useful information for further teaching, evaluation, and readmission
- indicates that the patient has the information he needs for self-care or to get further help
- shows that you've met the Joint Commission on Accreditation of Healthcare Organization's documentation requirements for collaboration with other disciplines and for patient teaching
- helps safeguard you and your employer against malpractice charges.

Association of Operating Room Nurses, and the Emergency Department Nurses' Association have developed guidelines, standards, or recommendations concerning the content and technique of nursing documentation.

Typically a health care facility has integrated the appropriate laws, regulations, and standards into its own policy and procedure manual. Your best assurance of following the law may be to adhere to the institution's policy, which usually describes who is to maintain each portion of a patient's record and by which technique. (See *Managed care: Implications for documentation,* page 246).

The courts and hospital policy

In a dispute, the law will frequently support an institution's policies and procedures with regard to documentation. Consider the case of *Stack v. Wapner* (1976).

The plaintiff was admitted to the hospital to give birth. At 2:45 a.m., according to her chart, intravenous oxytocin was started to induce labor. Accepted medical practice requires continuous monitoring of patients receiving oxytocin to prevent complications of excessive uterine contractions, such as subsequent fetal distress or uterine rupture. However, the labor room record didn't document monitoring of her clinical status until 5:15 a.m.

Managed care: Implications for documentation

Because managed care balances the importance of a medical procedure or treatment against its cost, it requires greater standardization of plans of care as well as continuous monitoring of health care outcomes. To improve outcomes, several tools have been developed.

Clinical practice guidelines

Practice guidelines are standards developed to help practitioners and patients make decisions regarding appropriate care in specific clinical circumstances.

Practice parameters

Practice parameters are educational tools that enable doctors to obtain the advice of clinical experts, keep abreast of the latest clinical research, and assess the clinical significance of often conflicting research findings.

Clinical pathways

Clinical pathways (also called critical paths) are clinical management tools that help to organize, sequence, price, and time the major interventions of nurses, doctors, and other health care providers for a particular case type, subset, or condition.

Care maps

Care maps are elaborate critical pathways that show the relationships of sets of interventions to sets of intermediate outcomes along a time line. They merge standards of care with standards of practice in a cause-and-effect relationship.

After delivery, the patient developed heavy uterine bleeding. Unable to stop the bleeding, the doctor performed a total hysterectomy. The patient later sued, claiming that her complications resulted from improper administration and monitoring of oxytocin.

Both the attending doctors testified that they had monitored the administration of the drug. However, they had no defense against evidence that hospital policy required them to document on the patient's chart all information that supported the diagnosis and treatment as well as the patient's response to treatment. The patient was awarded damages.

Hazards of improper nursing documentation

In the following cases, nurses or other health care providers made documentation errors that contributed substantially to the legal outcome. The cases reviewed here include faulty record keeping, failure to include information, charting after the fact, misplaced records, and failure to follow set standards of care when using charting by exception. All these cases contain important lessons about the courts' determination to uphold standards of documentation.

Faulty record keeping

Rogers v. Kasdan (1981) involved a woman who died of brain damage 7 days after admission for injuries sustained in an accident. The Supreme Court of Kentucky ruled against the doctor and the hospital, based on the patient's medical record: the emergency department records were incomplete, fluid intake and output was incorrectly tallied, and other records contained discrepancies or were illegible or incomplete.

Absence of information

St. Paul Fire and Marine Insurance Co. v. Prothro (1979) involved a claim in which the patient, after undergoing a total hip replacement, was injured while being lowered into a Hubbard tank by an orderly. The metal basket holding him collapsed, struck his hip, and reopened the wound. The orderly stopped the bleeding and took the plaintiff to his room, where a nurse treated the wound. However, the nurse failed to document the incident. The wound subsequently became infected, necessitating removal of the prosthesis and leaving the patient with a permanent limp. The court ruled in the patient's favor and noted that a determining factor was the absence of critical information on the patient's chart, which would have helped the doctor and staff provide proper care.

Charting after the fact

In *Thor v. Boska* (1974), a rewritten copy of a patient's record was suspected of being an altered record. This lawsuit involved a woman who had seen her doctor several times because of a breast lump. Each time, the doctor examined her and made a record of her visit. After 2 years, the woman sought a second opinion and learned that she had breast cancer. She sued her first doctor. But rather than producing his records in court, the doctor brought copies of the records, and said he had copied the originals for legibility. The court reasoned that he was withholding incriminating evidence and ruled in favor of the plaintiff.

Missing records

The case of *Battocchi v. Washington Hosp. Center* (1990) underscores the significance of missing records. In this case, parents brought a medical malpractice suit against the hospital and a doctor for injury to their son during forceps delivery.

The nurse had immediately documented the delivery and posted the record in the chart. Later the hospital's risk management personnel apparently lost the nurses' notes. The court ruled in favor of the hospital and doctor, saying that the jury couldn't presume negligence and causation simply because the hospital lost the nurses' notes. But the appeals court sent the case back to the trial court to determine whether loss of the record stemmed from negligence or impropriety.

Good charting, poor communication

Although thorough documentation is crucial, it's not always enough. Unless you report any significant findings you document, exemplary charting can be worthless. In a 1995 Nebraska case, a couple sued a hospital, claiming that the staff's negligence caused brain damage to their newborn son. Jeffrey Critchfield was born at 7:30 a.m., weighing 4 lb 10 oz. According to the admission assessment, Jeffrey had chest wall retractions, cyanosis, pallor, a weak cry, and flaccid muscles. He was admitted to the neonatal intensive care unit, where nurses documented his grunting, pallor, and chest retractions. At about 7:45 p.m., a nurse documented that Jeffrey was lethargic.

At the trial, a pediatric neurologist testifying for the Critchfields stated that lethargy was a sign of neurologic changes and that nursing observations recorded throughout the night indicated that Jeffrey had signs of acute brain damage from lack of oxygen and blood to the brain. He also said that the nurses should have reported these findings to the attending doctor during the night and early morning hours. Another expert testified that the hospital should have had a policy requiring expert consultation and that if nurses had reported Jeffrey's problems, his brain damage could have been ameliorated. The court ruled in favor of the Critch-

Distinguishing between subjective and objective charting

The most common error nurses make when they chart is writing value judgments and opinions – subjective information – rather than factual, or objective, information. Subjective information reflects how the nurse feels about the patient's condition, not the patient's condition itself. Here are some subjective entries, with their objective alternatives.

SUBJECTIVE CHARTING	OBJECTIVE CHARTING
She is drinking well.	Drank 1,500 ml liquids between 7 a.m. and noon.
She reported good relief from Demerol.	Pain in R hip decreasing, now described as "like a dull toothache."
Dorsalis pedis pulse present. Good pedal pulses.	Peripheral pulses in legs 2 + /4 + bilaterally.
Moves legs and feet well.	Leg strength 5 + /5 + bilaterally all major muscle groups. Sensation intact to light touch, pin; denies numbness or tingling. Skin warm and dry. No edema.
Voiding qs.	Voided 350 ml clear yellow urine in bedpan.
Patient is nervous.	Patient repeatedly asks about length of hospitalization, expected discomfort, and time off from work.
Breath sounds normal.	Breath sounds clear to auscultation all lobes. Chest expansion symmetrical – no cough. Nail beds pink.
Bowel sounds normal.	Bowel sounds present all quadrants – abdomen flat. NPO since 12:01 a.m.
Ate well.	Ate all of soft diet.

fields, reasoning that the hospital had a duty, through its nursing staff, to report medically significant changes in a patient's condition to the attending doctor without delay.

Avoiding documentation errors

Besides their potential impact on patient care, charting errors or omissions, even if seemingly harmless, will undermine your credibility in court. Especially avoid the following.

Omissions

Include all facts that other nurses will need to assess the patient. Otherwise, a court may conclude that you failed to perform an action missing from the record or tried to hide evidence.

Personal opinions

Don't enter personal opinions. (See *Distinguishing between subjective and objective charting*.) Record only factual and objective observations and the patient's statements (*Brookover v. Mary Hitchcock Memorial Hospital*, 1990).

Vague entries

Instead of "Patient had a good day," state why: "Patient did not complain of pain."

Late entries

If a late entry is necessary, identify it as such and sign and date it.

Improper corrections

Never erase or obliterate an error. Instead, draw a single line through it, label it "error," and sign and date it.

Unauthorized entries

Only you should be keeping your records (*Henry By Henry v. St. John's Hospital*, 1987).

Erroneous or vague abbreviations

Use only standard abbreviations, and follow institutional policies.

Illegibility and lack of clarity

Write so that others can read your entry. Use a dictionary if you're unsure of spelling or usage.

Signing your documentation

Sign all notes with your first initial, full last name, and title. Place your signature on the right side of the page as proof that you entered all the information between the previous nurse's signature and your own. If the last entry is unsigned, request that the nurse who made the entry sign it. Draw lines through empty or remaining spaces to prevent subsequent amendments or additions. (See *Signing your nurses' notes* and *Countersigning: Important guidelines*, page 250.)

Avoiding suspicious changes and potential legal traps

In the event of a legal challenge, or if the medical record has been requested for examination in a trial, avoid making

Signing your nurses' notes

To discourage other nurses from adding information to your nurses' notes, draw a line through any blank space after your entry and sign your name on the far right side of the column.

```
p: will continue plan and
request diabetic nurse
specialist to assess patient's
knowledge of diabetes
mellitus 3rd or 4th post-op
day. ——— J. Fallon, R.N.
```

If you don't have enough room to sign your name after the last word in the entry, draw a line from the last word to the end of the line. Then, drop down to the next line, draw a line from the left margin almost to the right margin, and sign your name on the far right side.

```
and hyperglycemia.
a: excellent knowledge of
disease and management.
p: see no need for
additional follow-up. ———
——— J. Fallon, R.N.
```

If you have a lot of information to record and you anticipate running out of room on a page, leave room on the right side of the page for your signature. Sign the page, continue your notes on the next page, and then sign that page as usual.

```
pt. drowsy and relaxed on
(continued) J. Fallon, R.N.
```

```
departure for O.R. ———
——— J. Fallon, R.N.
```

Countersigning: Important guidelines

If you're an RN, you need to be aware of the legality of countersigning notes made by LPNs, LVNs, or nurses' aides when you haven't supervised their actions.

Meaning of your signature

To protect yourself, begin by finding out what your hospital's policy says. Does the hospital interpret countersigning to mean that the LPN, LVN, or nurses' aide performed her nursing actions in the countersigning RN's presence? If so, don't countersign unless you were there when the actions occurred.

If your hospital acknowledges that you don't necessarily have time to witness your co-workers' actions, then your countersignature implies that:
• the notes describe care that the LPN, LVN, or nurses' aide had the authority and competence to perform
• you have verified that all required patient care procedures were actually carried out.

Legal risks of signing another nurse's notes

What should you do if another nurse asks you to document her care or sign her notes? In a word, "Don't." Unless your hospital policy authorizes or requires you to witness someone else's notes, your signature will make you responsible for anything put in the notes above it.

In addition, many lawyers advise against keeping personal notes about a questionable patient care incident. Personal notes that you may use to prepare for a deposition or trial can be obtained by the plaintiff's attorney; in a trial, if you deny using them—or any other source of information other than the patient's record—to refresh your memory, you are perjuring yourself. If you admit you did use personal notes, the notes may be used to incriminate other defendants.

Documenting doctor's orders

Doctor's orders fall into three groups: correct as written, ambiguous, and apparently erroneous. Follow your hospital's policy for clarification of orders that are vague or possibly in error. If your hospital lacks a policy, contact the prescribing doctor, and always document your actions. Then ask your *nursing administrator* for a step-by-step policy to follow in this situation, so that if it happens again, you'll know what to do.

An order may be correct when issued, but improper later because of changes in the patient's status. When this occurs, delay the treatment until you've contacted the doctor and clarified the situation. Follow your hospital's policy for clarifying an order. In *Poor Sisters of St. Francis Seraph of the Perpetual Adoration, et al. v. Catron* (1982), a hospital was held liable for negligence because a nurse failed to question the doctor's use of an endotracheal tube for an excessively long period. The patient's voice box was irreparably damaged.

Guidelines

Ambiguous orders must be clarified with the doctor. Document your efforts to clarify the order and whether or not the order was carried out.

changes, corrections, or additions to it beforehand. To do so would raise suspicion, even if you have legitimate reasons and the best intentions.

If you believe a doctor's order is in error, you should refuse to carry it out. Make a record of your refusal together with the reasons and an account of all communication with the doctor.

If the order is correct as written, initial and checkmark each line. Below the doctor's signature, sign your name, the date, and the time.

Handling verbal orders

As a general rule, verbal and telephone orders are acceptable only under acute or emergency circumstances, when the doctor cannot promptly attend to the patient, or according to institutional policy. Record the order on the doctor's order sheet, note the date and time of the order, and record the order verbatim. On the following line, write "v.o." for verbal order or "t.o." for telephone order and record the doctor's name, followed by your signature and the time. To avoid liability, be certain the doctor *countersigns* the order within the time specified by hospital policy.

Preprinted *standing orders* or *protocols* and standing order admission sheets are usually checkmarked and signed by the doctor, cosigned by the nurse, and retained in the chart according to institutional policy.

Controlled substances

You're responsible for proper storage of *controlled substances* in the nursing unit, as well as for maintaining detailed records of each dose dispensed and the remaining quantities.

The legal consequences of improper charting are especially significant when administering narcotics and other controlled substances and maintaining controlled substance records. Be familiar with your hospital's policy when *dispensing* these drugs. Also be aware of controlled substance acts (federal and state laws that control the distribution, classification, sale, and use of drugs). Consult your institution's policies or contact your state board of nursing for information about these laws. If you have a specific question about the propriety of a policy or procedure in your hospital, talk to your hospital's attorney or write to the state board of nursing and request a formal board opinion or a declaratory ruling.

Administering narcotics

For proper, accurate documentation of narcotics, use the special narcotics records — the control sheet and the check sheet — provided by your hospital pharmacy and follow the procedure described below.

Before you give a narcotic:

• Verify the count in the narcotics drawer.

• Sign the narcotic control sheet to indicate you removed the drug.

• Get another nurse to sign the control sheet if you waste or discard all or part of a dose.

At the end of your shift:

• Record the amount of each narcotic in the drawer on the narcotic sheet while the nurse beginning her shift counts the narcotics out loud.

• Sign the narcotic check sheet only if the count is correct. Have the other nurse countersign.

• Identify and correct any discrepancies before any nurse leaves the unit.

For your own protection, conform to all hospital, nursing department, and pharmacy policies and procedures if an ordered dose of a controlled substance is not administered, or if it is wasted or discarded.

Computerized medical records

Like the manual record system, the computerized medical record provides a detailed account of the patient's clinical status, diagnostic tests, treatments, and medical history. But unlike the manual system, the computerized record stores all the patient's medical data in a single, easily accessible source.

Using computers to maintain and access records dramatically increases efficiency and precision. Computerization improves the quality and accuracy of the documentation, makes the patient record more complete, and keeps patient information more current. The computerized record also allows practitioners to rely less on human recall, which helps to increase accuracy. Computers prove especially useful in areas that benefit from automated patient monitoring, such as the *intensive care unit* (ICU) and the *coronary care unit.*

Hospital computer systems

Senior hospital officials usually introduce computers for the sake of controlling health care costs. A hospital's computer system typically consists of a large, centralized computer to store information, which is linked to smaller video display terminals (VDTs) in each work area. Ideally, there should be a computer terminal at each bedside.

To use the system, a nurse signs in by typing on the keyboard a signature code, or password, that gives her access to a patient's records. The computer recognizes by the signature code that she has authorized access to the information stored in its memory. After a patient's *code* number is entered, the computer displays the patient's records on the screen. The nurse may access care plans, vital signs, medication records, general progress notes, laboratory and diagnostic test results, assessment findings, discharge plans, and other information. The nurse can also order a printed copy of the patient's record.

Benefits of a computerized system
Just how computer technology will change the nursing profession remains to be seen. Some experts predict a paperless chart. Health care reform may further transform the documentation process with the creation of a universal medical record that follows a patient through life. At best, integrating computers into your practice will free you to spend more time meeting the needs of your patients. The computerized medical record can save time spent filing, searching for, and retrieving information about a patient. By improving legibility, computers reduce the risk of misinterpretation. Computers also reduce misinterpretation by offering standardized, structured input formats and mandatory charting fields for assessment reports, flow charts, and care plans. And time-stamping can minimize scheduling errors.

Disadvantages
Many critics fear that computers will diminish the personal satisfaction that nurses derive from practicing their profession. They argue that technical advances tend to have a dehumanizing effect on the workplace. Relying on computers may mean less opportunity for interaction and communication with co-workers and patients. In addition, patients may be less truthful in providing medical histories and details about illnesses if they know that the information is going into a computer, which could be used to improperly divulge their medical information.

Another disadvantage of a computerized medical record system is the need for backup records in case computers break down, thereby making information unavailable. Ensuring completeness and continuity in charting requires a backup system. Poorly designed computer systems or human error can also scramble entries and disseminate flawed data.

Verifying computerized records

Verification is one way of reducing errors in the computerized record. It serves the same purpose as signing off on the manual record of a doctor's order. To use verification, the unit secretary enters the doctor's order into the computer. The order is held in a "suspense file" until a nurse reviews the entry, verifies the order, and adds it to the active record file.

Legal concerns

The legal implications of computerized medical records are evolving. (See *Computer charting: Minimizing your legal risks*.) Most computer records are legitimate substitutes for manual records. But some state laws require written records as well.

The most pressing legal questions concern the threat to patient *privacy* and *confidentiality.* With traditional records, information is restricted simply by keeping the record on the unit, but computer records can be called up at any terminal in the facility. The primary safeguard is the signature code, which limits access to the records. For example, a nurse's code would call up a·patient's entire record, but a technician's code would produce only part of it.

Various laws protect the privacy of a patient's medical records. The Federal Privacy Act of 1974 protects the confidential medical information of patients in veterans' hospitals, and some state nurse practice acts impose an ethical *duty* to guard patients' privacy. However, no one can fully guarantee that unauthorized persons won't gain access to computerized records.

Care must also be taken to safeguard patient information sent by facsimile (fax) machines. In particular, policies and procedures should be established to prevent confidential patient information, such as a positive human im-

---

Computer charting: Minimizing your legal risks

Your liability when working with computer documentation is exactly the same as when working with a manual system. You may be liable for any patient injuries associated with charting errors.

To minimize your legal risks:
● Always double-check all patient information entered.
● Don't divulge signature codes.
● Inform your supervisor if you suspect that someone is using your code.
● Indicate whether the doctor's order is written, verbal (in person), or verbal (by telephone) and when the entry is made.
● Know your state's rules and regulations and the hospital's policies and procedures regarding privileged data, confidentiality, and disclosure. To learn about state rules and regulations, consult your hospital's policy and procedure manual, check with your hospital's attorney, or consult your state board of nursing or the state statutory and administrative codes.

---

munodeficiency virus report, from being transmitted by a fax machine — especially one that's centrally located and available to many staff members.

In addition, hospitals must show that their computer systems are reliable enough to be used in court. For example, the software that's used should automatically record the date and time of each entry and each correction, as well as the name of the author or anyone who modifies a record. When an error is corrected, the software should preserve both the original and corrected versions and identify each author.

Challenging a computer record in court

In 1977, a patient in New York charged that use of a computerized record system was an invasion of his privacy. In *Whalen v. Roe* (1977), the patient challenged the constitutionality of a state law that required patients who bought certain prescription drugs to list their name, address, age, the drug, dosage, and prescribing doctor's name for the state's database. The Supreme Court upheld the law but acknowledged the threat to privacy implicit in the system. The court reasoned that the central storage and easy accessibility of computerized data vastly increase the potential for abuse of that information.

Tammelleo, A.D. "Charting by Exception: There are Perils," *RN* 57(10):71-72, October 1994.

Tammelleo, A.D. "Court Holds Charting by Exception Policy Negligent," *The Regan Report on Nursing Law* 34(12), May 1994.

Tammelleo, A.D. "Good Charting-Bad Communications: Recipe for Disaster," *The Regan Report on Nursing Law* 36(2), July 1995.

Selected references

Accreditation Manual for Hospitals. Chicago: Joint Commission on Accreditation of Healthcare Organizations, 1995.

Andreola, N., and O'Neill, P. "Managed Care: The Great Debate," *Nursing Spectrum* 6(15):4-5, July 25, 1994.

Bergman, R. "Getting the Goods on Guidelines," *Hospitals and Health Networks* 68(20):70, 72, 74, October 20, 1994.

"Clinical Pathways and Risk," *QRC Advisor* 11(8):1, 6-7, June 1995.

Dandry-Aiken, T.D., and Catalano, J.T. *Legal, Ethical, and Political Issues in Nursing.* Philadelphia: F.A. Davis Co., 1994.

Gobis, L.J. "Computerized Patient Records: Start Preparing Now," *Journal of Nursing Law* 2(2):39-43, Winter 1995.

"Implementing Charting by Exception: Nursing Project #3," *Health Care Advisory Board: Issue Tracking Service.* NUI-005-003, May 1995.

Mastering Documentation. Springhouse, Pa.: Springhouse Corp., 1995.

7

Nurses' rights as employees

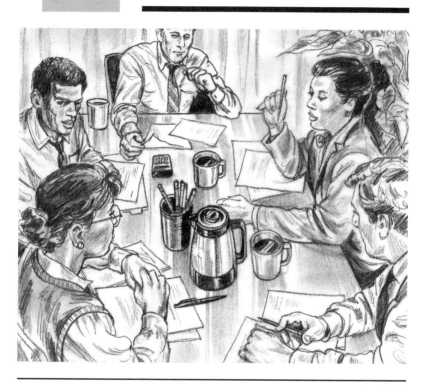

Decent wages mean financial security for you and your family. Optimal working conditions can mean improved job security, enhanced job satisfaction, and the opportunity to deliver the best possible care to your patients. But to achieve the wages and working conditions you deserve, you need to understand your rights as an employee. You also need to be prepared to fight back if your employee rights are violated.

Becoming familiar with the information in this chapter will help you assert your employee rights. The focus is on two crucial issues: how to read and understand an employment contract and the pros and cons of joining a union. You'll learn about types of contracts, implied conditions, and what to do if your employer commits a breach of contract. You'll also learn about the strategies unions use to protect the rights of nurse-members, including *collective bargaining, grievance procedures,* strikes, and *arbitration.*

Understanding employment contracts

Most nurses are hired without the benefit of a written employment contract. Usually, an application or a résumé is submitted and an agreement is reached as to starting date, position, benefits, and starting pay. This arrangement is no less *legal* than a written contract. It does, however, present certain problems if, at a later date, some portion of the employment agreement is disputed by either party.

If you do sign an employment contract, read it carefully to make sure it adequately defines your *duties,* authority, and *benefits.* Learning to interpret contract terms will help you function within the contract's specified limits. Also be sure to read carefully the procedure for terminating the contract.

Currently, labor attorneys try to draft most employment agreements as *at-will* contracts, meaning that either party can end the agreement for any reason or for no reason. This is in contrast to the less common *just cause* agreements, in which the employer has to have just cause to fire you (and avoid penalties for a wrongful termination, after a court case). You can understand the benefits of the at-will contract for an employer. Of course, the employer risks having the employee quit without any reason at any time.

Types of contracts

A contract is a legally binding promise between two parties that can be enforced in court. According to U.S. and Canadian law, a contract is legally binding if all of these provisions apply:

• You've accepted an offer, verbal or written, to perform in a certain capacity.

• You and the other person are legally competent (of legal age and without mental impairment).

• You both understand the agreement.

• Terms of the agreement are lawful.

• You receive something of value, such as money, for fulfilling the agreement.

In general, agreements regarding conscience, morals, and social activities aren't legally binding. If you break a lunch date, you can't be fined or taken to court. But if you violate any term in a legally binding contract, you might face consequences.

Formal contract

Usually, your contract with an employer is a formal, written contract. It may be an individual contract, which you *negotiate,* or a *collectively bargained contract,* agreed to by a nurse negotiation committee and a labor organization or union. In either contract, wage increases may be awarded automatically or may be linked to merit or experience.

Oral express contract

An employment agreement is usually an oral contract, offered and accepted verbally. Most states allow parties to orally agree to employment relationships, and those contracts are just as legal and enforceable in court (assuming state law allows them). However, because the judge and jury will not have a written contract to consider, other documents (handbook, notice of a physical examination, welcoming letter, pay stubs, and so on) would play a major role in proving that such an oral contract existed and in verifying its content.

Finally, witnesses who may have overheard the offer extended to the nurse and the nurse's acceptance may be called to testify at any hearing before the magistrate to prove the existence of an oral employment agreement.

Pitfalls of oral contracts

Contracts need not be in writing to be legally binding; a handshake over a deal may constitute a contract. But oral contracts can cause legal problems. Memories fail and witnesses move away. The needs of the parties may change under new administrators. Consequently, if the original agreement is not in writing, the subjective and fallible memories of the parties may have to reconstruct it. If the matter must be litigated, more time and money will be spent to prove what could have been simply put into writing.

If an employer does not offer you a written contract, you can write a letter to the person with whom you spoke, confirming that you accept their offer and repeating the facts you heard. Confirm the starting date and say that you look forward to working with them. Be sure to put all important, agreed-to terms and conditions in the letter. At the end, ask the employer to notify you in writing about any omissions or disagreement about the facts in your letter. Send it, but first make a copy for your file at home. Hopefully, you'll never need to refer to it.

Implied conditions

Most contracts contain *implied conditions* — elements that aren't explicitly stated but are assumed to be part of the contract. For example, your employer assumes that you'll practice nursing in a safe, competent manner, as defined by your *nurse practice act,* and that you'll maintain the hospital's standards and policies. You assume, based on implied conditions, that the employer will staff your unit adequately with qualified personnel and ensure a safe working environment with the necessary supplies and equipment.

Components of a legal contract

To be legal, a contract must include the following components.

A promise
Two or more legally competent parties must promise each other to do or not do something.

Mutual understanding
The parties involved must clearly understand the terms and obligations the contract imposes on them.

Compensation
The parties involved must agree that, to fulfill the contract, only lawful actions will be performed in exchange for something of value.

Offer and acceptance

In any contract, there must be an offer and an acceptance. An offer must be definite and communicated by words or actions. If you fail to respond, the employer can't interpret your silence as acceptance, but he may withdraw his offer without penalty. Although you may verbally accept an offer or simply report for duty, a written acceptance is recommended. The employment contract should be as specific as possible about wages, hours, and the terms and conditions of the relationship. (See *Components of a legal contract.*)

Breach of contract

Unjustified failure to perform all or part of your contractual duty is a *breach of contract,* and substantial breaches are never lawful. If the breach is substantial, the entire agreement may have been broken and legal damages may result. If only part of the agreement has been breached, the remaining contract may be in effect, and both parties may want to continue the relationship with some clarification. Breaches can be avoided where both parties carefully consider the terms and conditions of the contract and know what they are promising each other.

Employee breach of contract

When you agree to do (or not do) something in an employment contract and you don't perform as promised, you may be in breach of contract and subject to litigation forcing you to perform as promised. You may even be required to reimburse your employer for the cost of hiring someone to do the job and to pay for his court costs and legal fees.

Of course, the terms and conditions of a contract can be changed or modified by verbal or written agreement. For example, your organization may need you to work at a different location. Agreements can be renegotiated or verbally modified. Certainly, it's far better to change a contract than to breach it. Good communication may prevent a perceived breach and renegotiation is cheaper than litigation.

Employer breach of contract

An employer also may breach a contract. If, for example, he fails to give you the vacation time agreed to, he has breached the contract. If you discover a breach, follow the procedures in your employee handbook. Often, misunderstandings can be cleared up by talking with the appropriate persons in the chain of command (in a professional and nonemotional manner). If documents are involved, they are important proof. If you have a union contract, tell your union representative as soon as you're aware of a breach.

If you exhaust all channels of appeal, you may need to discuss the problem with an attorney with contract expertise. You'll need a written log of your attempts to rectify the situation, including statements made, dates, and times.

Canadian law

Because the laws vary between Canada and the U.S., it's best to check with local legal counsel about procedures and deadlines. If you work as a nurse in Canada, you may find that the provincial government offers free contract processing services.

When is a contract invalid?

A nursing employment contract is considered invalid when the agreement concerns actions that are illegal or impossible to carry out, or when any of the following applies:

- An applicant has lied about qualifications.
- A nurse is forced to sign a contract.
- The agreement involves theft or other crimes.
- A *minor* or *mentally incompetent* person signs the contract.

Note that if you become physically or mentally disabled it does not automatically void an employment contract. You may be protected under the Americans with Disabilities Act, which requires the employer to make reasonable accomodations in certain instances.

Terminating a contract

When you *terminate* a contract, you've either fulfilled or absolved yourself of all your obligations. Since most employment contracts don't specify termination dates, you can end them at any time, if you follow proper notification procedures. You also can end contracts with termination dates if your employer agrees. Follow the contract's procedures for giving written notice (most require 2 to 4 weeks).

Employer discharge

Your employer can terminate your contract if he determines that you're incompetent or that you've behaved unprofessionally on the job. Before discharging you, he'll probably give you several warnings about the quality of your work. Then he might confront you with several examples of your shortcomings from previous written evaluations of your performance. If you don't want to lose your job, you should discuss areas of improvement and a *probation period.*

If you disagree with your employer's complaints, you can request an evaluation by someone else who supervised your work, or you can request a transfer to another unit where you'd be reevaluated after an agreed-upon length of time. However, your employer isn't obligated to agree to either request. If he doesn't, you can seek written support from your co-workers that will refute your employer's complaints. You can also seek support from your employee union, if you have one. It may file a *grievance* on your behalf.

Most hospitals operate on an employment-at-will basis, in which there is either no employment contract or the existing contract fails to specify the job's duration. However, the hospital can't violate a bargaining agreement mandating proof of just cause for discipline or discharge.

Some state courts have broadened employee rights by prohibiting certain discharges of at-will employees if the discharge violates public policies — for example, the firing of a nurse who reports the hospital's illegal drug distribution procedure.

Unions

Although individual contracts provide significant legal protection, employees in many areas — from farmworkers, laborers, and truck drivers to actors, teachers, and musicians — have found that they are better off signing a contract negotiated for them as a group. Their union representatives engage in collective bargaining for contract conditions. When necessary, they use arbitration, strikes, and threats of strikes to enhance their terms of employment and enforce contracts.

Nurses' unions

Until 1974, only nurses working in for-profit hospitals or *nursing homes* could join unions. That year, Congress amended the National Labor Relations Act to allow the employees of private, not-for-profit health care institutions and agencies to unionize. Since then, the number of unionized nurses has increased dramatically.

The National Labor Relations Act now applies to employees of hospitals and other health care facilities with an annual revenue of at least $250,000 and to nursing homes, visiting nurses' associations, and related facilities with an annual revenue of at least $100,000. Also, many states now have collective bargaining laws patterned after the National Labor Relations Act that control public sector bargaining in the state.

In 1991, the U.S. Supreme Court decided, in *American Hospital Association v. NLRB,* that it is appropriate for collective bargaining units in acute care facilities to bargain for RNs, doctors, and other health care professionals. After the 1991 decision, unions began campaigns to organize nurses, but when hospitals began to downsize, union growth was dampened. Today, state affiliates of the American Nurses' Association (ANA) serve as the bargaining agent for most unionized nurses (more than 140,000).

Where nursing unions exist, management occasionally challenges them

Nurses' associations and collective bargaining

Most RNs choose their state nurses' association as their collective bargaining representative. Because nurses' associations are professional associations—not just labor organizations—their role in the collective bargaining process is controversial.

Arguments in favor of collective bargaining

Proponents contend that state nurses' associations are the natural labor representatives for nurses, who come to the bargaining table concerned about much more than just their salaries and working conditions. Indeed, Plank 9 of the American Nurses' Association's (ANA's) Code of Ethics states: "The nurse participates in the profession's efforts to establish and maintain conditions of employment conducive to high-quality nursing care." Hence many nurses believe that their state nurses' associations provide the appropriate channel for working effectively, ethically, and with professional dignity in the collective bargaining process.

Arguments against collective bargaining

Nonetheless, association members who oppose this activity wonder whether collective bargaining itself is professional, or whether it's an appropriate role for their professional associations to play. Members of some associations think not, and consequently their associations don't engage in collective bargaining.

Employers and other unions also question whether associations represent the interests and needs of staff nurses. They contend that so many association members are supervisors and administrators that the associations are management dominated and, therefore, inappropriate employee bargaining representatives. Some employers discourage their nurse-managers from participating in their state nurses' associations because of the associations' labor activities. However, hospital associations have not successfully sustained a management domination claim against a state nurses' association since 1983, when the state associations were restructured to insulate the managerial and supervisory membership from collective bargaining.

Activities

Once a state nurses' association becomes involved in collective bargaining, its activities are the same as any other bargaining agent's. The association represents its members in contract negotiations and in resolving grievances.

on the grounds that nurses perform in supervisory capacities. So far, the National Labor Relations Board has ruled that nurses who work in charge positions, and who direct others, do so based on professional knowledge and skill, which does not make them supervisors. (See *Nurses' associations and collective bargaining*.)

Joining a union: Pros and cons

Union officials have targeted the hospital field as one of the last large industries ripe for organizing. Unionization continues to spark debate within the nursing profession. According to Sandra Houglan, RN, MS, director of the Center for Labor Relations of the ANA, some 500,000 registered nurses are potential union members. Whether the union movement in health care can gain momentum remains to be seen. (See *Joining a nurses' union.*)

Pros

Union proponents argue that unionization gives nurses a strong voice in such bread-and-butter issues as wages, benefits, and pensions. Unionization, they argue, assures fair grievance procedures and more influence in patient care decisions. Unionization also gives nurses more control over working conditions, such as scheduling and staffing, and equalizes bargaining power between employer and employee.

Cons

Critics argue that unionization tarnishes the image of the nursing profession by shifting emphasis away from patient care to economic advancement. Many nurses are reluctant to depend on an organization for their economic and professional well-being. Still others object to the cost of union dues, as well as the expenditure of time and effort that unions require of their members. Some nurses fear the potential disruption of picketing and strikes. Others argue that unionization creates antagonism between nurses and their employers, preventing effective cooperation.

Questions to consider

Before deciding whether to participate in collective bargaining, ask yourself these questions:
- Will collective bargaining help my professional and economic status?
- Can I address my professional concerns through collective bargaining?
- Can I devote the time and effort that such organized activity demands?
- Can I change my working conditions as an individual, or do I need to organize with other nurses?

If you believe that organizing a union is necessary to improve the professional or economic status of the nurses

---

QUESTIONS ABOUT THE LAW

Joining a nurses' union

For most nurses, the decision to join a union is a difficult one. Here are some answers to frequently asked questions about unionization.

Can I join a labor union?
Yes. Congress amended the National Labor Relations Act in 1974 to allow employees of private, not-for-profit hospitals and health care institutions to unionize. The law covers all private hospitals that provide at least $250,000 worth of health care services a year and all related facilities that provide services worth at least $100,000. Most hospitals and nursing homes fall into these categories.

Can I be forced to join a union?
If you work under a "union shop" contract, you must join the union within a specified time to remain employed. If the contract provides for an "open shop," you can choose not to join the union and still keep your job.

Can the hospital where I work fire me for helping to organize a union?
Federal regulations strictly forbid your employer from firing you or taking any other reprisal against you for union organizing.

What consequences do I face if I refuse to participate in my union's strike?
As long as you continue working, your hospital or health care facility will pay your wages and benefits. No union can force you to strike. But you might face some antagonism, even retaliation, from those colleagues who do strike.

Recognizing unfair labor practices

You have a legal right to participate in union activities. If your employer infringes on that right—through interference, domination, discrimination, or refusal to bargain—you can charge your employer with unfair labor practices.

Interference

Employers may interfere with a union election by unilaterally improving wages or benefits during a union campaign to encourage employees to vote against the union. Other types of interference include:

- making coercive statements about participation in union activities
- threatening to close down the facility if a union is elected
- questioning employees about union activities
- spying on—or implying the possibility of spying on—union meetings.

Domination

Management may attempt to dominate a union by paying a union's expenses, giving union leaders special compensation or benefits, or taking an active part in organizing a union.

Discrimination

This unfair labor practice may involve discharging, disciplining, or threatening an employee for joining a union or for encouraging others to join. Other types of discrimination include:

- refusing to hire anyone who belongs to a union
- refusing to reinstate or promote an employee because she testified at a National Labor Relations Board hearing
- enforcing rules unequally between employees who are involved in union activities and those who aren't.

Refusal to bargain

To weaken union participation, management may refuse to take part in collective bargaining. One strategy involves taking unilateral action to alter employment conditions that either are covered in an existing contract or are included among legally mandated areas of bargaining. Other unfair labor practices include:

- refusing to meet with a union representative
- refusing to negotiate a mandatory issue
- demanding to negotiate a voluntary issue.

in your institution, the full force of the law will protect your efforts.

Protecting the right to unionize

In the United States, regulations governing union organizing among nurses in private-sector employment come under the jurisdiction of the National Labor Relations Board (NLRB), the agency that enforces federal labor laws.

The NLRB protects your right to organize a union, join a union, or decertify a union (vote the union out), and may defend you against *unfair labor practices.* The NLRB also helps employers by enforcing regulations that control picketing and strikes, and by providing remedies for any unfair union practices.

If you decide to organize a union, the NLRB supervises procedures for elections. These procedures enforce rules that both the union and management must follow. The NLRB works to investigate any unfair labor practices that may arise during the election process. (See *Recognizing unfair labor practices.*)

Initiating a union drive

To organize a collective bargaining unit at your facility, begin by contacting your state nurses' association, if it engages in collective bargaining, or the union of your choice.

An experienced worker, usually a former hospital employee, will be assigned by the union to help you organize your campaign. The union may support your efforts by supplying stationery, printing, legal advice, organizational guidance, and encouragement. The union can also arrange for meeting halls and publicity, and can file the proper election petitions with the NLRB.

Management's rights and limitations during a union drive

To protect your right to organize and belong to a union, the NLRB places the following limitations on management:

• Management can't interfere with your organizing activities.

• Management can't discriminate against you for participating in union activities, for testifying against management, or for filing a grievance.

• Management can't dominate a union by gaining undue influence over it, such as by paying union expenses or giving union leaders special benefits.

• Management can't refuse to bargain in *good faith.*

• Management must assume responsibility for any unfair labor practice committed by a supervisor. (See *The NLRB: Protecting your right to organize a union,* page 264.)

Management also has rights protected by the NLRB. Under the law, management can:

• tell you the disadvantages of belonging to a union

• explain to you your election rights, such as your right to refuse to sign an *authorization card*

• encourage you to vote "no" in a union election (provided they don't use threats or coercion of any kind).

Limitations placed on the union

The union must also comply with certain limitations. The NLRB ensures that the union:

• bargains in good faith

• assumes responsibility for any unfair labor practice committed by union officials

• doesn't threaten or force you to support the union

• doesn't demand that your employer do business only with companies that have unions.

Neither management nor the union can interfere with your individual rights as guaranteed by federal or state law. Federal laws that help protect employee rights include the Fair Labor Standards Act, the Civil Rights Act, and the Age Discrimination in Employment Act. States may also enact protective legislation, such as so-called "whistle-blower" statutes, equal employment opportunity acts, or public employee collective bargaining laws.

Union election

In the initial step toward a union election, nurses or union representatives distribute authorization cards. Nurses who want a union election sign an authorization card. In the United States, if at least 30% of the eligible nurses sign the cards, you or the union can ask the NLRB to authorize and supervise an election. If 50% or more of the eligible nurses sign the cards, U.S. law allows the employer to forgo the election process and simply recognize the union, but this rarely occurs. In Canada, more than 50% of the nurses must sign the cards to authorize an election.

The NLRB: Protecting your right to organize a union

If your hospital punishes you solely because you're involved in union organizing activities, the federal government, in the form of the National Labor Relations Board (NLRB), will protect you. The board enforces the National Labor Relations Act, which explicitly sets forth your rights to form and join a union.

An example

For instance, suppose you're working as a hospital pediatrics nurse, and you support unionization of the hospital's nurses. Union organizers ask you to distribute pro-union pamphlets to your colleagues. You begin giving out pamphlets in the nurses' lounge, but a hospital administrator orders you to stop. He says the hospital's solicitation policy prohibits anyone from distributing literature inside the hospital. You remind him that the hospital has allowed nurses to distribute other information, such as literature to recruit volunteers for the local cancer society. You

ignore the administrator's order and resume handing out the pamphlets.

The next day you're called into your nursing supervisor's office and fired. Stunned, you ask for an explanation. The supervisor gives you two reasons: violating the hospital's nonsolicitation policy and disobeying the administrator.

You file an unfair labor practice charge with the NLRB. After a hearing, the board concludes that the hospital can't prevent you from distributing the pamphlets on your own time in a nonwork area. The board also concludes that the hospital was discriminatory in applying the nonsolicitation policy.

A likely ruling

In this situation, the board would order the hospital to reinstate you, pay your back wages, and refrain from punishing you or any other nurse who was active in the union drive.

(See *What happens when nurses decide to unionize.*)

Union and management may disagree about which nurses are eligible to vote. Either side can challenge a nurse's eligibility. In the United States, the NLRB will settle an eligibility dispute by reviewing the nurse's job description, her duties and responsibilities, and her supervisory functions, if any.

To win the election, the union must get a majority of the votes of those nurses who actually voted, not those who are eligible to vote.

In a rare case, more than one union may be on the ballot. This can happen when, after the first petitioning, the union demonstrates that 30% or more of the eligible nurses want an election.

If this occurs, other unions can get on the ballot provided they can obtain a show of interest from 10% of the nurse-employees.

If elected, the union will negotiate a contract addressing mutually agreeable wages, benefits, and work rules and other professional issues. The contract will be devised by the negotiators and ratified by members of the bargaining unit.

Maintaining perspective

If you commit yourself to a unionization drive, be prepared to expend a great deal of energy. Don't let your commitment prevent you from nurturing good relations with supervisors and co-workers who oppose the union. Keep in mind that, regardless of the election's

What happens when nurses decide to unionize

The decision to unionize initiates a step-by-step process. First, organizers distribute leaflets and authorization cards. At least 30% of all the proposed union employees must sign those cards to authorize a union election.

Steps in the election process

After the employees sign the authorization cards, the following occurs:

1. The union organizer notifies the National Labor Relations Board (NLRB), and an NLRB representative steps in to referee and organize the election.

2. The NLRB holds a hearing to decide who's eligible to join the bargaining unit. The employer may challenge any employee's eligibility. For example, an employee in a supervisory position may not be considered eligible according to the employer's interpretation of the law.

3. The NLRB determines the place and election date. The employer and the union can then begin campaigning.

4. Within 7 days of the NLRB announcement of the election date and place, the employer provides the NLRB with a list of the names and addresses of all eligible employees. The NLRB gives this list to the union.

5. On election day, employees vote by secret ballot to accept or reject the union. If more than one union is on the ballot, employees can select one of the unions or vote for no representation at all.

6. The NLRB representative tallies the votes. The results depend on the majority of ballots cast, regardless of what percentage of eligible employees actually vote. (If only a minority of eligible employees vote, those few employees will decide the question of unionization for all.)

The outcome

If a majority of the voting employees choose the union, that union is legally required to represent all eligible employees, even those who didn't vote. The NLRB will certify the union as the employees' collective bargaining representative.

If a majority of the voting employees reject the union, the law prohibits another election involving any union for 1 year.

---

outcome, everyone will continue to work together. If the union wins, both management and labor will have to adjust to new rules spelled out in the contract. If the union loses, management should correct the problems that led to the organizing campaign, or expect to face a renewed union effort.

Legal issues in collective bargaining

In collective bargaining, the employer and the employees' representatives meet to confer about employment issues and put their agreements in writing. According to the National Labor Relations Board (NLRB), two or more people who share employment interests and conditions may constitute a bargaining unit. (See *Landmarks in the history of collective bargaining*, page 266.)

The NLRB's role in collective bargaining

In the U.S., laws governing collective bargaining are outlined in the National Labor Relations Act and the Labor Management Relations Act (LMRA, also called the Taft-Hartley Act). The NLRB is the federal agency authorized

Landmarks in the history of collective bargaining

Since winning the right to unionize, nurses have made great strides in collective bargaining. Today, nurses across the country are improving their professional and economic status through active participation in collective bargaining units. The following is a summary of major legislative landmarks in the struggle for collective bargaining rights.

1935: Congress passes the National Labor Relations Act. This act requires employers to bargain with their employees and provides for the formation of the National Labor Relations Board (NLRB) to enforce the provisions of the act.

1946: The American Nurses' Association (ANA) launches its Economic Security Program to establish national salary guidelines for nurses. ANA takes an active role in supporting nurses' right to bargain collectively.

1947: The Labor Management Relations Act (LMRA) – known as the Taft-Hartley Act – says that nonprofit organizations, including nonprofit hospitals, don't have to bargain with their employees.

1962: An amendment to the LMRA gives federal employees, including nurses, the right to bargain collectively.

1974: The Taft-Hartley Amendment, officially named the 1974 Health Care Amendments to the Taft-Hartley Act, explicitly grants employees of not-for-profit health care institutions and agencies the right to bargain collectively.

1991: In *American Hospital Association v. NLRB*, the U.S. Supreme Court upholds NLRB regulations that make it easier for unions to organize hospital workers.

State law

Before passage of the 1974 Health Care Amendments to the Taft-Hartley Act, several states had passed legislation requiring not-for-profit hospitals to bargain with their employees. Consequently, nurses who worked for such hospitals in Connecticut, Idaho, Massachusetts, Michigan, Minnesota, Montana, New Jersey, New York, Oregon, Pennsylvania, and Wisconsin had some bargaining rights all along.

State legislatures have also passed laws defining the rights of nurses who work for state, county, and municipal health care institutions. Some states gave these government employees the right to organize and bargain, but not the right to strike. Other states assigned a specific arm of the state government to negotiate labor concerns or mandate pay scales for state-employed nurses.

to administer and enforce these laws. (See *Appealing to the NLRB.*)

The NLRB's responsibilities include determining appropriate bargaining units for employee groups, resolving disputes between labor and management, and conducting elections for employee bargaining representatives. The NLRB will not assert jurisdiction over labor laws for minimum wages, over-

time pay, termination, or discrimination unless those issues have been written into the employees' labor contract and the contract doesn't provide for *binding arbitration* of alleged violations. If arbitration is provided for, the NLRB usually declines its jurisdiction and defers to the *arbitrator*.

Appealing to the NLRB

If you're organizing a union and feel that management is engaging in unfair labor practices, begin by telling your union representative. If she believes your charges are valid, either you or the union can appeal to the National Labor Relations Board (NLRB).

NLRB response

The board will ask you for a sworn statement concerning the dates and times of the alleged events, the names and positions of management staff involved, and the names and addresses of other employee witnesses. Your statement will serve as a legal affidavit that will supply the NLRB with the information it needs to carry out an investigation.

Should the NLRB investigate and find that management is engaging in unfair labor practices, it will issue a formal complaint against your employer. The employer may appeal the board's complaint, but if the court upholds it, then the employer must comply with the board's penalty—usually reinstating employees, issuing back pay, or restoring other benefits.

An example

While nurses at Good Faith Hospital were organizing a union campaign, supervisors asked them for the names of nurses who attended meetings sponsored by the organizers. Also, one supervisor suggested to her staff that if a nurses' union was organized, the union might try to force management to increase wages—which, because of the hospital's precarious financial position, could result in layoffs. Several nurses complained about the supervisor's remarks at a subsequent union meeting. The union organizers agreed that management was interfering with union organization—an unfair labor practice—and consequently filed a charge with the NLRB.

Canadian law

In Canada, the provincial labor relations boards handle local labor issues, and the Canada Labour Relations Board deals with labor issues at the federal level, as in the case of military hospitals.

Bargaining units

Bargaining units usually represent different groups of workers in the same hospital. The National Labor Relations Act empowers the NLRB to decide what's an appropriate bargaining unit. This gives the NLRB considerable power. It's much easier to unionize employees if there's a bargaining unit for each kind of job classification; employees in each bargaining unit will have more shared interests.

In 1987, the NLRB issued rules permitting eight bargaining units for acute care hospitals. Since its establishment in 1935, this was the first time the NLRB had drafted rules defining permissible bargaining units for an entire industry. These bargaining units are:
- *registered nurses* (RNs)
- doctors
- professionals, except for RNs and doctors
- technical employees
- skilled maintenance employees
- business office clerical employees
- guards
- all other nonprofessional employees.

In response to these 1987 rules, the ***American Hospital Association*** (AHA), which represents management, filed suit. In *American Hospital Association v.*

NLRB (1991), the AHA claimed that the NLRB rules were illegal, arguing that the Taft-Hartley Act requires determination of appropriate *bargaining units* in each individual hospital.

The U.S. Supreme Court unanimously rejected the AHA's interpretation and ruled that the NLRB has the power to promulgate rules for all hospitals, not just on a hospital-by-hospital basis. This ruling makes it easier for unions to organize hospital workers and is considered a blow to management.

Other NLRB functions

In addition to rule-making, the NLRB resolves disputes by interpreting provisions of the LMRA. The NLRB hears cases on the supervisor's role and the employee's right to solicit new members or picket. The NLRB also determines whether labor or management has committed unfair acts during a campaign or the term of a contract. For example, in *NLRB v. Baptist Hospital* (1979), the NLRB upheld its rule against soliciting new members in upper-floor hospital halls and sitting rooms near patients, but upheld the employees' right to talk about the union in first-floor lobbies and other areas away from patients.

If a hospital or bargaining unit disagrees with an NLRB decision, either party can appeal in a federal *appellate court.* Canadian courts won't interfere with a professional organization's decision unless it has acted outside its jurisdiction or violated *common law.*

Mandatory bargaining issues

The NLRB has broadly interpreted the *mandatory bargaining issues* (issues an employer must address during bargaining) to include wages and hours; seniority; leaves of absence; work schedules and assignments; breaks, holidays, and vacations; benefits; promotion and layoff policies; and grievance and discipline procedures. (See *Perils of not bargaining.*)

Voluntary issues

Bargaining on other issues may occur if both parties voluntarily agree. The NLRB considers *voluntary bargaining issues* to include all other possible legal employment issues. Because nurses can't force an employer to bargain over voluntary issues, whether negotiations occur usually depends on how committed nurses are to their professional concerns and on management's willingness to be flexible.

Negotiations

Before bargaining begins, negotiators should prepare for the procedure by understanding the beliefs and attitudes of the people they represent and developing a system of communication between negotiators and the bargaining unit. They should also consider in advance how management may respond to various issues.

The actual bargaining involves good faith negotiations (an honest desire to reach an agreement) between the union's and management's negotiating teams. Proposals may be exchanged for study before the first session. Each proposal and counterproposal is talked over, and disagreements are discussed in detail, sometimes with teams taking time-outs to privately reconsider their positions. When disagreements persist and outside mediation fails, union members may decide to strike. But if all issues are resolved, the written agreement is taken to the union members with a recommendation that they ratify the terms.

Decision to strike

Collective bargaining doesn't guarantee that the bargaining parties will reach an agreement. If the parties arrive at a stalemate, employees may decide to strike in hopes of forcing the employer to make concessions. A strike

COURT CASE

Perils of not bargaining

A hospital can't avoid collective bargaining by refusing to recognize its nurses' union. The law, strengthened by court decisions, requires a hospital to bargain in good faith with duly elected unions. A key court case, *Eastern Maine Medical Center v. NLRB* (1981), illustrates this principle.

An anti-union stand

Nurses at Eastern Maine Medical Center voted 114 to 110 to be represented by the Maine State Nurses' Association, the state's largest nurses' union. In response, the hospital administration adopted a strong anti-union stand, refusing to meet with the nurses for collective bargaining talks. Moreover, the administration gave substantial wage-and-benefit increases to nonunion employees and withheld the increases from the unionized nurses.

The administration's policy of not bargaining with the union made the union nurses bitter and frustrated. The union filed unfair labor practice charges against the hospital administration.

NLRB ruling

The National Labor Relations Board (NLRB) concluded that the hospital had violated the National Labor Relations Act by refusing to bargain in good faith and by discriminating against the unionized nurses. The board directed the hospital administration to negotiate with the union and to pay the wage-and-benefit increases withheld from members of the bargaining unit.

Appeals court ruling

In upholding the actions of the NLRB, an appeals court ruled that the hospital's refusal to negotiate violated the nurses' collective bargaining rights.

---

decision is an extreme measure, so labor laws have established provisions that require any curtailment of services to be orderly, thus protecting the employer and the public.

In the United States, negotiating parties must follow this timetable—and series of steps—before a strike can be called:

• The side wanting to modify or terminate the contract must notify the other side 90 days before the contract expires (or labor or management proposes that changes take place).

• If, 30 days later, the two sides don't agree, they must notify the Federal Mediation and Conciliation Service (FMCS) and the corresponding state agency of the dispute.

• Within 30 days, the FMCS will appoint a mediator and, in rare cases, an inquiry board. Within 15 days, the mediator or inquiry board will give both sides its recommendations.

• If, after 15 more days, the parties don't agree, the employees may plan to strike. If the union didn't have employees vote earlier, it will hold a vote to to decide whether or not to send a strike notice.

• If a majority of employees vote to send a strike notice, the union must send management the strike notice at least 10 days before the scheduled strike, specifying the exact date, time, and place of the strike. The strike cannot be scheduled before the contract expires.

In most cases, union and management representatives, with the assistance of a mediator, schedule additional negotiations during this period. A strike vote is held before the walkout is scheduled to begin.

Note that, in many states, public-sector employees are prohibited from striking. If an impasse occurs, labor and management must resolve their differences through binding arbitration.

Canadian law

Some Canadian provinces prohibit health care employees from striking. In these provinces, compulsory arbitration is imposed when employees and employer fail to reach an agreement. The arbitrator can then draft and impose contract terms.

Wildcat strikes

Employees who ignore the strike provisions and engage in illegal strikes lose the protection of the National Labor Relations Act. They may be discharged by their employer. Unions that sanction or encourage illegal strikes may have their certification revoked by the NLRB.

Delaying a strike

Employees may delay a strike for up to 72 hours if they feel the extra time would enable them to come to terms with management.

To delay the strike, they must give management written notice at least 12 hours before the time the strike was scheduled to start. If the initial strike date passes during the negotiations, the union must issue another 10-day strike notice. If the contract expires during the negotiations, the employer and employees remain bound by the contract.

Grievances and arbitration

When an employee's dispute isn't resolved, tempers flare, morale declines, and apparent injustices smolder. That's why union and management officials give grievance and arbitration procedures high priority when they negotiate collective bargaining agreements. Even if your workplace isn't unionized, understanding these procedures can help you create fair work rules and grievance procedures where you work.

Resolving disputes

When unionized employees and management sign a labor contract, they agree to abide by certain rules and policies. A contract can't cite every potential dispute, so it includes grievance procedures, specific steps that both sides agree to follow. Usually, the grievance process moves from discussions to formal hearings with written statements of times, dates, details, and witnesses. If matters can't be resolved, the aggrieved party requests arbitration.

Recognizing a grievance

Some contracts define a grievance as any complaint that reflects dissatisfaction with union or management policies. But most contracts define a grievance as a complaint that involves *contract violations.*

As a staff nurse, you or your union representative can file a grievance against your employer. Your union can file a grievance against management. Management can file a grievance — usually called a disciplinary action — against any employee. Most grievances are filed against management because of management's decision-making role.

Distinguishing between gripes and grievances

Smooth labor relations require both sides to honor the contract's terms and to show good faith in using the grievance procedures.

Union representatives must often defuse complaints before they become formal grievances. An effective union representative will be able to distinguish between a legitimate grievance and a gripe. A grievance is a substantive complaint that involves a contract violation; a gripe is a personal problem unrelated to the contract.

Sometimes union or management representatives pursue a groundless grievance (that is, a gripe) for political or harassment purposes. A nurse's self-interest or her resentment of authority can lead to a groundless grievance. So can a supervisor's poor decision or misuse of her authority.

Types of legitimate grievances

Most grievances fall into one of two classifications:
• unfair labor practices
• violations of a contract, a precedent, or a past practice. (See *Legitimate grievances,* page 272.)

Unfair labor practices are tactics prohibited by state and federal labor laws. For example, under federal law, an employer who discriminates against you because you're involved in union activities commits an unfair labor practice. Violations of a contract, precedent, or past practice are actions that break mutually accepted work rules. For example, suppose your contract says a supervisor must give you 2 weeks' notice before making you rotate to another shift. If a supervisor assigns you to another shift without giving you notice, you can file a grievance.

Most common grievances

Grievances can involve an almost infinite number of complaints, but some occur frequently. Management often takes disciplinary action against employees who:
• allow personal problems to interfere with their jobs
• fail to perform their assigned duties

• show poor work habits, such as tardiness or unreliability
• take an antagonistic attitude toward management in labor relations when serving in union positions.

Employees commonly file grievances against supervisors who dispense discipline inconsistently, show favoritism, or treat employees unfairly. Other common sources of grievances include management's selection policies for promotions, favored shift assignments, disciplinary actions, and merit salary raises. Staff nurses sometimes file grievances when they're temporarily assigned head nurse responsibilities without getting commensurate pay.

Many grievances result from unwitting contract violations (such as poorly thought-out workload decisions) by first-level or mid-level managers. Personnel and labor relations departments can resolve many actions that would otherwise lead to grievances by answering labor questions and offering advice.

Grievance procedures

The elements of a grievance procedure vary from contract to contract. Key elements always include:
• reasonable time limits for filing a grievance and making a decision
• procedures to appeal a grievance to higher union-management levels if the grievance isn't resolved
• assigning priority to crucial grievances (such as worker suspensions or dismissals)
• an opportunity for both sides to investigate the complaint.

The first step is usually an informal discussion between nurse and supervisor. The nurse may then submit her complaint in writing. If the supervisor doesn't or can't resolve the grievance, the nurse can ask for a union representative, or *steward,* to assist her. The representative will meet with the su-

Legitimate grievances

Not all complaints against an employer meet the definition of a legitimate grievance. If your complaint fits into one of the following categories, chances are that it's a legitimate grievance that can be acted upon by your union.

Contract violations

Your employment contract is binding between you and your employer. If your employer violates it, you have a valid grievance. The following examples describe violations that would likely be prohibited in an employment contract:
• You're performing the charge nurse's job 2 or 3 days a week but still receiving the same pay as other staff nurses.
• You've had to work undesirable shifts or on Sundays more often than other nurses.
• Your supervisor doesn't post time schedules in advance.
• Your employer fires you without just cause.

Federal and state law violations

Any action by your employer that violates a federal or state law would be the basis of a grievance, even if the employment contract permits the action. For example:
• You receive less pay for performing the same work as a male nurse.
• You don't receive the overtime pay you're entitled to.
• Your employer doesn't promote you because of your race.

Past practice violations

A past practice—one that's been accepted by both parties for an extended time, but that's suddenly discontinued by the employer without notification—may be the basis for a grievance. The past practice need not be specified in the contract. If the practice violates the contract, either party can demand that the contract be enforced. If the practice is unsafe, an arbitrator may simply abolish it. Examples of past practice violations might include:
• Your employer charges you for breaking equipment when others haven't been charged.
• Your employer revokes parking lot privileges.
• Your employer eliminates a rotation system for float assignments.

Health and safety violations

These grievances usually involve working conditions for which the employer is responsible. Legitimate grievances may be recognized even if the contract doesn't address the specific complaint. For example:
• You're required to hold patients during X-rays.
• You have no handwashing facilities near patient rooms.

Employer policy violations

Employers have the right to establish *reasonable* work rules and policies. These rules and policies are not usually specified in the employment contract. Your employer can't violate its own rules without being guilty of a grievance (note, however, that an employer can change rules unilaterally). For example:
• You haven't received a performance evaluation in 2 years, although your employee handbook states that such evaluations will be done annually.
• Your employer assigns you a vacation period without your consent, contrary to personnel policies.

pervisor to discuss the grievance's merits. If the supervisor stands firm, the nurse can then file a written complaint within a contract-specified time period. Subsequent hearings move to higher levels of management. The number of steps in a grievance procedure varies with each contract's provisions.

Arbitration

At times neither side can work out a settlement on a substantive issue. That's when arbitration enters the picture. During arbitration, the parties present evidence to a neutral labor relations expert. Parties who have negotiated a collective bargaining agreement or are covered by one with an arbitration clause are required to arbitrate contract disputes. Parties with no bargaining agreement (non-unionized) may agree to independent arbitration, hoping to resolve a matter short of litigation or termination of the relationship.

The side requesting arbitration gives a written notice to the other party. The requesting party then contacts one of several national agencies that supply arbitrators, such as the FMCS or the American Arbitration Association. Both sides must agree on a specific arbitrator; on the date, time, and place for the hearing; and that the arbitrator's decision will be final.

Arbitration hearing

This type of hearing resembles a courtroom proceeding, except that it's less formal. The party requesting arbitration has the burden of proof and must present evidence that the contract has been violated. (However, when a nurse challenges disciplinary action, management must prove its case first by presenting supporting evidence.) In any arbitration hearing, both sides may call and *cross-examine witnesses.* The requesting side makes a closing summary, followed by one from the opposing side. Each side can submit written briefs instead of making summary statements.

The arbitrator usually renders a written decision weeks or even months after the hearing. But if both sides request an immediate response, the arbitrator can issue an oral decision and withhold a written explanation of the decision unless requested by both parties.

In most cases, both sides prefer arbitration to a lengthy court fight because arbitration is speedier, less expensive, and may be conducted without attorneys. But when a dispute goes to arbitration, both sides lose control of the outcome because, in the United States, the arbitrator's decision is binding. Although the losing party can challenge the decision in court, the court rarely overturns an arbitrator's decision.

In Canada, the court may supervise the arbitration itself but it will never overturn an arbitrator's decision unless there is a question of jurisdiction.

Resolving complaints caused by unfair labor practices

Most grievances arising from contract violations follow contract-stipulated grievance and arbitration procedures. But allegations of unfair labor practices go to the NLRB. If a nurse who is not a member of a collective bargaining unit brings an allegation to the NLRB, the NLRB must determine if she is engaged in concerted action; that is, if her action is part of (or in concert with) a group effort. The NLRB will conduct a hearing to review evidence and then issue a decision. Either side can challenge an NLRB decision in court.

If a nurse has a complaint involving discrimination on the basis of race, religion, national origin, age, disability, or sex, she can file a charge of discrimination with the U.S. Equal Employment Opportunity Commission (EEOC) or a comparable state agency in addition to filing a grievance. The EEOC handles violations of:

• the Equal Pay Act of 1963, which forbids wage discrimination based on an employee's sex

• the Civil Rights Act of 1964, which forbids job and wage discrimination based on an employee's religion, race, sex, or ethnic background

• the Age Discrimination in Employment Act of 1967, which forbids discrimination based on an employee's age

• the Americans with Disabilities Act of 1990, which states that "no individual shall be discriminated against on the basis of disability in the full and equal enjoyment of the goods, services, facilities, privileges, advantages, or accommodations of any place of public accommodation...."

The EEOC will also prosecute disputes involving sexual harassment. Employees don't have to be union members to file a complaint with the EEOC.

Disciplinary hearings

A disciplinary hearing can be initiated at the complaint of an employer or a patient. The hearing may be based on allegations of incompetence or on alleged violation of state law pertaining to nursing practice.

If you are ever served with notice that you are being investigated by your state's licensing board, seek legal counsel and emotional and professional support. Do not approach these proceedings lightly or unprepared. The hearing process and the outcome can have a major impact on how you view yourself, how you practice nursing, and how you view your profession.

Before the hearing, do your homework, be aware of recent state laws, gather witnesses and evidence, and be prepared to stand up for your rights and your nursing license. Learn every-

thing you can from the experience. Finally, be prepared to support your colleagues who may also go through a disciplinary hearing.

Selected references

Adcock, G. "Negotiating an Employment Contract," *Nurse Practitioner* 20(6):22-23, June 1995.

Gerardi, D.S. "Ask the Experts: Is it Legal for Hospital Administration to Mandate Overtime?" *Critical Care Nurse* 15(3):142-43, June 1995.

Horsley, J. "Does a Criminal Past Rule Out a Nursing Future?" *RN* 57(10):74-75, October 1994.

Horty, J. "What Managers Should Know About the ADA," *OR Manager* 9(8):21-23, August 1993.

Makin, R. "A Bitter Blow," *Nursing Times* 90(9):26-28, March 2-8, 1994.

Meissner, J.E. "How's Your Job Security?" *Nursing* 24(3):57-58, March 1994.

Pietro, J. "The Legal Side: Overburdened with Overtime," *American Journal of Nursing* 95(8):60-61, August 1995.

Sullivan, G.H. "Your Rights When You're Disabled—and Afterward," *RN* 57(8):61-63, August 1994.

"Unsafe Conditions: Afraid to Complain," *Nursing* 24(10):70, October 1994.

"When Work Redesign Prompts Unionization Activity," *Nursing Management* 24(9):36, 38, September 1993.

8

Ethical decision making

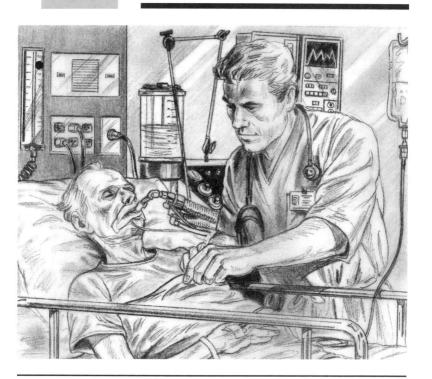

Every day, nurses make ethical decisions in their nursing practice. These decisions may involve patient care, actions toward co-workers, or nurse-doctor relations. At times, you may find yourself trapped in the middle of an ethical dilemma, caught among conflicting *duties* and responsibilities to your patient, to your employer, and to yourself. And even after you make a decision, you may wonder, "Did I do the right thing?"

There are no automatic guidelines for solving all ethical conflicts. Although such conflicts may be painful and con-fusing, particularly in nursing, you don't have to be a philosopher to act ethically or to make decisions that fall within nursing's *standards* of practice and ethical *codes.* Nonetheless, you do need to understand the principles of *ethics* that guide your nursing practice.

You are *legally* responsible for using your knowledge and skills to protect the safety and comfort of your patients. At the same time, you are *ethically* responsible for acting as a patient advocate to safeguard patients' rights. For instance, although you are not legally responsible for obtaining a patient's informed consent, you are ethically responsible for notifying the doctor if the patient misunderstands his treatment or withdraws consent. To be an effective advocate, you must know that a patient's consent isn't valid unless he understands his condition, the proposed treatment, treatment alternatives, probable risks and benefits, and relative chances of success or failure.

Law vs. ethics

Ethics is the area of philosophic study that examines *values,* actions, and choices to determine right and wrong. *Laws* are binding rules of conduct enforced by authority. In many situations, laws and ethics overlap. When they diverge, you have to identify and examine the fine lines that separate them.

Relationship between law and ethics

When a law is challenged as unjust or unfair, the challenge usually reflects some underlying ethical principle. That's because, ideally, laws are based on what is right and good. Realistically, though, the relation between law and ethics is complex. (See *Nursing ethics and the law.*)

Your role as patient advocate bridges law and ethics. For instance, most medical malpractice suits result from patients' dissatisfaction with the care they received. Such dissatisfaction may arise from a belief that staff members failed to show them respect or ignored or violated their rights. You can be pivotal in preventing such lawsuits by serving as your patient's advocate.

Moral dilemmas

A nurse who must decide whether to follow a doctor's orders to administer an unusually high dose of a narcotic drug faces a *moral dilemma* — an ethical problem caused by conflicts of rights, responsibilities, and values.

Such a dilemma carries with it a great deal of stress. As you grapple with the situation, trying to decide what to do, you'll probably experience psychological and emotional stress, provoked by fear or guilt. In addition, you may experience stress caused by external factors that are political or interpersonal; for example, you may be nervous about confronting the doctor with your doubts because you fear his anger.

Moral dilemmas call for ethical choices in the face of profound uncertainty. At times, you may not know what the right or ethical course of action is. At other times, you may believe completely in the righteousness of a particular action, and yet, for various reasons, find it difficult to act.

A moral dilemma may be further complicated by psychological pressures and personal feelings, especially when any choice is a forced one at best and, in many cases, results in an uncomfortable compromise. Many moral dilemmas in nursing involve choices about justice or fairness, when scant resources (such as bed space or limited staffing) must be divided among patients with equal needs. In other cases, a choice must be made quickly because the patient's medical condition is fluctuating or rapidly deteriorating. By and large, nurses who are compelled to make ethical decisions don't have the luxury of time.

Types of dilemmas

Most moral dilemmas in nursing can be identified according to the following classifications:
• Dilemmas of *beneficence* — dilemmas that involve deciding what is good as opposed to what is harmful; such di-

Nursing ethics and the law

The following diagram shows four types of situations that occur in nursing, each with a different relationship between ethics and the law.

Potential moral dilemmas

Certain actions are clearly unlawful and immoral (Type 4). Other actions are ethically or legally ambiguous (Types 2 and 3). In Types 2 and 3, determining whether the action described is legal or ethical may depend on a person's values or religious beliefs or how the law is interpreted. These types of situations present nurses with potential moral dilemmas.

Type 1 **Nursing actions are both ethical and legal.** *Example:* A nurse gives the right drug by the right route in the right amount to the right patient at the right time – as the doctor ordered.	**Type 2** **Nursing actions *may be considered* ethical but not legal.** *Example:* A nurse is caring for a terminally ill patient who is in unendurable pain. The nurse arranges, at the patient's insistence, to help him commit suicide with an overdose of a nonprescribed drug.
Type 3 **Nursing actions *may be considered* legal but not ethical.** *Example:* A nurse administers a large dose of a pain-relieving drug to an AIDS patient, as prescribed by the patient's doctor, even though she fears it may compromise respiration.	**Type 4** **Nursing actions are neither legal nor ethical.** *Example:* A nurse gives the wrong medication to the patient, does not inform the patient's doctor of the error, and does not make an incident report.

lemmas commonly arise when health care providers, patients, or family members disagree over what course of action is in the patient's best interest

• Dilemmas of ***autonomy*** – those that involve deciding what course of action maximizes the patient's right of self-determination; these dilemmas are similar to dilemmas of beneficence, especially when someone other than the patient must determine what's best for him

• Dilemmas of ***justice*** – dilemmas that involve dividing limited health care resources fairly

• Dilemmas of ***fidelity*** – those that involve honoring promises; such dilemmas may occur when a nurse's duties to a patient conflict with her other duties, such as those to the doctor

• Dilemmas of ***nonmaleficence*** – dilemmas that involve the avoidance of harm; these arise when a nurse believes other staff members' actions are compromising patient safety, impelling her to "blow the whistle"

• Dilemmas of *confidentiality* — those that involve respecting privileged information; these dilemmas often pit a patient's right to privacy against society's right to be informed of potential threats to public health

• Dilemmas of *veracity* — dilemmas that involve telling or concealing the truth, such as when a patient is not fully informed of his medical condition.

Types of decisions

In any of these moral dilemmas, the types of decisions facing nurses usually can be grouped into four categories:

• Active decisions — ethical decisions and moral judgments that lead directly to actions and bring about change

• Passive decisions — decisions that deny, delay, or avoid action and maintain the status quo by denying or shifting responsibility to avoid change

• Programmed decisions — decisions that use precedents, established guidelines, procedures, and *rules* to resolve anticipated, routine, expected types of moral dilemmas

• Nonprogrammed decisions — decisions that require a unique response to complex and unexpected moral dilemmas.

Most commonly, a nurse's programmed decisions also are active ones. For example, when a nurse and a doctor tell a patient what to expect in surgery and then ask the patient to sign a *consent form*, they're participating in a programmed decision process that involves ethical and legal practices (such as truth-telling) as well as patients' rights (such as self-determination).

The patient facing surgery — feeling unprepared to make a complex decision — may respond passively, saying, "I don't know what's best. Should I risk the complications of having surgery or the danger of not having it? I'll do whatever you tell me."

In this situation, the doctor and nurse must make a choice. They must either relieve the patient's stress by telling him what's "best" for him, or ensure the patient's autonomy by removing themselves from the decision-making process.

Whenever you're faced with a moral dilemma, you must make moral judgments that lead to decisions about right and wrong courses of action. Even passive decisions — for example, deciding to protect oneself by remaining silent or not taking a stand on an issue — are based on moral judgments. (See *Approaching ethical decisions*.)

Values and ethics

Values are strongly held personal and professional beliefs about worth and importance. (The word *value* comes from the Latin "valere" — to be strong.) The remarks that follow are examples of value statements:

• "Nursing is a meaningful profession."

• "Nurses make a difference to their patients by comforting, caring, and teaching."

• "Nurses should be paid more for what they do."

• "The nursing profession must change radically to survive in today's health care system."

• "If you want recognition and respect, don't become a nurse."

• "HMOs put too much pressure on professional health care employees."

• "Doctors should make important health care decisions, not hospital administrators."

• "A new emphasis on preventive medicine will make nursing a more valuable and respected profession."

Not all nurses would agree with every one of these value statements. Value conflicts are common among nurses, doctors, patients, families, and hospital *administrators.*

Clarifying your own values is an important part of developing a professional ethic. A person may become more aware of his values by consciously examining his statements and behavior. (See *Developing value awareness,* pages 280 and 281.)

Moral relativism

The question arises: Are certain values intrinsically best, or are values always a matter of personal interpretation? A theory of ethics known as *moral relativism* holds that there are no ethical absolutes, that whatever a person believes is right, is right for him or her at that moment.

Consider what would happen if everyone practiced moral relativism.
• There would be no objective way to resolve moral dilemmas.
• A person could never question or disapprove of another's moral judgment.
• Professional standards, such as nursing standards, would become meaningless.
• Law and order in society would disappear.
• People and cultures would be unable to grow morally.

Although different people and cultures have different values, moral relativism doesn't provide an adequate basis for ethical decision making. Because you will probably face numerous moral conflicts in the course of your career, you need to develop consistent ethical standards to guide your behavior.

Ethical theories

As the basis for professional codes of ethics, ethical theories attempt to provide a system of principles and rules

> ### Approaching ethical decisions
>
> When faced with an ethical dilemma, consider the following questions:
> • What health issues are involved?
> • What ethical issues are involved?
> • What further information is necessary before a judgment can be made?
> • Who will be affected by this decision? (Include the decision maker and other caregivers if they will be affected emotionally or professionally.)
> • What are the values and opinions of the people involved?
> • What conflicts exist between the values and ethical standards of the people involved?
> • Must a decision be made and, if so, who should make it?
> • What alternatives are available?
> • For each alternative, what are the ethical justifications?
> • For each alternative, what are the possible outcomes?

for resolving ethical dilemmas. Ethical theories consist of fundamental beliefs about what is morally right or wrong, and propose reasons for maintaining those beliefs.

Teleology and deontology

In nursing, two types of ethical theories—*teleology* and *deontology*—frequently are used as guides in ethical decision making. (For a description of some other types of ethical theories, see *Alternative ethical theories,* page 282.)

Teleologic ethical theories determine what is right or wrong based on an action's consequences. (One such teleologic theory, called utilitarian eth-

Developing value awareness

At times, some nurses, like all people, tend to rely on hearsay, opinions, or prejudice instead of developing a strong sense of their own values. Infrequently do they stop to reflect on the values that are mirrored in their conversation and behavior.

Consider the following dialogue, in which three nurses express various value judgments. As you read, ask yourself: What values does each nurse express? Do the values of the three conflict? Are individual nurses expressing consistent values? Do they show a high regard for patient autonomy?

Shop talk

Kate: I can't believe it. I have to float to the ICU—and it's only my second week on the job. I hate floating, especially to intensive care.

Dean: So do I. The last time I floated to ICU, I was assigned to a 300-pound patient who had been driving drunk and hadn't been wearing a seat belt. The guy was badly hurt, and I had to do all the positioning myself because the unit was so short-staffed. I just about killed my back. It's not fair that they always assign the male nurses to obese patients.

Pat: Floating is really a tough issue. I try to see it from the patient's side, though. I mean, maybe you were assigned to care for this patient because you are a good nurse and could give him the best care.

Kate: What bugs me is having to care for patients like that drunk driver, who obviously don't care how they live. They don't watch their weight, they drive drunk, they don't use seat belts—and we get pulled from the work we're comfortable with to care for them. I can't even find time for a cigarette break.

Pat: Don't forget, Kate, we're supposed to take care of patients regardless of their health habits or life-style. No one's perfect, after all.

Kate: Yeah, I guess you're right, but floating makes me nervous anyway. I'm scared I'll really mess up because everything's so unfamiliar.

Dean: Let me give you some advice. No matter what you think about floating, don't say anything. If you're pegged as a complainer around here, your career is over.

Pat: You sound like you think nurses shouldn't ever speak out if something's wrong with the system. I think nurses do have the power to change things for the better, but that won't happen if we aren't willing to take some risks.

Dean: You're an idealist. I'm a realist. I ask, what's worth risking your job for?

Pat: I think being a nurse means not being willing to compromise your standards of care just to keep a job.

Kate: What happened to the 300-pound patient? Is he still in ICU? Do you think I might get assigned to him?

Dean: Well, no. It's the craziest thing. He was a quadriplegic after the accident. So we put all this time and effort into getting him stable and keeping him infection-free, and one day he decides it's not worth it. So the docs just turned everything off. Now I ask you, is that right?

Examining values

The nurses in this scenario make a variety of moral judgments. By analyzing their attitudes you can come to a better understanding of your own values.

Developing value awareness continued

• Kate criticizes the health habits of an obese trauma patient but insists on her own right to have time for a cigarette break. What values are guiding her opinions? Do you think her outlook is consistent?

• Dean thinks that Kate should take on an assignment for which she isn't prepared rather than risk losing favor with the administration. Do you think that this attitude is irresponsible or merely realistic?

• Pat is accused of being an idealist. Is that a fair judgment?

• What values are mirrored in each nurse's attitude about floating?

• At the end of the conversation, Dean mentions that the doctor decided to withdraw treatment from the quadriplegic patient. If the three nurses were to discuss the ethical questions raised by the doctor's decision, how do you think each nurse would respond?

• Would these three nurses have similar or conflicting views about what it means to be a patient advocate?

Values clarification

Values clarification refers to the process of raising unconscious values to consciousness so that value conflicts can be resolved. Exercises (such as analyzing the dialogue among Kate, Dean, and Pat) offer one way to clarify values. Reflecting on one's own statements and actions is another. You're likely to encounter many conflicting sets of values in the course of your professional career. You must choose among competing values to establish your own ethical beliefs. Then you need to incorporate chosen values into your everyday thoughts and actions. You will then be better prepared to act on chosen values when you're confronted with difficult ethical choices.

Making ethical decisions need not be haphazard. By clarifying your own values and checking to see if they're consistent with the established ethical standards of the nursing profession, you can enhance your ability to make responsible moral judgments.

ics, requires decision makers to determine and choose those actions that will result in maximized good — that is, the greatest good for the greatest number of people.)

In teleologic theories, ethical decisions most often are made through a process called risk-benefit analysis. For example, you may help patients and their families evaluate several courses of treatment to decide which one will produce the greatest amount of relief (benefit) with the least danger of suffering (risk).

The fact that teleologic theory assumes that good and harm can be quantified and evaluated can make it a less than ideal approach to resolving health

care issues. Determining the "greatest good" is highly subjective, and can result in inconsistent decisions.

Deontologic ethical theories emphasize moral obligation or *commitment.* Deontologic theories give most weight to obeying moral laws such as "Always tell the truth" and "Never harm a patient." According to deontologic theories, honoring ethical obligations ensures good, even though actions may be difficult and consequences painful.

Because deontology centers on duty or obligation to others, many experts consider it the only acceptable theory for ethical decision making in health care. Nevertheless, complications can arise when duties conflict with one an-

Alternative ethical theories

In addition to deontology and teleology, other ethical theories may guide decision making, but each has its limitations.

Egoism

Egoism considers self-interest and self-preservation as the only proper goals of all human actions, insisting that the only right decision is the one that maximizes the autonomy of the decision maker.

Limitations

• Egoism ignores moral principles or rules outside one's own point of view.
• Inconsistencies arise from one decision to the next, even in similar situations.
• Because it ignores the rights of others, egoism is unacceptable for most ethical decisions in health care.

Obligationism

Obligationism attempts to resolve ethical dilemmas by balancing *distributive justice* (dividing equally among all) with *beneficence* (doing good and not harm). This theory holds that benefits and burdens should be distributed equally to all people, according to their merits and needs.

Limitations

• The two basic principles of obligationism—justice and beneficence—may conflict in certain situations.

• The theory can be useful in determining public policy but is not practical for decisions affecting one person.

Social contract theory

Social contract theory is based on the concept of *original position:* The least advantaged people (such as children and the handicapped) are considered the norm. Whether an act is right or wrong is determined from the norm's point of view.

Limitations

• Without specific guidelines, this theory is useless in day-to-day health care decisions.
• Social inequalities will persist.

Theological ethics

This theory is based on ethical, moral, and legal principles derived from religious traditions—for instance, *Good Samaritan acts,* which are based on the biblical concept of altruism and selflessness.

Limitations

• Religious beliefs and teachings may be out of touch with contemporary social issues and health care dilemmas.
• Various cults and sects may interpret traditional religious beliefs and teachings in different ways.

other and you have to decide which duty takes precedence.

For example, suppose someone proposes keeping a **brain-dead** patient on a ventilator while recipients for a kidney transplant are found. Several staff members object because the patient had expressed a wish to die naturally, without artificial support.

On the one hand, you may favor maintaining the patient on a ventilator be-cause you recognize how useful his kidneys will be to others. On the other hand, if you resolve this dilemma by deciding which course of action best supports the patient's rights, you would probably give more weight to his right of self-determination. This would lead you to oppose maintaining the patient on a ventilator. So, as you can see from this example, duties can conflict, and you'll have to determine which duty takes precedence.

Nurses usually combine aspects of both teleologic and deontologic theories when making ethical decisions. To avoid becoming confused, you should develop orderly, systematic, objective decision-making methods. Otherwise, your decision making becomes subjective and arbitrary, and results in moral relativism.

Basis of ethical decisions

Ethical decision making most commonly involves reflection on the following:

• options or courses of action available
• options that seem unavailable
• consequences, both good and bad, of all possible options (teleology)
• rules, obligations, and values that should direct choices (deontology)
• who should make the choices
• desired goal or outcome.

Equally important is the process of self-reflection. This involves uncovering, sharing, and discussing:

• personal and professional values relevant to the situation (values clarification)
• prejudices or biases that affect objectivity
• previous experiences with similar situations and decisions
• limitations that affect skills or understanding
• motives and intentions, particularly those of self-interest and convenience.

All these elements should come together when you're making an ethical decision. The best way to ensure this may be to use a method with which every nurse is familiar: the *nursing process.*

Applying the nursing process to ethical decision making

The nursing process is a continuous, interdependent, systematic organization of cognitive behaviors designed to resolve problems and promote well-being. The essential steps of the nursing process include assessment, planning, *implementation,* and *evaluation.*

Assessment begins with the nurse's initial contact with a patient. It involves collecting systematic data, identifying the patient's needs, and determining the *nursing diagnosis.*

Planning includes assigning priorities to nursing diagnoses based on acuity, determining goals of nursing actions, identifying appropriate nursing actions necessary to attain goals, establishing outcome criteria, and developing a *nursing care plan.*

Implementation involves coordinating, performing, or delegating activities specified in the nursing care plan, and recording results.

Evaluation includes collecting data, measuring outcomes against outcome criteria, and altering the nursing care plan by continuation of the nursing process.

You can effectively use the same type of continuous, systematic, rational approach when making ethical decisions.

Assessment

• Gather facts, perceptions, and opinions about the ethical problem. Read the patient's chart. Talk with the patient and his family, other health care providers, and anyone who may be familiar with the patient's values.
• Identify the people involved in the problem and assess their roles, responsibilities, authority, and decision-making abilities.
• Identify available resources. These may include the hospital ethics committee, chaplain, nurse ethicist, coun-

selors, and facilitators. Resources also may include hospital policies, as well as literature on similar cases.

• Help decision makers participate in values clarification.

Planning

• Identify the types of moral dilemmas involved — beneficence, autonomy, justice, fidelity, nonmaleficence, confidentiality, or veracity. Identify the specific issues involved by examining the rights, duties, and values that are in conflict.

• Identify possible courses of action, along with their probable and possible risks and benefits (teleology).

• Formulate and assign priorities to the ethical goals or objectives desired by the people involved.

• Determine the ethical obligations of those involved and the ethical principles that shape their actions (deontology).

Implementation

• Develop an ethical goal that maximizes good, working with others involved, as appropriate.

• Determine the course of action that will produce results closest to those of the ethical ideal.

• Determine if that course of action violates legal or moral principles. (If so, modify or change the course of action until it does not do so.)

• Carry out the agreed-on course of action.

Evaluation

• Determine whether the results approximate the ethical ideal.

• If the results fall short of the ideal, determine what new moral dilemmas have been created.

• Reenter the decision process in the assessment phase to resolve additional moral dilemmas.

Although this process imposes the structure and objectivity necessary for resolving a moral dilemma, it does not provide all the answers. Because human beings are fallible, it is impossible for anyone to gather all the facts or to be completely without bias. Psychological and emotional factors can play havoc with fairness and impartiality.

Communication skills

When it comes to making fair and ethical decisions, personality conflicts, political forces, and power plays can sabotage even the best intentions. For this reason, you should use communication skills and management techniques to help promote collaboration and prevent divisiveness. In addition, you should observe the following rules of behavior:

• Act within professional bounds, following the appropriate codes of ethics. (See *Ethical codes for nurses.*)

• Don't make ethical decisions alone. Seek counsel and advice from other professionals.

• Validate information. Don't base ethical decisions on rumors, innuendo, hearsay, first impressions, or snap judgments.

• If religious faith and spiritual values are important to you or others involved in the ethical dilemma, include prayer in the decision-making process.

Acting as a patient advocate

One of your most important moral obligations is your role as a *patient advocate.* When a patient must make an ethical decision, you should help him resolve his moral dilemma in ways that enhance personal values, priorities, freedom, dignity, and *quality of life.*

As an advocate, you must never impose personal agendas or values on a patient. There may be times when you will have to set aside one important nursing value (beneficence, or doing

Ethical codes for nurses

Two of the most important ethical codes for registered nurses are the American Nurses' Association (ANA) code and the Canadian Nurses' Association (CNA) code. Licensed practical and vocational nurses (LPNs and LVNs) also have an ethical code. The International Council of Nurses, an organization based in Geneva, Switzerland, that seeks to improve the standards of and status of nursing worldwide, has also published a code of ethics.

ANA code of ethics

The ANA views both nurses and patients as individuals who possess basic rights and responsibilities, and whose values and circumstances should command respect at all times. The ANA code provides guidance for carrying out nursing responsibilities consistent with the ethical obligations of the profession.

According to the ANA code, the nurse:
- provides services with respect for human dignity and the uniqueness of the patient unrestricted by considerations of social or economic status, personal attributes, or the nature of health problems
- safeguards the patient's right to privacy by judiciously protecting information of a confidential nature
- acts to safeguard the patient and the public when health care and safety are affected by the incompetent, unethical, or illegal practice of any person
- assumes responsibility and accountability for individual nursing judgments and actions
- maintains competence in nursing
- exercises informed judgment and uses individual competence and qualifications as criteria in seeking consultation, accepting responsibilities, and delegating nursing activities to others
- participates in activities that contribute to the ongoing development of the profession's body of knowledge
- participates in the profession's efforts to implement and improve standards of nursing
- participates in the profession's efforts to establish and maintain conditions of employment conducive to high-quality nursing care
- participates in the profession's efforts to protect the public from misinformation and misrepresentation and to maintain the integrity of nursing
- collaborates with members of the health professions and other citizens in promoting community and national efforts to meet the health needs of the public.

CNA code of ethics

The CNA code consists of four sources of nursing obligations.

Patients

- A nurse is obligated to treat patients with respect for their individual needs and values.
- Based on respect for patients and regard for their rights to control their own care, nursing care should reflect respect for patients' right of choice.
- The nurse is obligated to hold confidential all information about patients learned in the health care setting.
- The nurse has an obligation to be guided by consideration for the dignity of patients.
- The nurse is obligated to provide competent care to patients.
- The nurse maintains trust in nurses and nursing.

(continued)

Ethical codes for nurses continued

Health team
• The nurse recognizes the expertise and contribution of colleagues from nursing and other disciplines.
• The nurse takes steps to ensure that patients receive competent and ethical care.

Social context of nursing
• Conditions of employment should contribute in a positive way to patient care and the professional satisfaction of nurses.
• The nurse is obligated to work toward securing conditions of employment that enable safe, appropriate care for patients and contribute to the professional satisfaction of nurses.
• The nurse advocates patients' interests.
• The nurse represents the values and ethics of nursing before colleagues and others.

Responsibilities of the profession
• Professional nurses' organizations recognize their responsibility to clarify, secure, and sustain ethical nursing conduct. To fulfill these tasks, professional nurses' organizations must respond to the rights, needs, and interests of patients and nurses.

Code for LPNs and LVNs
The code for licensed practical nurses (LPNs) and licensed vocational nurses (LVNs) seeks to provide a motivation for establishing, maintaining, and elevating professional standards. This code requires these nurses to:

• regard conservation of life and disease prevention as a basic obligation.
• promote and protect the physical, mental, emotional and spiritual well-being of the patient and his family.
• fulfill all duties faithfully and efficiently.
• function within established legal guidelines.
• take personal responsibility for actions and seek to earn the respect and confidence of all members of the health care team.
• keep confidential any information about the patient obtained from any source.
• give conscientious service and charge reasonable fees.
• learn about and respect the religious and cultural beliefs of all patients.
• meet obligations to patients by staying abreast of health care trends through reading and continuing education.
• uphold the laws of the land and promote legislation to meet the health needs of its people.

International Council of Nurses code of ethics
According to the International Council of Nurses, the fundamental responsibility of the nurse is fourfold: to promote health, to prevent illness, to restore health, and to alleviate suffering.

The International Council of Nurses further states that the need for nursing is universal. Inherent in nursing is respect for life, dignity, and the rights of man. It is unrestricted by considerations of nationality, race, creed, color, age, sex, politics, or social status.

Ethical codes for nurses continued

Nurses and people
- The nurse's primary responsibility is to those people who require nursing care.
- The nurse, in providing care, respects the beliefs, values, and customs of the individual.
- The nurse holds in confidence personal information and uses judgment in sharing this information.

Nurses and practice
- The nurse carries personal responsibility for nursing practice and for maintaining competence by continual learning.
- The nurse maintains the highest standards of nursing care possible within the reality of a specific situation.
- The nurse uses good judgment in relation to individual competence when accepting and delegating responsibilities.
- The nurse, when acting in a professional capacity, should at all times maintain standards of personal conduct that would reflect credit upon the profession.

Nurses and society
- The nurse shares with other citizens the responsibility for initiating and supporting action to meet the health and social needs of the public.

Nurses and co-workers
- The nurse sustains a cooperative relationship with co-workers in nursing and other fields.
- The nurse takes appropriate action to safeguard the individual when his care is endangered by a co-worker or any other person.

Nurses and the profession
- The nurse plays the major role in determining and implementing desirable standards of nursing practice and nursing education.
- The nurse is active in developing a core of professional knowledge.
- The nurse, acting through the professional organization, participates in establishing and maintaining equitable social and economic working conditions in nursing.

good for patients) to honor another one (autonomy, or the patient's right to decide his own future).

By listening carefully to the patient and asking thoughtful questions, you may be able to help the patient and his family make ethical decisions. Consider asking the patient to describe the problem to you, and then ask him the following questions to help him clarify his thoughts.
- What has the doctor told you about the situation?
- What options are you considering?
- Have you considered making a list of the best and worst things for each option you're considering?
- What else would it help you to know as you're making the decision?
- Is there anyone you would like to speak with about this decision (for example, a clergyperson, counselor, social worker, trusted friend, or lawyer)?
- What is the hardest part about coping with this decision?
- What things in the past have helped you cope with difficult decisions or situations?
- What would make it easier for you and your family to talk about this situation?
- What do you think is the best thing to do?

Selected references

Bosek, M.S.D. "Nursing Ethics. What Does an Ethics Consultant Do?" *MedSurg Nursing* 4(1):55-57, February 1995.

Campbell, M.L. "Interpretation of an Ambiguous Advance Directive," *Dimensions of Critical Care Nursing* 14(5):226-33, September-October 1995.

Catalano, J.T. *Ethical and Legal Aspects of Nursing,* Second Edition. Springhouse, Pa.: Springhouse Corp., 1995.

Clarke, R.A. "Ethics and Midwifery Practice," *Midwives* 108(1291):270-71, August 1995.

Corley, M.C., and Selig, P. "Prevalence of Principled Thinking by Critical Care Nurses," *Dimensions of Critical Care Nursing* 13(2):96-103, March-April 1994.

Curtin, L.L. "Ethics in Management. Nurses Take a Stand on Assisted Suicide," *Nursing Management* 26(5):71, 73-74, 76, May 1995.

Curtin, L.L. *Nursing into the 21st Century.* Springhouse, Pa.: Springhouse Corp., 1996.

Edwards, B.S. "Ethical Dilemmas. Discomfort over a 'Death Sentence'," *American Journal of Nursing* 95(3):65-66, March 1995.

Gournic, J.L. "Ethical Issues: Responses of Clinical Nurses about What Is Moral in Nursing," *Nursing Connections* 7(4):33-37, Winter 1994.

Haddad, A. "Acute Care Decisions. Ethics in Action...a Nurse is Told by a Friend that a Colleague on Her Neonatal Intensive Care Unit is HIV-Positive," *RN* 58(3): 14-16, March 1995.

Kuhn, J.E. "A Nurse's Right to Refuse a Patient Care Assignment," *AORN Journal* 62(3):412, 414, 416+, September 1995.

Lutzen, K., et al. "Modifying Autonomy — a Concept Grounded in Nurses' Experiences of Moral Decision-Making in Psychiatric Practice," *Journal of Medical Ethics* 20(2):101-107, June 1994.

Mattiasson, A., et al. "Staff Attitude and Experience in Dealing with Rational Nursing Home Patients Who Refuse to Eat and Drink," *Journal of Advanced Nursing* 20(5):822-27, November 1994.

Maupin, C.R. "The Potential for Noncaring when Dealing with Difficult Patients: Strategies for Moral Decision Making," *Journal of Cardiovascular Nursing* 9(3):11-22, April 1995

Oldaker, S. "Legal and Ethical Issues. Entrepreneurial Ethics: A Contextual Perspective," *Journal of Professional Nursing* 11(1):6, January-February 1995.

Price, D.M., et al. "An Ethical Perspective. Nurses Are Always Responsible," *Journal of Nursing Law* 1(2):63-66, Winter 1994.

Salladay, S.A. "Ethical Problems. Sexual Misconduct: Flirting with Danger," *Nursing95* 25(5):82-83, May 1995.

Sim, J. "Moral Rights and the Ethics of Nursing," *Nursing Ethics* 2(1):31-40, March 1995.

9

Ethical conflicts in clinical practice

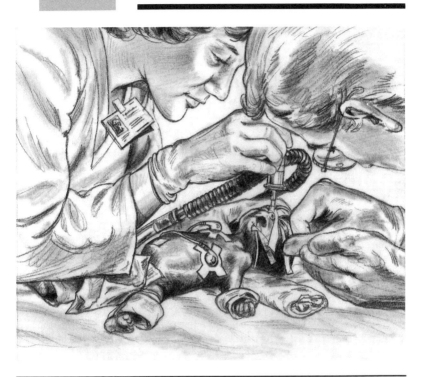

Rapid advances in medical research have outpaced society's ability to solve the ethical problems associated with new health care technology. For nurses, ethical decision making in clinical practice is complicated by sociocultural factors, legal controversies, growing professional *autonomy*, and consumer involvement in health care.

This chapter describes seven major areas of ethical conflict—the right to die, organ transplantation, critically ill neonates, acquired immunodeficiency syndrome (AIDS), abortion and reproductive technology, genetic engineer-ing and screening, and personal safety in the workplace. No matter what your *nursing specialty*, you'll probably encounter at least one of these conflicts in the course of your career.

Ethical dilemmas resist easy resolution. The choice often is between two equally desirable or two equally undesirable alternatives. By learning as much as possible about the underlying ethical principles, you'll be better equipped to take part in decision making. The more you practice ethical thinking, the more confident you'll become in your ability to make decisions.

Getting help

When ethical problems arise, be sure to discuss them candidly with other members of the health care team, especially the patient's doctor. Also consider calling on social workers, psychologists, the clergy, and members of the ethics committee to help you resolve difficult ethical problems. By learning as much as possible, you can facilitate the decision-making process for the patient, his family, and his doctor. (See *The ethics committee.*)

Right to die

The most difficult ethical decisions in health care involve whether to initiate or withhold life-sustaining treatment for patients who are irreversibly comatose or vegetative or suffering with end-stage terminal illness. Treatment decisions for these patients are often morally troubling. The patient, his family, and the health care team may be asked to choose between a potentially painful extension of life and immediate death. Surrogate decision makers— people who are designated to act when a patient is no longer capable of deciding his own fate — also face tremendous moral and emotional pressures.

Sometimes, the patient's expressed wishes to withhold life-sustaining treatment are ignored or overridden by doctors and family members. As a nurse, you may feel that you are caught in the middle, frustrated and demoralized by the demands of caring for an unresponsive patient.

Defining death

Part of the problem stems from a lack of consensus about what constitutes death. Some people define death as the loss of all vital functions, whereas others recognize neurologic criteria such as *brain death* — the irreversible cessation of brain functioning accompanied by ongoing biologic functioning in all other parts of the body, maintained by life-support measures.

Some people maintain a strong ethical belief in the absolute sanctity of life. Others argue that it is wrong and wasteful to continue life support when a patient's life is devoid of any dignity. To function effectively when caring for critically ill patients, you'll need to be aware of your personal feelings about death and quality-of-life issues.

Ordinary vs. extraordinary treatment

Ordinary means of medical treatment are medications, procedures, and surgeries that offer the patient some hope of benefit without incurring excessive pain or expense. In contrast, extraordinary means, sometimes called heroic measures, offer little hope of improving the patient's condition. Instead, these measures merely maintain or prolong a patient's life, usually at great expense and suffering. Because of the continuing advances in medicine and technology, the distinction between "ordinary" and "extraordinary" treatments is becoming less and less well-defined.

In 1983, the President's Commission for the Study of Ethical Problems in Medicine and Behavioral Research defined "ordinary" and "extraordinary" treatments in terms of their respective benefits and burdens:

"The Commission believes...that extraordinary treatment is that which, in the patient's view, entails significantly greater burdens than benefits and is therefore undesirable and not obligatory, while ordinary treatment is that which, in the patient's view, produces greater benefits than burdens and is therefore reasonably desirable and undertaken."

The commission further stated that *health care professionals* are not obli-

The ethics committee

The ethics committee addresses ethical issues regarding the clinical aspects of patient care. It provides a forum for patient, family, and health care providers to resolve difficult conflicts.

The functions of an ethics committee may include:

• policy development, such as developing policies to guide deliberations over individual cases

• education, such as inviting guest speakers to visit the hospital and discuss ethical concerns

• case consultation, such as debating the prognosis of a patient in a persistent vegetative state

• addressing a single issue – for instance, reviewing all cases that involve a no-code or "do not resuscitate" (DNR) order

• addressing problems of a specific population. For example, the American Academy of Pediatrics recommends that hospitals have a standing committee called the "infant bioethical review committee."

Pros and cons

Properly run, an ethics committee provides a safe outlet for venting opposing views on emotionally charged ethical conflicts. The committee process can help to lessen the bias that interferes with rational decision making. It allows for members of disparate disciplines, including doctors, nurses, clergy, social workers, hospital administrators, and ethicists, to express their views on treatment decisions.

Critics of ethics committees think that committee decision making is too bureaucratic and slow to be useful in clinical crises. They also point out that one dominating committee member may intimidate others with opposing views. Furthermore,

they contend that doctors may view the committee as a threat to their autonomy in patient care decisions.

Selection of committee members

Committee members should be selected for their ability to work cooperatively in a group. The American Hospital Association recommends the following ratio of committee members: one-third doctors, one-third nurses, and one-third others, including laypeople, clergy, and other health professionals. Regulations of the Joint Commission on Accreditation of Healthcare Organizations require that nursing staff members participate in the hospital ethics committee.

Nurse's role on ethics committees

Because of the nurse's close contact with the patient, family, and other members of the health care team, she frequently is in a position to identify ethical dilemmas, such as when a family is considering a DNR order for a relative. In many cases, the nurse is the first to recognize conflicts between family members or between the doctor and the patient or family.

Before ethics committees were widely used, nurses had no official outlet for voicing their opinions in ethical debates. In many situations, doctors made ethical decisions about patient care behind closed doors. Nursing supervisors frequently would call meetings to alert nursing staff of treatment decisions and to discourage protest. Now, ethics committees provide nurses with a means to express their views, hear the opinions of others, and understand more deeply the rationale behind ethical decisions.

gated to provide treatment that's considered useless or futile.

Discontinuing treatment

Despite the commission's recommendations, countless terminally ill patients continue to receive treatment that is unlikely to benefit them. Determining whether a particular treatment is futile is highly subjective. Not only are many such decisions based on incomplete information, they may also involve value judgments about quality of life. One tool under consideration as an aid in making these decisions less subjective is a computerized mortality prediction system called the Acute Physiology and Chronic Health Evaluation (APACHE) system.

When deciding whether to terminate life-sustaining treatment, health care providers face incredible emotional pressure; a patient can't be brought back once treatment is stopped. Nurses do have one ethically sound option: helping patients determine their own fate by educating them about their right to refuse extraordinary treatment.

Right to refuse treatment

The right to refuse treatment is grounded in the ethical principle of respect for the autonomy of the individual. This principle of autonomy has led to the concept of informed consent — the obligation of health care providers to inform the patient of the risk and benefits of a procedure and to obtain permission before the procedure is carried out. Terminally ill patients who receive life-sustaining treatment have an equal right to informed consent.

Because the nursing profession is oriented to saving and prolonging lives, you may find it difficult to go along with a patient's decision to withhold life-sustaining treatment. Keep in mind that limiting treatment doesn't mean abandoning the patient. Supportive mea-

sures are not considered extraordinary treatment. A patient who's chosen to forgo life-sustaining treatment still has the right to receive care that preserves his comfort, hygiene, and dignity. In particular, he has the right to adequate pain control.

Health care workers' rights

Although patients have the right to decide whether to accept or forgo heroic measures, they don't have the right to insist on treatments that provide no medical benefit. If you believe that you'll violate your own *values* by implementing a certain treatment, you have an obligation to arrange for the transfer of the patient's care to another provider. Likewise, if you believe that you'll be violating your values by withholding treatment, you should request the transfer. Known as the "conscience clause," this right applies to assisting in abortions as well as to noninitiation or withdrawal of life-sustaining treatment.

Documenting a patient's wishes

A patient who has a strong desire to request or reject aggressive treatment measures should document his wishes. He should also designate a surrogate decision maker to speak for him if he can no longer make his own health care decisions. Statements that indicate a patient's wishes in the event he loses his decision-making capability are known as *advance directives.* The patient's best means of ensuring that his wishes will be respected, an advance directive may include both a *living will,* which goes into effect when the patient can't make decisions, and *durable power of attorney,* which designates a surrogate decision maker with full authority to carry out the patient's wishes regarding health care decisions. The authority of this surrogate is based on the principle of substituted judgment — allowing the surrogate to make the same decisions the patient would, if he were able.

If a patient has both a living will and a durable power of attorney, the person with durable power should be in complete support of the patient's wishes; then, no family member or health care provider can override him.

Specific treatments can be requested in an advance directive. However, most people execute a living will to ensure that no extraordinary procedures are used to sustain or prolong life.

Advance directives, while useful, haven't ended the controversy over a patient's right to limit treatment. Critics contend that they represent the first step toward active *euthanasia,* or "mercy killing." These people believe that advance directives, such as living wills, should be restricted to a narrow range of circumstances. (See *When family members contest a living will,* page 294.)

Helping the patient plan ahead

Of the many professionals who care for the critically ill, nurses probably have the best chance to act as true *patient advocates.* The patient will probably look to you as well as his doctor for guidance. You can't make the ultimate medical decisions to initiate or limit treatment. But you can help the patient express his wishes concerning his health care and guide him in translating these desires into advance directives.

When you're discussing limiting treatment with a patient, consider these suggestions:
• Present options, such as do-not-resuscitate (DNR) orders, in a realistic but positive context. Reassure the patient that he'll continue to receive supportive care and pain medication. (See *DNRs and slow codes,* page 295.)
• Pay attention to the patient's questions and misunderstandings. Be especially alert for unexpressed fears.
• During your discussions with the patient, note his nonverbal cues and emotional responses.

Despite your best efforts to provide objective advice, the patient may not be able to reach a decision about initiating or terminating care. Remember that you must respect the patient's explicit refusal to participate in health care decisions.

When the patient shouldn't decide

At times, you may question whether a particular patient should be allowed to decide to refuse life-sustaining treatment. Consider whether the patients described below are capable of making life-and-death decisions.
• Joe Ryan suffered a stroke 2 years ago that left him paralyzed on the right side and unable to speak. He was admitted to the hospital with sepsis caused by infected stasis ulcers of his lower legs. Joe's doctor recommended bilateral above-the-knee amputations. As he was being prepared for the surgery, Joe became visibly agitated.
• Mary Kane suffered a severe head injury in a traffic accident that also left her a quadriplegic and dependent on a ventilator. Three months after the accident, she insisted that the ventilator be removed. A hospital psychiatrist determined that Mary was seriously depressed.
• George Bowen has Alzheimer's disease. He can't remember a recent conversation, the names of his three children, or how to find his bedroom, although he's still continent and responsive. When George was admitted to the hospital with his third heart attack, his wife told the doctor he had begged to be allowed to "meet his Maker."

When family members contest a living will

A living will isn't a guarantee that the patient's expressed wishes will be honored. The language in many living wills is vague and unclear. Patients who have added specific requests to a standardized form (for example, requesting termination of tube feedings) may not realize that such requests may conflict with state law. Sometimes nurses and doctors find it difficult to carry out wishes expressed years ago, before current treatment options became available.

The family's response to the living will also can create problems. Family members may not know about the living will or may choose to ignore it in their turmoil over "letting go." As the following case history demonstrates, health care workers, including nurses, can be caught in the crossfire.

Conflicting demands

Esther Summerson was brought to the emergency department in respiratory distress after a long history of chronic obstructive pulmonary disease (COPD). The emergency department staff asked Mrs. Summerson if she wanted help breathing, but they couldn't get a clear response before she lost consciousness. She was intubated and transferred to the intensive care unit.

When Mrs. Summerson's oldest daughter, Jean, arrived at the hospital, she was upset to find that her mother had been placed on a ventilator. She showed the staff a copy of her mother's living will, specifying that her mother not be placed on a ventilator or receive supplementary nutrition. Jean also produced a form giving her durable power of attorney. As her mother's designated decision maker, she demanded that her mother be removed from the ventilator.

Susan, Mrs. Summerson's younger daughter, reached the hospital about an hour after her sister. Although her mother was still unresponsive, Susan did not want her removed from the ventilator. "I don't know what I'd do without Mom," she sobbed. "I want you to do everything you can for her."

Implementing hospital policy

Fortunately, the hospital had developed procedures for resolving this sort of conflict. Mrs. Summerson's doctor, her primary nurse, her priest, and a representative of the hospital's ethics committee called a meeting with Jean, Susan, and Susan's husband, Bob. They explained the living will and Jean's role as the surrogate decision maker, emphasizing that Mrs. Summerson had clearly specified her opposition to the ventilator. Susan and Jean were informed that without the ventilator, their mother might breathe on her own or she might die. But if she did die, it would be from the lung damage caused by her long-standing COPD, not their decision to honor her living will. Each step of the procedure was carefully reviewed.

As a result of this discussion, Susan changed her mind and agreed to remove the ventilator. All three family members decided to be present when this occurred. After they had a chance to talk to Mrs. Summerson and express their love for her, the balloon was deflated and the tube removed. Mrs. Summerson died quietly 2 days later, with her daughters and her son-in-law by her side.

The concept of *informed consent* creates ethical dilemmas in situations in which the patient's ability to make an informed judgment about his treatment options is questionable. If the patient is nonverbal, depressed, demented, or semiconscious, can he truly consent to or refuse life-sustaining treatment?

It is important to remember that some patients may remain capable of expressing health care preferences even when they can't manage in other areas, such as personal care, eating, or speaking.

Standards for judging decision-making ability

Commonly used standards for judging decision-making capability include:
- the ability to indicate a choice
- a clear understanding of the issues at hand
- the ability to reason based on the information given
- an appreciation of the true nature of the situation.

If a patient is incapable of making a decision, it then becomes the duty of a surrogate decision maker or the health care team to act in his best interest.

Making decisions for the patient

Two ethical principles can be used in making decisions for an incapacitated patient. The *substituted judgment* test professes to make the same decision the patient would, if he were capable (the principle of autonomy). Alternatively, the decision may be based on the best interest standard, or deciding what is best for the patient, given his current circumstances (the principle of *beneficence*). Both principles are ethically valid. If the two are at odds, they can create dilemmas for family members, doctors, and nurses.

DNRs and slow codes

Cardiopulmonary resuscitation (CPR) is widely used to treat victims of heart failure, despite its limited usefulness in prolonging life. For example, a study of the resuscitations carried out at a major medical center over a 1-year period revealed that only 14% of those who received CPR actually survived to leave the hospital. Nonetheless, it's not uncommon for a patient to undergo several CPR attempts during a single hospitalization.

Most U.S. hospitals require CPR unless a specific medical order, known as a do-not-resuscitate (DNR) order (also called a no-code situation) is written to prevent this. In addition, the doctor usually must notify the patient and his family before writing a DNR order.

Slow codes

Sometimes slow codes, also known as Hollywood codes, are used when a doctor wants to write a DNR order but can't persuade the patient or his family to agree. Instead, the health care team forms a secret pact to respond slowly to a cardiac or respiratory arrest.

Ethical alternative

Regardless of the rationale behind such a decision, slow codes are morally unacceptable. You may find yourself in a moral dilemma if you're asked to participate in a slow code. To avoid this dilemma, you can insist that code status be part of the treatment plan for all patients, whatever their medical condition.

Hemlock Society: Euthanasia advocates

The Hemlock Society supports the option of active voluntary euthanasia for patients with advanced terminal or severe, incurable illnesses. Founded in 1980, the group claims 28,000 members. Its goals include promoting a climate of public opinion tolerant of the terminally ill person's right to end his own life in a planned manner. It also seeks to improve existing laws on assisted suicide.

The Hemlock Society does not encourage suicide for any primary emotional, traumatic, or financial reasons in the absence of terminal illness. The group in fact approves of suicide prevention work. To obtain further information, contact the Hemlock Society at (503) 342-5748.

Fostering communication

Effective communication is essential when helping families to decide whether to limit or withhold treatment. If you're helping family members or surrogates while they are making life-and-death decisions, the following guidelines can improve communication.

• Create a quiet, private, and unhurried environment — keep all communication simple, factual, and direct.
• Encourage questions.
• Express medical information in simple, clear language.
• Ask decision makers to summarize information, and check their responses.
• Clarify missing or misunderstood information.

Keep in mind that this may be the most heart-rending decision family members or surrogates will ever be asked to make. They need plenty of time, care, and understanding.

Mercy killing

Euthanasia (a term that means painless death) and assisted suicide further confuse the right-to-die issue. Although DNR orders and other decisions to limit treatment sometimes are referred to as passive euthanasia, the term *euthanasia* usually refers to active intervention (such as lethal injection) to bring about death (mercy killing). The issue of whether nurses or other health care professionals can ever ethically assist in taking a life is hotly debated. In 1994, Oregon voters legalized physician-assisted suicide. Enactment of the law was delayed in the courts, but similar bills were introduced in other states. The Oregon law states (with qualifying safeguards) that a terminally ill person may ask a doctor to prescribe a lethal oral medication, which the patient may take when he deems it appropriate.

Proponents of euthanasia and assisted suicide base their argument on the right to self-determination. They contend that if a terminally ill patient is in unendurable, uncontrollable pain, doctor-assisted suicide may be a humane alternative. Public reaction to cases of assisted suicide suggests that many people support a patient's right to control his own fate. Dr. Jack Kevorkian, who has assisted in more than 24 suicides, has many supporters — including Michigan jurors, who have acquitted him of criminal charges. (See *Hemlock Society: Euthanasia advocates*.)

Many people, however, find the concept of mercy killing repugnant. While some nurses believe that the family of a comatose patient should be allowed to withdraw food and fluids, most oppose more active forms of euthanasia.

Allowing euthanasia, they argue, eventually would lead to patients being selectively put to death without consent. The potential object of mercy killing — an Alzheimer's patient or a patient in a *persistent vegetative state* — has lost the capacity to express his wishes. Family members and health care providers do not know if the patient truly desires to die and do not have the moral right to make the decision for him.

Cost considerations

You may find the mention of cost considerations in the context of limiting treatment for the terminally ill offensive. Such considerations, however, are ethically legitimate. The necessity of conserving resources eventually will force the public to consider this issue. Health care resources — including organs available for transplants, beds in the *intensive care unit,* and experimental drugs — are limited in quantity and are costly. Some individuals have begun to debate the equity of giving a disproportionate share of the most expensive medical treatments and procedures to elderly patients who are gravely ill. *Medicare* pays out $21 billion, or 28% of its budget, for bills incurred in the final year of life. Some policy makers believe that the patient's age should be a valid ethical consideration in the delivery of medical care, especially when tremendous amounts of money are spent to achieve relatively small gains in life expectancy.

Like it or not, the truth is that health care in the United States is already rationed to a degree, through policies that discourage the poor from seeking medical attention. Unaffordably high insurance rates, underfinanced state medical programs, and crowded clinics, in effect, ration care.

Deciding how to ration lifesaving technology is an ethical dilemma of huge proportions. It ultimately will have to be resolved by society at large, using the ethical principle of justice.

Organ transplantation

The benefits of organ transplantation are widely recognized by both health care professionals and the general public. Nevertheless, organ transplantation poses serious ethical concerns. Transplant procedures affect families of the donor and the recipient, nurses, doctors, and even ambulance attendants at the deepest emotional level. In such a highly charged atmosphere, conflicts of rights easily can develop.
• If the donor is a child, the validity of informed consent may be questioned.
• Controversy may occur over when to declare a potential donor dead.
• The wishes of a potential donor's family may conflict with the needs of a transplant patient.
• Because the number of available donor organs is limited, difficult choices must be made about which patients should receive transplants.
• Many transplants are prohibitively expensive; questions arise as to whether subsidizing the procedure is a just allocation of health care resources.
• In light of the limited number of available donor organs and the high cost of the procedure, questions arise as to the patient's right to multiple transplants.

Even if you don't make the ultimate medical decisions about an organ transplant, you may play a critical role in resolving ethical conflicts.

Protecting the rights of potential donors

Some transplantation procedures pose few ethical problems. An autograft, in which tissue is transplanted from one part of the patient's body to another (such as a skin graft to treat a third-degree burn), is a good example. Certain types of transplants from one person to another (homograft), including blood transfusions and cornea or bone marrow transplants, also are widely accepted and ethically untainted.

The most difficult ethical issues surround the procurement of organs essential for life: hearts, kidneys, livers, and lungs. In these instances, organ procurement remains ethical only if steps are taken to assure that the donor's life or functional integrity aren't compromised.

Nonmaleficence

At first glance, removing an organ from a healthy person who has nothing to gain from the procedure seems to violate the ethical principle of *nonmaleficence*—the obligation to "do no harm." But when providing care, there are many instances in which the principle of nonmaleficence cannot be strictly applied. Some harm, in the form of an invasive or a potentially risky procedure, must be incurred in diagnosing and treating many diseases.

When a living person donates the organ, the key issue is informed consent. From both an ethical and a legal standpoint, informed consent requires the donor to be fully aware of all risks and benefits that can result from the transplant procedure. Because relatives, particularly identical twins or full siblings, typically provide the closest match for a transplanted organ, a great deal of emotional pressure can be exerted on a potential donor. Extreme guilt feelings and emotional distress may disturb a potential donor's ability to render informed consent.

Child donors

Special problems arise when the potential donor is a child. Because, in most cases, a *minor's* consent is legally invalid, the parents or *legal guardians* must give substitute consent. Sometimes the wishes of the child and the parents are clearly the same. A 13-year-old whose parents support her wish to donate a kidney to her 5-year-old brother can probably give valid informed consent. But what about a 3-year-old, who can't express his opinion? Can his parents ethically "volunteer" this child to donate a kidney? Parents have a moral obligation to protect the life and well-being of all their children. Sometimes it's unclear how to best uphold this obligation. Which are more important—the rights of the healthy child or the rights of the child who needs the kidney?

In a widely publicized 1991 case, doctors at the City of Hope Medical Center, in Duarte, Calif., transplanted bone marrow into Anissa Ayala, a 19-year-old girl with potentially fatal leukemia. The marrow came from her baby sister, Marissa. The parents said that they conceived Marissa to provide bone marrow to save Anissa's life. This marked the first time a family publicly admitted to conceiving a child to serve as an organ donor.

The case raised troubling ethical questions. Does conceiving a child as a source of donated organs violate the principle that children should be brought into the world and cherished for their own sake and no other motive? If prenatal tests indicate that the fetus is the wrong tissue type to serve as a donor, is an abortion justifiable? Selling organs is both unethical and illegal, but the legal and ethical status of conceiving potential donors remains unclear.

Cadaver donors

Harvesting organs from a deceased donor poses a different set of ethical problems. Perhaps the most fundamental issue involves the actual definition of *death.* Although some organs and tissues, such as bone, skin, cornea, and even kidneys, can be transplanted after complete cardiac arrest, other organs, including the heart, lung, liver, and pancreas, aren't viable unless they're taken from a brain-dead, or "beating heart," cadaver.

Most states recognize the definition of brain death set forth by the Uniform Determination of Death Act as the legal definition of death. In general terms, a patient is pronounced brain dead when all functional activity in every area of the brain, including the brain stem, stops. Significantly, this definition of death isn't universally accepted by health care workers, ethicists, or lay people. Many find it difficult to declare death when other aspects of bodily function continue, even if by artificial support.

The issue of declaring brain death must be approached cautiously. The determination that a person is brain dead should be made by neurologic consult and never by a doctor who's involved in organ removal. No request for organ donation should be made until the family understands what brain death is and that it is a final state.

Informed consent

The Uniform Anatomical Gift Act allows a person to donate specific organs or even his entire body for organ transplantation. A patient who before death indicated his willingness to be an organ donor could be considered to have given informed consent. True informed consent, however, requires that the patient have the option to withdraw consent at any time before a medical procedure. Therefore, the final decision is left up to the potential donor's family, even if it results in the loss of an organ donation.

Approaching a potential donor's family

Twenty-eight states have enacted required request acts. These laws require hospitals to ask families of potential organ donors to permit donation. The required request laws are intended to increase organ availability. (See *National Organ Transplant Act,* page 300.)

Most required request laws are fair to the families of potential donors. Family members are under no compulsion to grant permission to donate organs. Most required request acts grant an exclusion if the request will cause the family severe emotional distress.

These laws may create serious ethical conflicts, however, for a nurse who opposes organ transplantation or who finds the idea of approaching a grieving family offensive. Should a nurse be forced to request organ donation, regardless of her feelings? One solution to this dilemma is assigning the job of approaching the donor's family to a specially trained organ procurement team.

If you are making the request for an organ donation from a patient's family, approach family members tactfully and be sufficiently informed to answer their questions. You should be able to explain the potential good to others. Remember, the decision of the family must be respected.

Fetal tissue

Because the mother and the health care team carrying out an abortion are responsible for the death of the fetus, the transplantation of fetal tissue is far more controversial than transplantation from a cadaver donor (see *Fetal tissue transplant debate,* page 301).

Caring for a potential donor

If you're caring for a patient who's a potential donor, your ethical responsibility includes maintaining his dignity as a human being until he's declared legally dead. You'll want to follow nor-

National Organ Transplant Act

In response to widespread public interest in organ transplantation, Congress enacted the National Organ Transplant Act of 1984 (PL 98-507). This act:
• prohibits the sale of organs
• provides funding for grants to organ procurement agencies
• establishes a national organ-sharing system.

Task force on organ transplantation

This act also convened a 25-member Task Force on Organ Transplantation with members representing medicine, law, theology, ethics, allied health, the health insurance industry, and the general public. Representatives from the Office of the Surgeon General, the National Institutes of Health, the Food and Drug Administration, and the Health Care Financing Administration also were appointed to the task force. This task force examined the medical, legal, ethical, economic, and social issues created by organ transplantation.

In its final report, the task force concluded that the best way to close the gap between the small number of organ donors and the large number of potential transplant recipients was to actively solicit donations from bereaved families. As a result, the task force recommended that all state legislatures introduce and enact legislation requiring health care professionals to present organ donation as an option to families ("required request").

Assertive approach

Required request policies are legally mandated in many states. This assertive approach to organ procurement has proved highly successful; as many as 80% of families given the option to become donor families ultimately do so. Significantly, studies show that organ donation can facilitate the grieving process and speed recovery for the bereaved family.

---

mal cleansing and skin maintenance procedures and keep the body properly covered. You'll also need to adhere to the doctor's instructions for discontinuing medication and avoiding procedures that could damage the organ.

Maintaining a brain-dead patient until preparations for the transplant are complete raises additional ethical questions. If death is defined as brain death, doesn't the patient have the right to die when this determination is made? If not, how long can he be ethically maintained on a life-support system? One day? One week? Is this a justifiable allocation of resources? The effort and money spent to maintain a brain-dead organ donor for any appreciable period

might be better spent helping living patients.

Using organs from anencephalic infants

Anencephaly is the congenital absence of most or all of the cerebral hemispheres. Many anencephalic infants are stillborn, but others have a functional brain stem, and live for a short time after birth.

Anencephalic infants might seem to be ideal organ donors. Their immune systems are still immature, reducing the chance of rejection. In addition, their small organs can be readily used in children, who commonly encounter

Fetal tissue transplant debate

Although still in the research phase, transplants using tissue from aborted fetuses offer new hope for treating Parkinson's disease, Alzheimer's disease, diabetes, and other degenerative disorders. The immaturity of the fetal immune system reduces the chances of rejection, making fetal tissue ideally suited to transplantation. From an ethical standpoint, though, fetal tissue transplants are a cause for concern as well as hope.

Obtaining fetal tissue

When family members give permission for the donation of organs from a deceased loved one, they are not responsible for his death. In fetal tissue transplants, the mother, along with members of the health care team carrying out the abortion, is responsible for the death of the fetus. This makes questions about when and how tissue is obtained much more problematic.

Opponents of fetal tissue transplants point to the high risk of ethical abuses. For example, suppose a woman can no longer stand to watch her father, who has Alzheimer's disease, deteriorate. She decides to conceive and then abort a fetus to supply brain tissue for a transplant for her father. Although it's easy to understand her motives, few people would agree that this is ethical.

Clearly, guidelines need to be developed to ensure that women who provide tissue from abortions are adequately informed about fetal tissue transplants yet not encouraged to consent to an abortion they might not otherwise have.

Second-trimester abortions

The timing of the abortion is another critical issue. Most elective abortions take place during the first trimester, almost as soon as the mother finds out she's pregnant. Unfortunately, the best tissue for transplantation comes from second-trimester fetuses. Is it ethical for the mother to postpone the abortion? Some fetuses may be viable by the last stages of the second trimester.

Research ban

In 1988, the Department of Health and Human Services banned federal funding for research into the use of healthy cells from fetal tissue to replace defective cells in adults. However, President Clinton addressed the issue early in his presidency and, in 1993, lifted the ban.

---

the most trouble in locating a suitable donor.

The anencephalic infant, however, isn't a "beating heart" cadaver. Although severely debilitated, an infant with a functioning brain stem must be considered to be in a persistent vegetative state or a coma, not brain dead. Until an anencephalic infant meets the clinical criteria for brain death, using his organs for transplantation remains ethically controversial.

In the United States, laws have been proposed that would increase the supply of organs available for donation. One such law would broaden the definition of brain death, making organs from anencephalic infants available. In 1995, the *American Medical Association* came out in support of such legislation. Opponents of this legislation argue that if the definition of brain death is broadened to include anencephalic infants, other groups may be targeted for organ donation without consent, for example, people in a persistent vegetative state. (See *Organ donation and the concept of consent,* page 302.)

Organ donation and the concept of consent

Recent legislative initiatives to increase the supply of organs available for donation have sought to broaden the definition of consent. One recent proposal is based on the concept of presumed consent — the assumption that all sane and rational persons would consent to donate organs if they had the chance to do so.

Under this legislation, every person would be considered an organ donor unless they carried a card stating they did *not* want to donate their organs. Rather than being asked if they wished to have their loved one's organs transplanted, family members would be asked if they had any objections to transplantation.

A violation of informed consent?

Although the doctrine of presumed consent is applied to other aspects of health care law, when applied to organ donation, presumed consent is a controversial idea. Opponents argue that it is coercive and violates the right to informed consent. It contradicts the widely-held belief that an individual should have free choice in all decisions related to his own body.

Selecting transplant recipients

The number of potential transplant recipients far exceeds the number of available donors. How should one determine who receives a transplant?

Medical and physical factors rule out some matches. For example, the donor and recipient must have compatible blood and tissue types and be fairly close in size and age.

Beyond such limitations, the selection of transplant recipients depends entirely on value judgments. This means the potential for serious value conflicts and unethical behavior is tremendous. (See *Choosing between potential transplant recipients.*)

To ensure that transplant recipients are selected as fairly as possible, most medical centers have adopted the following guidelines.

Coordinating transplants

A regional organ donation center should coordinate the matching of transplant recipients and potential donors. The principle of "first-come, first-served" should form one criterion for selection.

All transplant decisions should be made by a committee under the auspices of an impartial organization, such as the Red Cross. The committee should include a doctor, nurse, lawyer, religious leader, and well-informed layperson.

Determining need

The selection procedure should be based on need as well as the potential for survival. Patients with the greatest need (those closest to death) and best survival potential receive the highest priority.

Determining potential for survival

Survival is a more complex issue than need. For example, the potential for survival doesn't necessarily decrease as a patient ages. A health-conscious elderly patient may represent a better transplant risk than a younger patient who has neglected his health.

A patient's life-style changes, medication regimens, and diet restrictions can influence survival. Life-style factors may raise questions about a patient's suitability as a transplant recipient. Should a heavy smoker who refuses to quit be given a heart-lung

CASE STUDY IN ETHICS

Choosing between potential transplant recipients

One concern about organ transplantation is the potential for elitism when choosing one recipient over another. Consider the following situation, in which the committee on organ donation and transplantation at a major teaching hospital had to choose between two potential liver recipients.

Patron's daughter

Jodi Morgan, a 5-year-old girl, had received a liver transplant 18 months earlier. Although her initial response was promising, she'd recently been hospitalized again with signs of irreversible hepatic failure.

Jodi was born with multiple birth defects. Besides biliary atresia, which led to her need for a transplant, she had only one functioning kidney and a cyanotic heart defect. She was mildly retarded, still unable to speak, and had only recently mastered toilet training.

Jodi's father, Jack, was a prominent local businessman and politician, as well as a patron of the hospital. He wanted Jodi placed at the head of the transplant registry for a second liver transplant. She'd spent 4 months on the registry before her first transplant. Nonetheless, rumors had spread that Mr. Morgan had "bought" Jodi's first transplant by making a sizable donation to the hospital's new cardiology wing.

Mother of three

Brenda DiStefano, a 22-year-old mother of three young children, headed the list of potential liver recipients. In chronic hepatic failure for nearly 2 years, she'd been on the transplant list most of that time and was now near death. She was unemployed and had no health insurance. Because the federal government will not reimburse liver transplants, the hospital stood little chance of being paid for her surgery.

Committee decision

According to state law, Jodi couldn't receive a second transplant unless she was returned to the registry. But should she be placed at the head of the list?

The committee struggled with many ethical questions:
● Mr. Morgan would probably exert a great deal of political and financial pressure on the hospital. Could committee members realistically ignore this factor?
● How might past rumors that Mr. Morgan bought Jodi's first transplant influence the present thinking of committee members?
● Brenda's inability to pay would probably create a financial hardship for the hospital. Should this influence their decision?
● Do risk-benefit calculations justify another procedure for Jodi Morgan? Because of her underlying cardiac pathology and renal dysfunction, even if the transplantation is successful, her prognosis is poor. The potential for success of the transplant is less than it would be for healthier patients.
● Should a child like Jodi be given automatic preference over an adult? What about Brenda DiStefano's children? Should their right to have a mother be an overriding consideration?

After much debate, the committee decided to return Jodi to the transplant list, behind Brenda. Once a donor was found for Brenda, Jodi could have a second chance at life.

transplant? Should a person with a long history of alcohol abuse receive a liver transplant, as did baseball legend Mickey Mantle in 1995?

The principle of *distributive justice* could work either way in such cases. On the one hand, to ensure equal treatment, everyone should have equal access to a new organ. On the other hand, the scarcity of donor organs argues for reserving organs for people with healthful life-styles who are more likely to sustain them.

Determining potential value to the community

The selection procedure also can take into account a potential recipient's value to the community. A good case could be made for assigning a higher priority to a mother of two young children than to a convicted drug dealer.

Avoiding manipulation

Neither the donor nor his family ought to play a role in selection. Because of the potential for manipulation (a payoff by the recipient), such participation isn't compatible with an ethical selection procedure.

Drawing lots

When other criteria fail to establish priority, the final selection should be made by lot.

Cost considerations

Organ transplants are prohibitively expensive. A kidney transplant costs about $35,000; a heart transplant may exceed $100,000. Liver and pancreas transplants are even more costly. The federal government will pay up to 80% of the costs for kidney and heart transplants, but does not subsidize liver or pancreas transplants, which are still considered experimental. For the patient whose life depends on receiving a liver transplant, the current reim-

bursement policy would appear unjust.

One might pose an even more challenging question: Is it fair for one person to receive that great a share of the limited funds available for health care? The cost of a heart transplant would finance inoculations for several thousand children or prenatal care for hundreds of women. Utilitarian ethical theory would claim that the rights of hundreds of potential patients to a quality life exceed the right of one person to a heart transplant.

Multiple transplants

The issue of multiple transplants is closely related to the concept of distributive justice. It might seem unethical, or at least unfair, for the same person to receive three or four transplants. However, nurses and doctors caring for a transplant recipient may believe that everything possible must be done to keep the patient alive, including performing another transplant.

Perhaps the most equitable course of action is to place a repeat-transplant patient back on the regional transplant center register for a fair evaluation.

Perinatal ethics

Twenty years ago, an infant born at 26 weeks' gestation had almost no chance of surviving. But today, such infants can and do survive, thanks to spectacular advances in neonatology, such as intrauterine surgery.

Many people argue that this lifesaving technology has gone too far. Doctors and nurses who treat critically ill neonates, they say, act too aggressively, frequently overriding the wishes of the infant's parents. Treatment leads to even greater suffering for the infant and places an enormous financial burden on society. Ethical questions are complicated by lack of knowledge about the long-term outcome of heroic measures.

Sanctity of life vs. quality of life

Without life, other values are irrelevant. As a result, society holds the sanctity of life in high regard. The belief that all human lives have meaning and ought to be respected supports the notion that a critically ill infant should be kept alive at any cost.

But what about *quality of life?* A utilitarian ethic would support a decision to withhold treatment for a severely handicapped newborn when the prospect for an acceptable quality of life is poor. But what is an "acceptable quality of life"?

One measure of the value of a person's life is his ability to achieve certain goals. Thus, if an infant has little hope of achieving anything but sheer survival, it may be ethically acceptable to terminate treatment.

The "best interest" criterion is another measure of the quality of life. Unfortunately, not everyone agrees on the exact meaning of "best interest." Is death ever in anyone's best interest?

Still another definition considers the patient's potential to establish some type of human relationship. According to this view, an infant who has little chance of recognizing and relating to his family has such a poor quality of life that withholding treatment is both compassionate and ethical. There are two objections to the "human relationship" standard. First, this criterion suggests that medical treatment be withheld from adults who have a limited capacity for human relationships. You'd almost certainly find it morally unacceptable to refuse to perform an emergency appendectomy on a psychotic patient or to withhold medication

from a comatose automobile accident victim.

Some experts argue that the infant isn't the only one with a right to an acceptable quality of life. The financial and emotional cost of sophisticated perinatal technology places an enormous burden on the family, as well as society in general. Is this too great a price for a few extra months or years of life?

Who should decide

The best-qualified person to make a quality-of-life decision is the patient himself. But who's best qualified to give *proxy* consent for a premature infant born at 25 weeks' gestation?

Parents

Although no one knows the infant's true desires, legal and ethical precedent suggests that his parents ought to be the chief decision makers. Others argue that the parents' ability to make a wise and rational decision on short notice in such an emotionally charged atmosphere is limited. In addition, few parents have the necessary medical knowledge to make an informed decision. The combination of time pressure, ignorance, prejudice, and religious or moral beliefs can force parents into a decision that's at odds with the opinions of the medical team caring for their infant.

Health care team

Not only are members of the health care team more objective, but they also are better informed about the potential outcomes of the various treatment options. Ethically, however, this paternalistic approach is unacceptable. After all, the health care team won't bear the burden of raising the child.

Hospital ethics committee

Unfortunately, the slow pace of most committee decisions isn't compatible with the rapid decisions required when treating seriously ill neonates. In addition, using this approach might simply substitute the biases of the committee members for the biases of the parents, doctors, and nurses.

Courts

As the designated protector of individual rights, the legal system typically takes a narrow view of the issues. For example, up to the time of birth, greater weight is given to the rights of the mother. But during or after birth, the courts often have decided that the rights of the infant supersede those of the parents.

"Baby Doe" regulations

Court-mandated settlements to perinatal ethical conflicts have created significant debate. The best-known case involved an infant born with Down's syndrome and a tracheoesophageal fistula. The family opted to forgo surgical treatment of the fistula and withhold supplemental nutrition, reasoning that the child's quality of life was too severely compromised. A nurse caring for the child disagreed. She contacted the authorities, but during the ensuing legal battle, the infant died.

On the basis of this and similar cases, the federal government instituted regulations standardizing the care of critically ill or severely handicapped newborns. Enacted under the umbrella of the Child Abuse Protection and Treatment Act, these "Baby Doe regulations" prohibited doctors and nurses from denying treatment to disabled infants. The only exceptions were infants in an irreversible coma; those for whom treatment would prolong dying, not life; and those for whom treatment would be futile or even in-

humane. Violators could be prosecuted for *negligence* or *malpractice.*

Some lawmakers opposed the constitutionality of the Baby Doe regulations. The Supreme Court agreed, and in June 1986, struck down federal laws requiring the treatment of all handicapped newborns. In addition, it reinforced the right to *privacy* by denying access to Baby Doe's *medical records.* Unfortunately, because many states backed up the federal laws with their own Baby Doe regulations, it's still possible to be prosecuted for withholding treatment.

The major ethical problem with these regulations is their failure to address the quality-of-life issue. In addition, they are based on the mistaken assumption that a set of rigid laws can take the place of the ethical decision-making process.

Nurse's role

The repeal of federal Baby Doe regulations hasn't clarified the ethical issues surrounding the care of critically ill infants. If anything, by creating a conflict between the federal government and state and local laws, it's made the situation even more complicated.

To help the parents of an extremely premature or critically ill neonate reach ethically sound decisions, you'll need to present all available options in a compassionate, unbiased manner, using simple terms. By carefully considering the pros and cons of both initiating and withholding treatment, you can help family members come to terms with their child's condition and reach a decision they will be able to live with. (See *Critically ill neonate.*)

Critically ill neonate

If you care for extremely premature or severely handicapped infants or their mothers, family members will look to you to assist them in life-and-death decisions. Your attitudes and opinions can have a powerful effect on their course of action. Consider the nurse's role in the case study discussed below.

Grim prognosis

Matthew Klein, a microcephalic infant with transposition of the great arteries, was born more than 6 weeks prematurely. He also had spina bifida. The news of his condition was devastating to his parents, an older professional couple who had eagerly anticipated their first child.

The attending pediatrician asked a noted neurosurgeon and a pediatric cardiologist to consult on Matthew's case. These experts concurred that without immediate corrective surgery, he might live as long as 1 month on life support. Even with surgery, he probably wouldn't live beyond age 20. During that time, the doctors explained to Mr. and Mrs. Klein, Matthew could be expected to suffer from seizure disorders, paralysis, and episodes of congestive heart failure. He'd be highly susceptible to infection and severely retarded. In fact, he faced a grave risk just from the surgery.

Treatment options

Mr. and Mrs. Klein were given two options. They could choose aggressive surgical intervention for their child. If Matthew survived, he'd need additional surgery at age 4 and again at age 10. Alternatively, the Kleins could elect a conservative treatment plan, which included antibiotics, nutrition, and comfort measures, but no heroic treatment.

Angelica Perez, an RN with more than 3 years of experience in caring for seriously ill newborns, was assigned to Matthew as his primary nurse. Ms. Perez soon realized that Matthew's parents were overwhelmed. She knew that as a result, their decision-making ability was compromised.

Ms. Perez strongly believed in the sanctity of life. Yet her practical experience gave her an appreciation for quality-of-life issues. In her professional opinion, the quality of Matthew's life was likely to be poor, and the conservative treatment option would be best.

She carefully reviewed both treatment plans with Matthew's parents, analyzing the possible outcomes and explaining unfamiliar medical terms. Ms. Perez pointed out that even with surgical intervention, Matthew might be too severely brain damaged to ever recognize or interact with them. Mrs. Klein would have to quit her job to care for Matthew, and his medical expenses would pose an enormous financial burden. Eventually, he was almost certain to require institutional care.

Ms. Perez recognized that the conservative option presented problems for the Kleins as well. Deeply religious, both husband and wife strongly opposed mercy killing. They had difficulty seeing the distinction between allowing their son to die and actually causing his death.

Even after extensive counseling, the Kleins couldn't reach a decision. At this point, Ms. Perez suggested that the couple discuss their feelings with the doctor, a social worker, and their minister. As a result of these discussions, Mr. and Mrs. Klein accepted the conclusion that conservative treatment was best for Matthew. The baby survived for 3 weeks and died in his mother's arms.

AIDS

Nurses have always honored their professional responsibility to care for all patients, regardless of personal attributes, life-style, or nature of the illness. Today, AIDS challenges this long-standing professional ethic. No other contagious illness incites such emotionally charged ethical debate.

AIDS touches on two highly controversial social issues: sexuality and drug use. It isn't surprising that many nurses experience value conflicts when working to meet their professional obligations. (See *Ethical issues and AIDS: Where do you stand?*)

Prejudice, fear, and misunderstanding surround AIDS. A human immunodeficiency virus (HIV)-positive test result often means the loss of a job, medical insurance, financial security, and even housing. Family and friends, as well as the public at large, may shun the AIDS patient. As a result, maintaining *confidentiality* is a serious concern for people with AIDS.

Mandatory testing

As many as 90% of the estimated 1.5 million Americans infected with HIV don't know about it. Lack of awareness can seriously undermine both patient care and prevention efforts. Testing for HIV isn't like testing for other infectious diseases. The patient with a positive gonorrhea culture doesn't face the same likelihood of discrimination as the patient who is HIV-positive.

Some organizations, including the military and prisons, and many insurance companies insist on mandatory testing. Several states attempted to institute mandatory testing to obtain a marriage licence and then abandoned the policy because of high costs and the low percentage of positive results.

Most states now mandate written consent for testing, as well as pretest and post-test counseling.

Does mandatory testing violate the ethical principles of autonomy (the patient's right to control his own fate) and justice (his right to be treated fairly)? Does it violate his right to privacy? Many nurses believe that it does not. Health care workers, they argue, have a right to protect themselves and need a complete picture of the patient's health status to deliver quality care.

Public health officials contend that mandatory testing would improve our understanding of the spread of the disease and aid in prevention. Hospital *administrators* say that knowing a patient's HIV status could lower health care costs by pinpointing those who require universal precautions.

Opponents of mandatory testing emphasize the risk of discrimination and the high cost of screening all patients. They also believe testing would drive away patients who need care because many people fear being tested. Mandatory testing also can backfire. An exposed person can take 12 weeks or longer to develop HIV antibodies. During this time, he's contagious, but seronegative.

Case history

The following example illustrates some of the ethical problems raised by mandatory testing.

Karen Owen, a trauma nurse, was accidentally exposed to a patient's blood during emergency surgery to treat a gunshot wound. Many AIDS patients are treated at Karen's inner-city hospital. As a precautionary measure, hospital *policy* dictated HIV testing of source patients when an employee was exposed to blood or body fluids. But Karen's patient strongly objected. She argued that she was equally likely to have contracted AIDS from Karen. She demanded that Karen be tested as well.

Ethical issues and AIDS: Where do you stand?

Acquired immunodeficiency syndrome (AIDS) raises numerous ethical issues for nurses and other health care professionals. These issues range from personal safety to societal obligations. Read and answer the questions below to help you articulate your ethical positions on AIDS.

• Should all health care professionals have the right to refuse to treat human immunodeficiency virus (HIV)-positive patients?

• Should AIDS patients receive "heroic" life-sustaining treatments?

• Should pregnant HIV-positive patients have abortions rather than risk the chance of passing the virus to their unborn children?

• Should health departments obtain lists of all sexual contacts of people diagnosed as HIV-positive and notify those on the lists of their risk of exposure?

• Should the U.S. government provide free medical insurance to HIV-positive patients who are no longer able to buy health insurance?

• Should pregnant drug abusers who acquire HIV and infect their infants be charged with child abuse?

• Should costly, limited intensive care unit (ICU), neonatal ICU, and pediatric ICU resources be tied up in the care of AIDS patients if other patients with better prognoses for survival are being deprived?

• Should hospitals and nursing homes routinely test all new admissions for HIV infection?

• Should hospitals and nursing homes test all current and new employees for HIV infection?

• Should states and provinces enact special laws allowing terminally ill AIDS patients to request and receive a lethal, painless injection?

Is this a legitimate request, and must the hospital honor it? What about Karen's right to privacy? If she proved HIV-positive, would she lose her job? If she was HIV-negative, did she have to consent to be retested at a later date?

Out of concern for her own health, Karen agreed to be tested. Also, the hospital noted on the patient's consent form that the test was due to worker exposure, not because she was in a high-risk group. Fortunately, both nurse and patient proved to be HIV-negative.

Public's right to know

Many people believe that all health care providers should be routinely tested for HIV. The public, they argue, has the right to know a nurse's or doctor's HIV status.

After at least three patients contracted HIV from a Florida dentist, the *American Medical Association* and the American Dental Association recommended that HIV-positive doctors and dentists perform no invasive procedures and tell their patients of their HIV status.

Lawmakers have considered proposals to prevent HIV-positive doctors from performing surgery and other risky procedures. Such proposals are highly controversial. In 1991, a New Jersey court upheld the right of a Princeton hospital to ban a surgeon with AIDS.

Some people question the need for restrictions based solely on HIV status. Rules covering impaired health care workers, whether due to drug addiction, mental status, or physical illness, seem fairer and reduce the chance of HIV-based discrimination.

Testing guidelines

Following the guidelines below can help to ensure that HIV testing is carried out in an ethically responsible manner.

• The sole purpose of any screening program should be to prevent the spread of HIV.

• The confidentiality of the test results must be assured. If it's necessary to disclose the results (when a blood donor tests positive), the affected person should be notified.

• The patient should receive adequate pretest and post-test counseling.

• The diagnostic laboratory must be as reliable as possible.

• Informed consent should be obtained before a patient is allowed to participate in a voluntary screening program. (See *Correcting a flawed HIV testing policy.*)

Universal precautions

The **Centers for Disease Control and Prevention** (CDC) contends that mandatory testing isn't necessary to protect nurses if health care workers follow universal precautions for all patients. This means using gloves, gowns, and goggles to prevent contact with a patient's blood or body fluids and strictly adhering to safety measures when handling needles, scalpels, or other sharp instruments.

Unfortunately, few nurses follow these precautions all the time. Some hospitals fail to provide enough supplies. Some nurses complain that gloves and gowns make it more difficult to perform certain procedures. Nurses working in the emergency department may not have time to adhere meticulously to precautions. In addition, many white, middle-class patients are automatically assumed to be seronegative.

Universal precautions are time-consuming, expensive, and obstructive.

Nonetheless, following these precautions means that nurses can protect themselves without forcing patients to undergo mandatory testing.

Refusing to provide care

Dorothy, a critical care nurse, struggled for many months with her prejudices against AIDS patients. Although she was deeply committed to her career, her religion taught that both homosexuality and drug use were sins. She also was apprehensive about the danger of contracting AIDS. Finally, she begged her supervisor to avoid assigning her to AIDS patients.

Marie, who works on the surgical floor of a large teaching hospital, also wants to avoid AIDS patients. But she has a different reason. She's just learned that she's pregnant, and she wants to avoid exposure to cytomegalovirus (CMV), a common opportunistic infection in AIDS.

Ethical solutions

The **American Nurses' Association** Ethical Code for Nurses states that "the nurse provides services...unrestricted by considerations of social or economic status, personal attributes, or the nature of health problems." Thus, Dorothy's refusal to care for AIDS patients because this duty conflicts with her religious beliefs isn't ethically viable. No matter how strong your personal feelings, you can't allow them to interfere with your moral obligation to provide care.

This obligation isn't absolute, however. If the risk to you is greater than the potential benefit to the patient, you can ethically refuse to take that risk. Marie, for instance, is justified in refusing to treat patients with a CMV infection because of the risk to her unborn child. But she can't avoid caring for patients with *Pneumocystis carinii* pneumonia or Kaposi's sarcoma.

CASE STUDY IN ETHICS

Correcting a flawed HIV testing policy

Regardless of whether human immunodeficiency virus (HIV) testing is voluntary or mandatory, careless procedures can ruin lives and increase liability. Consider the case study discussed below.

Surgeon's request

Mike Robertson, a robust, athletic 25-year-old, suffered a herniated disk in a bicycling accident. When bed rest and anti-inflammatory drugs didn't relieve his pain, he was referred to an orthopedic surgeon. The doctor recommended surgery but insisted that Mike undergo HIV testing before the operation.

"I don't understand why I need an HIV test," Mike told Sherry Waters, the nurse counselor who performed his preadmission counseling.

Sherry explained that the doctor's request was legal and that it was probably a routine practice. She reviewed the details of the test procedure, emphasizing that a positive result did not mean that he had AIDS, although he faced a high risk of developing the disease and could infect others. Finally, she pointed out to Mike that his test results would remain confidential, but if he preferred, she could refer him to an anonymous testing site.

"No, that's OK," Mike replied. "I want to get this done and get my back fixed next week. It's really been killing me."

Devastating results

Mike's surgery was scheduled for the following Tuesday. Sherry set up an appointment for Monday afternoon to give him the test results. To her dismay, he was HIV-positive. Worse, he didn't keep his appointment. Later that day, he called to reschedule the appointment for the morning of the surgery.

Sherry became frantic. Should she tell Mike the test results just before surgery, when the information could be dangerously upsetting? Should she wait until after surgery, when he would still be somewhat sedated and might not really understand?

Sherry finally reached Mike's surgeon just an hour before the operation. Even though Mike had already received preoperative sedation, the doctor immediately canceled surgery. He recommended that Sherry explain Mike's test results as soon as he woke up. She agreed, knowing that Mike would need an explanation for the cancellation.

Mike was devastated by the news. He was disappointed and angry that the surgery hadn't taken place and even more horrified to learn that he was HIV-positive. He felt that his doctor had abandoned him, leaving him with two untreated medical problems: his back and his HIV status.

Changing hospital policy

Sherry also was disappointed and angry. Fortunately, she was able to capitalize on her feelings to improve her hospital's HIV testing program. She discussed Mike's case with the director of nursing, stressing that in the future, she would refuse to carry out a test unless ample time was provided for post-test counseling. In response, the hospital established new guidelines for HIV testing. Doctors who requested the HIV antibody test before any medical procedure had to verify that post-test counseling had taken place before the procedure could be performed. In addition, the doctor was required to specify whether he would continue to care for a patient who tested positive. If not, he'd need to designate another doctor who would do so.

ANA guidelines: Your obligation to provide care

In 1986, the American Nurse's Association (ANA) Committee on Ethics reviewed the nurse's obligation to care for patients with infectious diseases, including acquired immunodeficiency syndrome (AIDS). The committee concluded that a nurse must provide care when four criteria are met:

● The patient is at significant risk of harm, loss, or damage if the nurse does not assist.

● The nurse's intervention or care is directly relevant to preventing harm.

● The nurse's care will probably prevent harm, loss, or damage to the patient.

● The benefit the patient will gain outweighs any harm the nurse might incur and providing care does not present more than minimal risk to the nurse.

Moral option

The last criterion presents you with a moral option when a particular patient poses a significant risk to your health or emotional well-being. If the AIDS patient is purposefully uncooperative, you have the right to refuse to provide care. Although you can't abandon such a patient, ethically or legally, you can find someone else to care for him.

You also may refuse to perform procedures on a patient who deliberately puts you at risk. For example, if a patient deliberately moves his arm while you're drawing blood, you have the right to refuse to carry out the procedure. You may even be justified in refusing altogether to care for this patient, but you cannot abandon the patient. Ethically and legally, you're required to find

someone else to care for him. (See *ANA guidelines: Your obligation to provide care.*)

What if an AIDS patient becomes violent or threatens to bite you? If the patient's decisional capability is in doubt, the use of chemical or physical restraints may be justified. If the patient makes threats because of anger, warn him that his aggressive behavior must stop or treatment can't continue. You and the doctor should document the patient's behavior, stating, if necessary, that because treatment cannot be administered at this time, the patient is being discharged.

Contact notification

The patient's right to privacy may conflict with your duty to prevent the spread of the disease. The patient may balk when you request that he inform his partner that he's HIV-positive. You must respect the patient's right to confidentiality. You should try to impress on him, however, how crucial it is for the other person to know they've been exposed to the AIDS virus. Anonymous contact notification programs may provide assistance. For example, with the patient's consent, you can refer the problem to the county health department. They'll attempt to locate and inform contacts of their exposure.

Many married patients are reluctant to notify their spouses, especially if the infection can be traced to an extramarital affair. Legally, you can't compel the patient to tell his wife. But you can explore options that may make it easier for him to do so. For example, ask the patient if he would feel more comfortable if a family doctor gave her the news. A counselor also could work with the patient to reduce his anxiety about informing his wife, as well as to support him when he tells her.

AIDS and the pregnant patient

Mandatory HIV testing of pregnant women gained support when studies showed that giving a woman the drug zidovudine (AZT) markedly reduces the risk of HIV transmission to the fetus. In addition, giving AZT to newborns of HIV-positive women helps these at-risk infants.

Those who favor mandatory testing argue that the potential reduction in HIV transmission overrides the mother's autonomy. Those who oppose mandatory testing and AZT treatment worry that women who fear being tested will avoid prenatal care — which could cause more harm to infants in the long run.

Economic burden of AIDS

With the AIDS population rapidly growing, the cost of providing care will cause society to rethink questions about whether health care is a right or a privilege. Nurses must provide care regardless of the patient's ability to pay for it. But what about the rest of the health care system? Must hospitals and government agencies bear the burden of AIDS patients who cannot handle the financial burdens imposed by their illness?

The right to health care is, at best, a tentative and unenforceable right with no legal foundation, although nearly everyone agrees that a patient who enters the health care system has a right to receive treatment appropriate for his illness. Still, health care resources are limited. In the face of such limitations, the best you can do is to refer patients to the appropriate social service agencies and support legislation that guarantees equal access to health care.

Abortion and reproductive technology

Abortion poses a complex and painful ethical dilemma for nurses and their patients. Consider the cases described below.

● Ashley, a pregnant 14-year-old, quietly wept with her mother sitting next to her. They were waiting in the short procedure unit for Ashley's turn in the operating room. When the nurse took her aside to talk privately, Ashley began to cry harder. She told the nurse that she didn't really want an abortion, but her parents had placed so much pressure on her she had no real choice.

● Loretta was pregnant with her fourth child. Recently fired from his job, her husband had begun drinking heavily and on more than one occasion had become emotionally abusive. One of her three children is hyperactive and having trouble in school. Loretta believed that she couldn't handle another child or cope with going through a pregnancy and giving the child up for adoption. To get to the abortion clinic, she had to pass through a picket line of *pro-life* protesters, who harassed and taunted her. During her initial interview with the nurse, she is visibly shaken and says that she can no longer cope with the stress in her life.

● Lynnette works in a women's health center that provides general family planning, treatment for vaginal infections, counseling, health care for teens, and abortion services. Although she was fervently *pro-choice* when she took the job, over the months her feelings about abortion have changed. She wants to continue working at the center but without participating in abortions. She fears that this would create tension as well as extra work for her colleagues. The primary wage earner for her family, Lynnette is considering resigning for ethical reasons.

The U.S. Supreme Court has handed down more than 20 decisions related to the abortion issue. Court rulings, however, cannot answer the ethical questions about abortion that nurses encounter in their daily practice.

Is the fetus a human being?

The status of the fetus as a human life is an important element in the abortion controversy. Should the fetus be considered a human being, or a potential human being? Even if the early embryo isn't considered a human being (at least not in the same sense as a newborn), does its potential to become a human being guarantee a right to life?

This confusion is complicated by the fact that the age of fetal viability — the age at which a fetus can survive outside the womb — has decreased to about 20 to 24 weeks.

Many bioethicists use measurable criteria of human body development (such as fetal movement and the existence of a heart and nervous system) to determine when the fetus is alive. But this hasn't ended the debate.

Political battle

Abortion has become the focal point of a long and bitter political struggle.

Pro-life position

Opponents of *legal abortion* argue that human life begins at conception, and therefore abortion is murder. This position is most clearly identified with the Roman Catholic Church. In 1869, Pope Pius IX condemned all abortions as a form of murder. Before then, the church had imposed no penalties for abortions within the first 40 days of pregnancy.

Anti-abortion groups also contend that tolerance for the murder of unborn children will imply tolerance for as-

sisted suicide, death by neglect, or murder of other categories of "undesirable" people, such as the retarded, seriously ill, and deformed.

Pro-choice position

Those who support legal abortion argue that an embryo or young fetus represents the potential for human life but should not be considered a human being at the time. They view abortion as a type of surgery necessary for the physical and psychological well-being of certain women. Abortion, they point out, will always be part of human society, whether legal or not. Legal abortions reduce the number of mutilations and deaths associated with *illegal abortions.* Further, they argue that legal abortions help to reduce the number of unwanted children, forced marriages, and economic stress on some families.

Some take a third position: Abortions should be allowed, but only when the life of the pregnant woman is in danger or in cases of incest or rape.

Continuing debate

The furor over abortion is unlikely to go away anytime soon. An abortion-inducing pill, mifepristone (RU-486) has sparked new controversy. Taken in the first 7 weeks of pregnancy, mifepristone blocks progesterone receptors, allowing prostaglandins to stimulate uterine contractions and detach the conceptus. Mifepristone has been available in France since 1988 and is used in Great Britain and Sweden. In the United States, the drug has undergone clinical trials and was moving toward FDA approval for use by late 1996.

In 1995, a regimen of two common prescription drugs — methotrexate, used to treat cancer, and misoprostol, an anti-ulcer agent — was found to induce abortion safely and effectively. First, methotrexate is given to stop the division of fetal cells. Then, 5 to 7 days later, a misoprostol suppository is administered to induce contractions and expel the fetus. One researcher believes the regimen could be administered by nurse-practitioners under a doctor's supervision, enhancing availability and lowering the costs of abortion. Clinical trials were to begin in 1996 for possible FDA approval by 1997.

While many manufacturers may not supply RU-486 for fear of reprisals from anti-choice organizations, methotrexate and misoprostol are too well established to be forced off the market. Anti-abortion leaders, meanwhile, have targeted mifepristone and vow they will not ignore the newest method.

Mother's rights

The ethical principle of autonomy (self-determination) is an important part of the abortion debate. This principle upholds a woman's right to control her own body. From the mother's point of view, that right includes choosing whether or not to have an abortion. Many women may think they should not be forced to undergo the physical, emotional, and financial hardships of pregnancy.

Abortion opponents believe that pregnancy involves two persons with a right to autonomy — the mother and the fetus.

Resolving your views about abortion

A nurse who is ethically or morally opposed to abortion can't be forced to participate in the procedure. On the other hand, her employer can insist that she provide nursing to all in her care.

To reach your own ethical resolution to the abortion issue, you'll need to examine your views honestly. You'll also want to periodically reevaluate your position, in light of new medical information and your own experience. If you feel strongly about the issue, you should work for a facility that endorses similar views.

Post-abortion care

Every nurse has an ethical obligation to provide competent, compassionate care. Even nurses who strongly oppose abortion should not allow their personal feelings to interfere when caring for a post-abortion patient. Nor is it appropriate to impose your values on the patient. If the patient expresses guilt or regrets over her decision, an appropriate therapeutic response might be, "You made a decision that you thought was right. I want to help you live with your decision and rebuild your life." Offering to find a clergyperson is another way to help.

Prenatal screening

Thanks to diagnostic procedures such as amniocentesis, ultrasound, alpha-fetoprotein screening, and chorionic villus sampling, it's now possible to detect inherited disorders and congenital abnormalities well before birth. In a minority of cases, the diagnosis has paved the way for repair of the defect *in utero*. But because it's easier to detect genetic disorders than to treat them, prenatal screening often forces a patient to choose between having an abortion or taking on the emotional and financial burden of raising a severely handicapped child.

Even those who are opposed to abortion may waver after seeing a child afflicted with Tay-Sachs disease or Duchenne muscular dystrophy. Is the quality of these children's lives so poor that it would be more compassionate to prevent their birth? Is death ever more beneficial than life?

Some ethicists worry that this line of reasoning could cater to a desire for "perfect" children. How would this affect attitudes toward the handicapped?

How severe must a defect be for abortion to be considered an ethically acceptable option? For example, should a fetus with cleft palate, a surgically correctable defect, be aborted because of his handicap? What about a girl conceived by parents who desperately want a boy?

The diagnostic procedures themselves involve some risk to the fetus. Amniocentesis, for example, causes serious complications or death about 0.5% of the time. This risk creates a conflict between the rights of the fetus and the parents' right to know his health status. If testing is to be conducted ethically, patients must understand the associated risks before the procedure.

Patients also must comprehend what the test can and can't tell them, as well as all the available options. Thus, just as in AIDS testing, effective pretest and post-test counseling are essential parts of an ethical prenatal screening program.

In vitro fertilization

Infertility can have devastating effects on the emotional well-being of a couple who yearn for children. As a result, many such couples are willing to spend large amounts of time and money attempting to conceive or adopt a child. When medical procedures, such as fertility medications, hysterosalpingography (opening blocked fallopian tubes), and artificial insemination, fail and adoption proves impossible, infertile couples may resort to more controversial techniques, including *in vitro* fertilization (IVF).

IVF refers to the process of removing ova from a woman's ovaries, placing them in a petri dish filled with a sterilized growth medium, and covering them with healthy motile spermatozoa for fertilization. Three to five ova are reimplanted in the woman's uterus 10 to 14 days after fertilization, and the remaining fertilized ova are frozen for future use or discarded.

IVF can use the husband's sperm (homologous) or a donor's sperm (heterologous) to fertilize the ova.

Complex and expensive, IVF has resulted in the birth of hundreds of healthy "test-tube babies" since the first successful attempt in 1978. These parents have no doubts about the procedure—they're thankful for the opportunity to have children. Yet, *egoism* is not an acceptable basis for ethical decision making in health care. Worthy ends do not always justify the means, and many people question the morality of the IVF procedure.

Medical miracle or unnatural act?

Some people hail scientific manipulation of the ova and sperm as a medical miracle, but others denounce it as circumvention of the natural process of procreation. By concentrating on conception, IVF enables couples to sidestep other important aspects of a normal sexual relationship, including pleasure, respect, and love. Many religions maintain that a Supreme Being participates in the act of procreation. People with strong religious beliefs may contend that IVF diminishes the spiritual value of family life.

Question of degree

It's ethically acceptable to modify normal body functions to enhance natural actions. Thus, procedures such as hysterosalpingography pose few ethical problems. Is IVF the next logical step in fertility modification? Or is it an unnatural act that oversteps the bounds of standard medical intervention?

IVF and conflicts of rights

The long-term effects of IVF on the children, their parents, and society in general represent another serious ethical concern. Human society depends on the strength and integrity of the family. By distancing parents from the physical act of procreation, IVF could have a harmful impact on family life.

Leftover embryos

IVF would pose fewer ethical problems if only one embryo were needed to guarantee a successful pregnancy. Unfortunately, it doesn't work that way. From 15 to 20 embryos may result from a single fertilization effort. Three to five usually are reimplanted in the mother's uterus. The question arises: What should be done with the "leftover embryos"? Is it ethical to discard them, destroy them, or perform experiments on them?

In practice, leftover embryos usually are frozen. This raises questions with regard to parental responsibility for the frozen embryos. In 1989, for example, a divorcing Tennessee couple fought a custody battle over seven fertilized eggs that were frozen at an IVF clinic in Knoxville. Mary Sue Davis wanted custody for future implantation; her estranged husband, Junior Davis, insisted on having a joint say in the future of the embryos. In a controversial decision, a circuit court judge ruled that the embryos are people, not property, and should go to the mother.

Effects on child development

Parents may feel less responsible for IVF children born with congenital defects or conceived with donor sperm. Test-tube babies themselves may develop identity or adjustment problems after they learn the facts surrounding their conception. They're likely to feel insecure about their position in the family, especially if they have "naturally conceived" siblings.

Government regulation

One way to avoid potential abuses of IVF would be to allow hospitals, the courts, or government agencies to regulate the procedure. Although few existing professional practice acts or laws even mention IVF, this situation is likely to change.

Is IVF the best use of scarce resources?

As the cost of health care escalates, justice is probably best served by using available resources to treat common diseases and promote health. Infertility, although a real tragedy for affected couples, doesn't pose a serious health crisis to society as a whole. Thus, some ethical experts have argued that the money spent on IVF would be better spent controlling the spread of AIDS or preventing pregnancy in teenagers.

Conversely, if IVF is viewed as a medically essential procedure, the ethical principle of distributive justice holds that everyone—regardless of socioeconomic status—should have access to it. The cost of a publicly supported infertility treatment program based on IVF would be astronomical.

Surrogate motherhood

A surrogate mother is a woman who gives birth after carrying the fertilized ovum of another woman, or, more commonly, after being artificially inseminated with sperm from the biologic father. In this case, the infant is then legally adopted by the wife of the biologic father. Since the first surrogate birth in England in 1976, more than 1,000 babies have been born through this arrangement.

Surrogate motherhood offers hope to the 60% to 70% of infertile couples in which the woman is the affected partner. It's also an option for women whose age or health makes pregnancy risky. A surrogate birth poses no greater risk to the fetus (or the surrogate mother) than does any normal birth.

Surrogate motherhood vs. conventional motherhood

One concern about surrogate motherhood involves the true nature of mothering. Is "motherhood" merely the biologic act of bearing children? Many people believe that motherhood also implies a long-term commitment to the care and nurture of the child. By agreeing to give up the baby to the contracting couple, is a surrogate mother defaulting on a moral commitment? The advertising of services by potential surrogate mothers, with fees ranging from $50,000 to $150,000, suggests to some that surrogate motherhood represents a form of "baby selling."

Conflicts of rights

Surrogate motherhood also can produce conflicts among the rights of the surrogate mother, the infertile couple, the fetus, and society.

The basic dispute centers around who has the strongest claim to the child. Is it the surrogate mother, by virtue of her biologic connection? Or does the surrogate contract guarantee the infertile couple the right to the child? Courts of law usually have ruled in favor of the couple.

Surrogate mother contracts seemingly violate adoption laws, which prohibit a mother from surrendering parental rights before the infant is born. Such laws, enacted to protect a biologic mother from undue pressure, typically specify an initial waiting period of 10 days. In most cases, she can't terminate all parental rights until up to 6 months after the birth.

What if no one wants the child? This can become an issue if the infant is born with a handicap. Can the infertile couple or the surrogate mother refuse to take responsibility for such a child? What if the defect isn't apparent until the child is 4 years old? Can the infertile couple return the child to his biologic mother?

Clearly, the rights of the child to a normal family life mustn't be lost in the debate over custody. (See *Orphaned ova.*)

Exploitation

Both the infertile couple and the surrogate mother are highly vulnerable to exploitation. The couple, blinded by their longing for a child, are easy victims for financial and emotional blackmail. On the other hand, surrogate motherhood can be used to exploit poor women, who have few marketable skills other than their ability to bear children. "Womb renting" is as ethically unacceptable as "baby selling."

Your role in IVF and surrogate motherhood

You're unlikely to be directly involved in the IVF procedure or in drawing up a surrogate mother contract. But you may be called on to care for patients who choose these options. Before you can do so effectively, you'll need to examine your views on these controversial procedures and become familiar with the legal and ethical pitfalls they present.

You can't be forced to participate in procedures you find ethically and morally objectionable. But, according to the ANA Code for Nurses, you're obligated to care for all patients assigned to you, regardless of your beliefs or feelings. In any event, you have an ethical obligation to be aware of and report abuses of IVF or surrogate motherhood.

CASE STUDY IN ETHICS

Orphaned ova

Unanswered questions about *in vitro* fertilization and surrogate motherhood may come to haunt society in the not-too-distant future. Consider the case study below, which explores what could happen if a surrogate motherhood arrangement doesn't go as planned.

Orphaned before birth

Howard Belmont, age 39, owned a successful manufacturing company. He and his wife, Marsha, age 35, had been trying to have a baby for 2 years without success. After the Belmonts underwent a battery of infertility tests, their doctor concluded that Mrs. Belmont could ovulate and produce mature ova, but couldn't conceive or bear children. On the doctor's suggestion, the couple began to explore the possibility of *in vitro* fertilization and surrogate motherhood.

After lengthy consideration, Mrs. Belmont had her ova fertilized *in vitro,* using her husband's sperm. When some of the fertilized ova were frozen for implantation, the Belmonts located a surrogate mother, Hazel Towers. Ms. Towers agreed to sign a long-term contract, saying that she would bear a total of three children for Mr. and Mrs. Belmont. The contract stated that Ms. Towers would be paid $100,000 for the first child and $75,000 (already placed in trust) for the subsequent two children. Ms. Towers was successfully implanted with Mr. and Mrs. Belmont's fertilized ova. When Ms. Towers was near the end of her first trimester of pregnancy, Mr. and Mrs. Belmont were killed in an automobile accident.

Making an offer

Mr. Belmont's two brothers and one sister stood to inherit his company and assets worth $15 million. But, according to the Belmonts' will, if Ms. Towers had the baby, then the child would inherit the estate.

Mr. Belmont's brothers and sister offered Ms. Towers $500,000 if she would abort the fetus and refuse to be implanted with any more fertilized ova. In addition, the brothers and sister offered to make a $1-million donation for the construction of a new pediatric wing to the hospital where the frozen fertilized ova were stored if the administrator agreed to have the ova destroyed.

Hazel's dilemma

Ms. Towers was placed under a great deal of stress. She realized that she could base her actions only on her own ethical principles. The $500,000 offer was a temptation she'd have to ignore; she did not think that financial gain justified an abortion. According to the contract, she was to surrender the child to Mr. and Mrs. Belmont at its birth. She had serious misgivings, however, about surrendering it to the brothers or sister in light of the offer they made for her to have an abortion.

When they learned that Hazel Towers refused to surrender the child, the brothers and sister accused her of having the child for financial gain. They pointed out that the child would be heir to a large fortune; Hazel Towers would probably benefit from the estate in caring for the child.

Preborn siblings

Questions remained about production of the two other children agreed on in the contract. Was the contract still binding after the death of Mr. and Mrs. Belmont?

(continued)

CASE STUDY IN ETHICS

Orphaned ova continued

Because the money had already been set aside, could Ms. Towers be implanted with the ova, bear the children, and expect to be paid?

What about the hospital administrator and his role in destruction of fertilized ova? If he believes that the ova aren't human, he probably would not hesitate to carry out this request. But what if he believes that human life starts at the moment of conception? Then it would be betraying his ethical beliefs to destroy the ova.

Outcome

Over time, Hazel Towers began to think of the child in her womb as her own. She realized that her child would need to be loved and cherished for its own sake. She accepted the fact that she would

probably lose her surrogate mother's fee because the contract stipulated that she must turn the child over to the Belmonts. She decided to raise the child, regardless of the financial consequences.

Because of the severe emotional stress she experienced, Hazel decided to forgo having any more fertilized ova implanted. The Belmont family immediately initiated a legal action contesting her child's inheritance; eventually an out-of-court settlement was reached.

Hazel Towers experienced a bitter lesson in the moral uncertainty that surrounds *in vitro* fertilization and surrogate motherhood. Existing laws are not sufficient to answer the many questions raised by reproductive technology; future court rulings may provide better guidelines.

Genetic engineering and screening

Genetic engineering continues to contribute significantly to medical progress. Scientists are discovering new ways to identify and manipulate the genetic material of everything from single-celled organisms to human beings.

Each cell of an animal or plant carries a genetic blueprint for the entire organism. This information is encoded by the deoxyribonucleic acid (DNA) in its nucleus. By removing or adding DNA, scientists can program the cell or the entire organism to carry out new functions. Such manipulation can be highly beneficial. For example, it has given us new antibiotics and hormones (such as human insulin) and increased

our understanding of cancer cells. But genetic manipulation also gives researchers the potential to alter the gene pool in unethical ways or to create terrifying new biologic weapons.

Each of the estimated 100,000 genes found in nearly every human cell codes for a single protein involved in a specific body function. Even a small error in the gene produces a defective protein that can result in disease or deformity. More than 4,000 inherited disorders result from such genetic mistakes. Gene therapy, the introduction of healthy genes to overcome an inherited defect, may someday provide cures for diseases such as cystic fibrosis, muscular dystrophy, and hemophilia.

The identification of the genes responsible for inherited diseases and congenital malformations has spurred the development of screening tests. Genetic testing is now a fairly common component of prenatal care, facilitating the identification of fetuses with disorders like Down's syndrome and Tay-Sachs disease. The screening of newborns for phenylketonuria is legally required by most states.

Potential for discrimination

Researchers also have identified the genes responsible for adult-onset disorders such as Huntington's disease, polycystic kidney disease, and some forms of cancer. Ideally, the results of genetic screening could encourage patients to make life-style changes that reduce their risk of developing the disease. At the very least, the knowledge can help them prepare to deal with the disease. Unfortunately, this information also can lead to genetic discrimination, preventing people from obtaining health or life insurance or jobs or adopting children.

Ethics of genetic engineering

Genetic manipulation, or genetic engineering, has a tremendous potential for altering the course of human development. By themselves, genetic engineering techniques, including cloning, somatic alteration, germ cell alteration, recombinant DNA synthesis, and gene therapy, are ethically neutral. It's the application of these techniques that creates ethical problems. (See *Language of genetic manipulation*.)

Control over future generations

Do researchers have a greater obligation to help those currently alive, or to protect the interests of future generations? It would appear that the most ethical applications of genetic engineering should do both, and research should concentrate on solving long-term medical and environmental problems such as hereditary disease, cancer, pollution, and hunger.

Language of genetic manipulation

The following terms are associated with the science of genetic manipulation.

Cloning • production of an entire organism from a single cell

Eugenics • science of improving a species through control of hereditary factors by manipulation of the gene pool

Gene • fragment of deoxyribonucleic acid (DNA) that encodes a single protein

Gene-splicing • technique by which recombinant DNA is produced and made to function in an organism

Gene therapy • insertion of a normal gene into the nucleus of a cell to compensate for a defective one

Genetic marker • dominant gene or trait that serves to identify genes or traits linked with it

Germ cell alteration • changes in DNA structure during the earliest stages of cell growth (before differentiation)

Recombinant DNA synthesis • insertion of DNA segments from one species into the DNA of another species

Restriction fragment length polymorphisms • genetically variable DNA fragments usually used as *markers* for a nearby disease gene

Somatic alteration • *in vitro* isolation of a specific gene that is then synthetically reproduced in the laboratory

Safety

Genetic researchers have a moral obligation to take all necessary precautions to recognize and prevent harmful consequences of their work, such as the accidental release of new pathogens. Patients who participate in gene therapy trials must be fully informed of the potential risks, as well as the benefits. For example, the retroviral vectors used to introduce new genes also may increase a patient's risk of cancer.

Potentially dehumanizing effects

In the past, medical research has been limited to efforts to repair or halt the damage caused by disease and injury. But genetic engineering gives science the ability to recreate the human body. Is this unethical? If genetic engineering techniques are used to cure disease and improve the quality of life, society does stand to benefit. Imagine a society, however, in which genetically "perfect" children or genetically inferior servants could be created in the laboratory. Such unethical applications clearly violate human dignity and integrity.

Voluntary vs. mandatory genetic screening

Screening for genetic disorders isn't new. Progress in mapping defective genes to particular chromosomes has led to more sophisticated tests, which probe directly for the faulty gene or a nearby "marker" gene. Moreover, scientists are learning more about the genetic basis of diseases like diabetes, cancer, and hypertension.

Like genetic engineering, genetic screening is ethically neutral. Applications of this technology, however, may or may not be acceptable. Prenatal, neonatal, or adult screening can be used to improve treatment, guide personal decisions, and initiate prevention programs. Other applications are an ethical Pandora's box.

Mandatory screening

The ethical principle of beneficence requires that a procedure help the patient. Mandatory genetic screening can be beneficial, such as in the case of neonatal screening for phenylketonuria, in which early detection prevents mental retardation. But what about mandatory testing for incurable illnesses, such as Huntington's disease? No doubt some patients will want to know this information and can use it constructively. Others, however, could be seriously harmed psychologically. In this instance, voluntary screening is ethically acceptable, and mandatory screening is not.

Creation of a "biologic underclass"

Insurance companies have been among the first to be charged with genetic discrimination. From the company's point of view, it's a sound business decision to increase premiums or deny coverage to anyone with a serious medical condition or at high risk for developing such a condition. Unfortunately, predictive tests don't always tell the whole story. A single faulty gene may not cause trouble unless other related genes also are defective. Or the gene may never be expressed unless it's set off by an environmental trigger. A patient who's seen as "certain to become disabled" rather than "at risk" could easily join the ranks of the uninsured, with little legal recourse.

Employers represent another source of potential genetic discrimination. In times of increasing health care costs, employers may avoid hiring someone who's likely to incur large medical bills. Industry officials also argue that genetic screening can identify workers who might be especially sensitive to industrial toxins. A more ethical approach would be to clean up the workplace, so that all workers face a decreased risk.

Patient confidentiality

Preserving patient confidentiality may help to guard against abuses of genetic information. However, confidentiality isn't an absolute right. The confidentiality of health-related information, in particular, is protected by law only when the health and well-being of others aren't threatened. The law requires a doctor or nurse to report sexually transmitted diseases, gunshot wounds, and suspected *child abuse,* for example.

It's unclear whether the disclosure of genetic information represents a breach of confidentiality. Certainly the right to treatment of a child with phenylketonuria supersedes the parents' right to confidentiality. But what about a patient who has a positive test for the Huntington's disease gene? Here, confidentiality should be preserved, but the widespread use of computerized records makes this task increasingly difficult.

Justice and genetic screening

Justice, as an ethical principle in health care, requires equal sharing of the risks and benefits of diagnostic tests and treatments offered to patients. Genetic screening programs haven't always adhered to this principle. When large-scale screening programs for sickle cell carriers were initiated in the 1970s, for example, participants received little or no post-test counseling or follow-up care. In contrast, similar programs set up to screen for Tay-Sachs disease included teaching programs, support groups, and financial aid. All genetic screening programs need to incorporate this sort of thorough follow-up care.

The justice principle also impinges on the issue of health insurance coverage. Because patients with serious chronic diseases raise everyone's premiums, it would seem that justice is best served by asking those who pose a greater risk to bear more than the average share of the cost. The danger is that these people may never develop the disease. If so, they've been unfairly overcharged.

Your role in gene therapy

Genetic manipulation, including gene therapy, is still experimental. As a result, few nurses are directly involved in this aspect of genetic research. Nonetheless, you have an ethical obligation to stay informed and to support efforts to establish legal and technological safeguards.

You're more likely to be involved in genetic screening. If so, you have an important role to play in dealing with the related ethical conflicts. Your ethical responsibilities may involve:
• making sure that the patient understands the procedure and gives informed consent before the test
• thoroughly reviewing options for treatment or prevention of a genetic disease during post-test counseling
• refusing to take part in compulsory screening programs
• refusing to disclose test results to unauthorized people
• actively supporting legislation to prevent genetic discrimination by employers and insurance companies.

Right to know vs. right to safety

Seeking new knowledge is an essential part of human nature. Yet society tends to oppose the scientist's right to uncontrolled experimentation. This is particularly true with regard to genetic research. Many people believe in the sanctity of life and view genetic screening and manipulation as violations of that principle, especially when human beings are involved. The public also has a right to protection and personal safety. Thus, it seems likely that the federal government will be involved in regulating genetic research.

Scientists will remain suspicious of attempts to control their work, and a large segment of the public will oppose unregulated tinkering with the building blocks of life. Our hope is that both sides will remember that the dignity, value, and worth of human life must be preserved at all costs.

Personal safety in the workplace

Health care workers are entitled to work in as safe an environment as possible. The ethical principle of justice or fairness supports the position that employers enforce security measures. Without such safeguards, an ethical dilemma arises: Although you are obligated to care for patients, you also need to protect yourself.

Policies that address appropriate staffing levels, adequate training, and the use of security escorts minimize the ethical conflicts between providing care and ensuring employee safety. Federal safety and health standards require all employers to develop injury- and illness-prevention programs. However, it's up to the individual nurse to recognize and protect herself from hazards, such as the following:

• Infection: A particularly serious threat is the patient whose infection has not yet been diagnosed. Nurses who work in high-contact areas, such as emergency departments, are especially at risk for diseases such as tuberculosis. In addition, HIV has led to a host of new concerns. To address them, the CDC has mandated universal precautions to prevent HIV spread. Although it's up to the nurse to follow these pre-

cautions, employers must provide gloves, masks, sharps containers, and other equipment.

• Hazardous chemicals: Many potentially hazardous chemicals are routinely used in health care settings. For example, anesthetic gases increase the risk of birth defects and spontaneous abortions. New standards attempt to control anesthetics in operating rooms. Chemotherapeutic agents, radiation, and powerful cleaning solutions and disinfectants are other common hazards. Their use requires knowledge and vigilance by the nurse and strict supervision by the facility.

• Back injuries: Nurses lose more time from work due to back injuries than any other cause. Such injuries typically arise from lifting, turning, and supporting patients. To avoid injury, be assertive about your own safety. Getting enough help to safely care for patients shows sound judgment.

Selected references

Aiken, T.D., and Catalano, J.T. *Legal, Ethical, and Political Issues in Nursing.* Philadelphia: F.A. Davis Co., 1994.

Catalano, J.T. *Ethical and Legal Aspects of Nursing,* 2nd ed. Springhouse, Pa.: Springhouse Corp., 1995.

McPhersoon, E.C. "Ethical Implications of the Human Genome Diversity Project," *NursingConnections* 8(1):36-43, Spring 1995.

Richardson, D.S. "Oncology Nurses' Attitudes Toward the Legalization of Voluntary Active Euthanasia," *Cancer Nursing* 17(4):348-54, August 1994.

Stoeckle, M.L. "Issues of Transplantation: The Ethics of Potential Legislative Changes," *Dimensions of Critical Care Nursing* 12(3):158-66, May/June 1993.

Thomas, D.J. "Organ Transplantation in People with Unhealthy Lifestyles," *AACN Clinical Issues, in Critical Care Nursing* 4(4):665-68, November 1993.

10 Ethical conflicts in professional practice

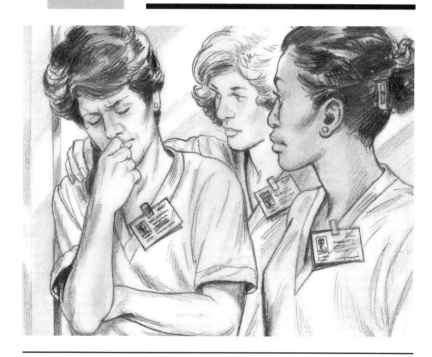

Today, the ethical commitment each nurse brings to her work affects patients and their families, colleagues, and the health care delivery system as a whole. As nurses gain power and influence, they are becoming a more visible force in resolving the ethical dilemmas that confront modern health care.

This chapter discusses three ethical responsibilities of the professional nurse: respecting the patients' autonomy, including the right to *confidentiality* and the right to refuse treatment; blowing the whistle on misconduct by colleagues; and responding to the problem of widespread substance abuse among nurses.

Respecting the patient's autonomy

A patient may refuse any treatment — whether ordinary or extraordinary. However, the decision to refuse ordinary treatment presents an especially complex ethical dilemma. This dilemma hinges on the conflict between *autonomy* and *beneficence.* If a patient can make an informed decision, he has a right to refuse treatment. But what if his decision doesn't serve his best interests? Which moral principle, autonomy or beneficence, should take precedence? (See *Saying no to rehabilitation.*)

Autonomy and its limits

One of the cornerstones of ethical decision making, autonomy refers to the right to make decisions about one's health care. But external and internal pressures can limit the patient's autonomy.

External pressures

Family members and health professionals can exert appreciable influence over the patient. Typically, this influence takes the form of persuasion or encouragement. Infrequently, it takes the form of coercion, in which the patient comes to believe he has no free choice.

Doctor-patient relationships are inherently imbalanced. The doctor possesses knowledge and skill, whereas the patient possesses a need for care. Because the patient has a need, he assumes a dependent and potentially vulnerable position. He must trust the caregiver. In so doing, he may feel that assertiveness isn't appropriate. You, however, can counteract this feeling by encouraging the patient to be informed and to ask questions.

Internal pressures

Doubt, and illness itself, can sap autonomy. For instance, the patient may see himself as too ignorant to make crucial decisions about his health. If he does, bolster his self-esteem; encourage him to take an active role in decision making, and support him in his efforts. The patient's signs and symptoms, such as dyspnea or pain, may distract him. If they do, try to relieve them so the patient can make thoughtful decisions.

Beneficence

When dealing with children or patients who are unable to make informed decisions, beneficence outweighs autonomy. Young children, for instance, don't understand the implications of not being vaccinated for measles or mumps and would simply prefer to avoid the pain of an injection.

For patients who can make an informed decision, though, the burden of proof for beneficence lies with the health care provider. Typically, a health care provider can advance these arguments in support of beneficence:
• The patient is under excessive stress and can't think rationally.
• The patient may change his mind later, when little or nothing can be done to restore his health.
• The patient needs to be protected from acting irrationally.

Underlying all of these arguments is a spirit of paternalism, of possessing superior or clearer knowledge than the patient has. Of course, the patient could and might change his decision, but this uncertainty doesn't constitute grounds for overruling a competent patient's decision.

Futility

Patient autonomy implies the right to demand treatment as well as to refuse it. Usually, patients select a course of action they believe is in their best interests. But patients sometimes make bizarre choices, demanding a futile treatment — one that is worthless and cannot possibly benefit them.

Unlike an ineffective or very questionable treatment, a futile treatment may achieve a short-term gain, such as improving carbon dioxide elimination

CASE STUDY IN ETHICS

Saying no to rehabilitation

One of the rewards of rehabilitative nursing is watching a patient with severe injuries come to terms with an altered body image and eventually go on to live a fulfilling life with a disability. But what happens when a patient turns down the help that nurses and therapists offer? Nurses may experience a bitter ethical conflict between the principle of patient autonomy – which includes the right to refuse treatment – and the principle of beneficence. Consider the case of Phillip Munson, a young quadriplegic who refused rehabilitative treatment, deciding that he preferred to die.

Wanting to die

Phillip, 30, was left a C3 quadriplegic after he broke his neck in an automobile accident. First admitted to the intensive care unit (ICU), Phillip was totally dependent on others for all activities and all aspects of his care. His only relatives were a brother and a sister-in-law, who visited regularly and planned to have him live with them after rehabilitation.

During his month in the ICU, Phillip told the nurses that he wanted to live. Shortly after being transferred to the rehabilitation unit, however, he changed his mind: He wanted to die and insisted on discontinuing his rehabilitation program. His brother made it clear that he wanted Phillip's wishes respected. A psychiatrist evaluated Phillip and concluded that he was competent and showed no evidence of psychosis or thought disorder.

Phillip understood his condition and his prognosis; he was aware that after rehabilitation, he would be able to operate a wheelchair and a computer. He also understood that he would be paralyzed from the neck down and would always need assistance with activities of daily living. Phillip said that he was not afraid of death and wanted no heroic measures taken. His brother helped him draft an extensive legal statement establishing the right to refuse specific treatments, including antibiotic and intravenous therapy. Plans were made to discharge him to a nursing home.

Ethical considerations

Many of the nurses and therapists on the rehabilitation unit were distressed by the decision to stop Phillip's program. Depression, anger, and refusal of treatment are common among young accident victims, and these health care professionals were skilled at encouraging, bargaining with, and even coercing patients to comply. They argued that Phillip's decision was misguided and that there was justification for intervention based on the principles of paternalism and beneficence.

Jim DiFrancesco, RN, a nurse on the rehabilitation team, pointed out that there was a significant difference between a young, recently injured quadriplegic and a terminal cancer patient who finally decides to "pull the plug." He believed that Phillip was under too much stress from the initial impact of the injury and would probably later change his mind and view life as worth living once again. He pointed out to members of the health care team that there are many examples of patients reversing their decision to die. Elizabeth Bouvia, a young woman incapacitated by cerebral palsy, received national publicity when she requested that the hospital discontinue her tube feedings and allow her to starve herself to death,

(continued)

Saying no to rehabilitation continued

but she later changed her mind and stated that she wanted to live.

Mr. DiFrancesco pointed out that many factors, such as depression, fear of treatment, hidden family dynamics, and ambivalence, complicated Phillip's ability to make an autonomous decision. Furthermore, Phillip was clearly ambivalent about his desire to die. His behavior was not always consistent with his expressed wish for death. For example, Phillip was cheerful on many days and took great interest in the positioning of his joints and measures taken to prevent joint contractures.

In fact, for a brief period, Phillip reneged on his wish to die. His best friend from high school learned about the accident and decided to devote a long visit to helping Phillip. When he learned his friend would be arriving soon, Phillip asked to start full therapy again. Although his high school buddy helped out tirelessly and offered to stay even longer, Phillip quickly became overwhelmed by the pain and hardship of his existence and requested that his previous statement outlining his wish to die be reactivated.

Respecting patient autonomy

Another nurse on the unit, Christina Walsh, RN, pointed out that the rehabilitation center's mission was to serve the patient's best interest, not meet the emotional needs of the staff. She believed that members of the health care team had their own vested interest in keeping Phillip alive. For example, the occupational therapist was excited about experimenting with the latest wheelchair control

devices. Many of her co-workers, accustomed to seeing their patients readjust to life, could not accept the fact that they would inevitably fail some of their patients. It was not right, asserted Ms. Walsh, to pursue every technological intervention regardless of the cost or burden to the patient.

An ethical struggle

During the time Phillip remained on the rehabilitation unit, the nurses who cared for him experienced an intense ethical struggle. It was difficult to agree not to perform routine tracheostomy care or range-of-motion exercises, or to care for the pressure ulcer that developed on the back of Phillip's head. It also was difficult, however, to do these things in good conscience for a patient who asked that they not be done. It seemed like a total usurpation of what little power and control Phillip still had. Each nurse had to struggle with questions about the rights of a patient who does not have the ability to leave the hospital against medical advice, protest his treatment, or even verbally complain without the assistance of another person.

Phillip's ordeal finally came an end when he was transported to a nursing home near the residence of his brother's family. After 2 months, he slipped into a coma and died. His existence was a lesson to the rehabilitation team: Most patients are grateful for the opportunity of a second chance at life; for some, however, the pain is too great. Ultimately, the decision to accept treatment belongs to the patient.

in a ventilated patient with chronic obstructive pulmonary disease. However, it does not lead to a true personal benefit (restoration of health). A treatment may be futile either because it lacks merit or because the patient's condition makes it futile.

A futile intervention differs from one that is harmful, impossible, or ineffective and should not be equated with hopelessness. A patient may maintain hope even in an impossible situation.

Many health care providers do not render care they deem futile. However, with the growing importance of patient autonomy and self-determination, such choices are being made less readily. Increasingly, patients believe they have a right to determine what constitutes a "benefit" to them. Nonetheless, nurses and doctors should be able to decide if a treatment is futile, based on their knowledge of the treatment and its anticipated effect on the patient's quality of life. Thus, the patient's right to choose is limited by the duty of nurses and doctors to provide quality care and to practice their professions responsibly.

Furthermore, ethicists argue that patient self-determination implies a right to refuse treatment or to choose from *medically justifiable* options — not to demand treatment. Also, with the growing emphasis on cost containment, futile treatment may not even be a patient option in the future. Treatment options may be determined by statistical measurement of probable patient benefits.

The Helga Wanglie case is a classic example of futile interventions. At age 85, Mrs. Wanglie suffered a myocardial infarction at the nursing home where she resided. Transferred to a hospital, she was resuscitated but remained unconscious and underwent mechanical ventilation. Doctors wanted to withdraw the life-sustaining support that they deemed futile, but her husband objected and had his wife transferred to another medical center. Doctors there diagnosed her as being in a persistent vegetative state and recommended removing the ventilator. Mrs. Wanglie's family objected.

The hospital asked the court whether medical professionals were obligated to provide treatment they believed to be unbeneficial and inappropriate. Mrs. Wanglie's husband then asked to be appointed conservator. The judge decided in his favor — but not on the basis of medical values and principles. Instead, he ruled that the husband was the proper surrogate and that his decisions about his wife's wishes were reliable.

Although individual rights and patient autonomy won out over the doctors' professional judgment of futility in this case, many health care providers reject the notion that patients have the right to futile treatments, especially when millions of Americans don't receive basic health care.

Confidentiality and the right to privacy

The American Nurses Association (ANA) Code of Ethics states that you must safeguard the patient's right to *privacy* "by judiciously protecting information of a confidential nature." Maintaining confidentiality is essential to preserving the trust necessary to provide effective nursing care. A patient must often reveal sensitive or embarrassing information during his assessment if an accurate diagnosis is to be made. The patient must have confidence that this information will be shared in a professional manner only with those who require it for his care. (See *Right to privacy,* pages 330 and 331.)

Right to privacy

When entering the hospital, most patients tacitly agree to sacrifice a considerable amount of privacy to enable doctors and nurses to plan and provide care. But occasionally, a patient refuses to cooperate. If his resistance hampers your ability to give good care, you may face an ethical dilemma, as the following case study shows.

Hidden medicine bottle

John Gordon is admitted to the hospital with chronic diarrhea. All diagnostic tests have been negative. His doctor, Marvin Stein, suspects that Mr. Gordon is causing the diarrhea by taking laxatives—a charge Mr. Gordon vehemently denies.

Mr. Gordon's nurse, Susan Morrison, is starting to think that Dr. Stein may be right: Yesterday, Mr. Gordon hid a medicine bottle in his satchel as she walked into his room. When she asked him what was in the bottle, he became defensive and refused to answer.

Dr. Stein asks Susan to "do a little detective work" by searching Mr. Gordon's room for laxatives the next time he receives visitors in the lounge. "After all," he tells her, "we can't help Mr. Gordon until we know for sure what's going on."

Ethical considerations

At first, Susan is willing to conduct a search of Mr. Gordon's room. Later, she begins to have doubts about whether such a search would be ethical. She decides to write down her concerns:

• Do we know Mr. Gordon is lying when he denies taking laxatives? Several possible explanations exist for his defensive behavior: Perhaps he doesn't know what

a laxative is and is reluctant to reveal his ignorance. Why did he hide the medicine bottle? He might be embarrassed to admit he's taking a home remedy. There may be several other reasons. What appears to be a medicine bottle could contain any number of things.

• Even if Mr. Gordon is lying, is a search justified? Can one person's unethical behavior justify another's? Dr. Stein, after all, is a medical authority, not a moral authority.

• Even if conducting an investigation is necessary, wouldn't openly searching Mr. Gordon's room without his permission be more ethical than conducting a secret search behind his back?

• What about Dr. Stein's role in this incident? Should I allow him to delegate this distasteful duty to me?

• Even if Mr. Gordon is indeed lying and is taking laxatives, who—besides himself—is he harming? Doesn't he have the right to treat himself with an over-the-counter medication against his doctor's advice?

• How would a search affect my nurse-patient relationship with Mr. Gordon? If he thinks that I violated his trust, it will probably destroy it forever.

• Will the search really help us to accomplish our goal—to help Mr. Gordon get better? Unless we find out why he's taking a laxative, he'll probably continue taking it.

Presenting alternatives

Susan decides that she has too many ethical misgivings to cooperate with the search. Before telling Dr. Stein of her decision, she outlines the ways in which she is willing to help. Her first recommenda-

---

CASE STUDY IN ETHICS

Right to privacy continued

tion is to call a conference with the patient. She's willing to discuss with Mr. Gordon the need for the health care team to know about all of his medications, including over-the-counter and home remedies, and to again ask him to identify the medication he takes. If Mr. Gordon still refuses to discuss the problem, she'll make it clear that she's willing to listen if he should change his mind.

She's also willing to arrange to be in Mr. Gordon's room during morning care. If, for example, she opens his drawer to get his toothbrush and finds a medicine bottle, she can then ask about it. But that's as far as she will go. She will not participate in a search without the patient's consent, even in his presence. She realizes that, as Dr. Stein said, this might limit the ability of the health care team to help Mr. Gordon, but a competent patient has the right to forgo help.

Underlying principles

Underlying confidentiality are two key ethical principles: autonomy and fidelity. Autonomy includes the patient's right to maintain control over his life; this extends to the right to maintain control over personal information. *Fidelity* refers to one's faithfulness to agreements that one has accepted. The temptation to gossip is very strong. To maintain confidentiality, the nurse's ethical belief in the patient's right to maintain autonomy must outweigh the temptation to gossip. If a nurse pledges to keep a confidence, she must recognize the seriousness of this obligation. After all, it's normal to share confidential information in the course of developing a therapeutic relationship. Without fidelity and respect for confidentiality, meaningful nurse-patient relationships cannot survive.

Breaches of confidentiality

Confidential information can ethically be disclosed in certain circumstances, for example, the failure to disclose information could cause serious physical harm to the patient, his family, the hospital staff, or any other identifiable

third party. However, knowing when confidentiality may be appropriately breached isn't always easy. Consider the three case studies below. For each case, decide whether or not you agree with the ethical decision made by the nurse.

Preventing harm to the patient

Kitisha Jefferson, RN, was caring for Will Cooke, a 33-year-old electrician who broke his femur in a fall at a construction site. She had established a good nurse-patient relationship with him. However, Mr. Cooke had seemed bored and edgy for the past day or so. When Ms. Jefferson checked his room, she found his curtain drawn halfway around his bed. She walked to the open side and saw Mr. Cooke hurriedly closing a plastic bag that contained white powder. "What are you doing?" she asked him.

"All right," Mr. Cooke replied. "Since you're a good nurse, I'll level with you. I was doing coke. I know I shouldn't, but it gets boring when you're in traction with nothing to do but watch the tube. Please, don't tell anybody. If my wife finds out, I'm finished."

Ms. Jefferson patiently explained that cocaine can have severe effects, especially when taken with other drugs. She advised Mr. Cooke to discontinue using cocaine — at least while he's hospitalized.

After taking these measures, Ms. Jefferson still faced ethical dilemmas. What should she write in the patient's chart? Should she tell Mr. Cooke's doctor? Should she recommend that Mr. Cooke tell the doctor?

After careful consideration, Ms. Jefferson decided to tell Mr. Cooke that she had an obligation to let the doctor know about his cocaine use — unless Mr. Cooke wanted to tell the doctor himself. Her decision was based on the ethical principle of beneficence; she believed the risk of cardiac arrest caused by the combination of cocaine and other medications was an overriding factor.

Protecting hospital staff

Steve Walcott, RN, was reviewing Tamara Smith's chart before giving her a preoperative sedative when he realized that one of his colleagues had been discussing her at lunch the day before. This colleague, who worked in the lab, didn't mention Ms. Smith by name. But the age and admission date gave away the patient's identity. She had said that Ms. Smith tested positive for human immunodeficiency virus (HIV) infection but that the results weren't being noted on the chart. Should Mr. Walcott inform the surgical team of Ms. Smith's test results?

Mr. Walcott felt a strong temptation to make protecting his co-workers the first consideration. However, he also realized that his colleague was remiss in discussing Ms. Smith's test results. Therefore, he reasoned that he would be remiss in further violating the confidentiality of this information. He also feared stigmatizing the patient. He further reasoned that the surgical team should employ universal precautions for all patients, not just those who test positive for HIV. After all, patients who have not had the test can also carry the antibody.

Protecting the patient's family

Jenny Chu, RN, was caring for Susan Schaffer, a 32-year-old mother of five scheduled for a tubal ligation. She wanted to be sure her patient understood the effects of this surgery, so she asked Mrs. Schaffer to explain the procedure. Mrs. Schaffer did so eagerly and added, "I'm so happy I won't have to worry about getting pregnant again. Five kids is more than I can handle as it is."

Satisfied, Ms. Chu left Mrs. Schaffer and continued her rounds. Later that day, she met Mrs. Schaffer's husband, Matt, at the nurses' station. He asked for a box of tissues and said, "I hope the surgery fixes Susan's problem. Did she tell you we've been trying to have another baby for over a year? I really want to have a few more kids."

What should Ms. Chu do: protect Mrs. Schaffer's confidentiality or tell Mr. Schaffer the truth? Ms. Chu felt that her first obligation was to protect Mrs. Schaffer's confidentiality. The urge to tell Mr. Schaffer about his wife's deception was compelling, but he wasn't in danger of physical harm from her action. Ms. Chu felt badly that Mr. and Mrs. Schaffer couldn't talk to each other frankly, but she also felt this wasn't an excuse for breaching confidentiality. Nonetheless, Ms. Chu decided to discuss the matter with the surgeon, especially since hospital policy required a spouse's signature on the *consent form* for a sterilization procedure.

Whistle blowing

Whistle blowing refers to an employee's disclosure of illegal, immoral, or unethical practices under an employer's control. The ANA Code of Ethics outlines the nurse's obligation to report acts of *negligence* or *incompetence* by other health care providers. It states that "the nurse acts to safeguard the patient and public when health care and safety are affected by incompetent, unethical, or illegal practice by any person." As a *patient advocate,* you must be willing to take appropriate action — in short, to blow the whistle.

The 1994 ANA guidelines on reporting incompetent, unethical, or illegal practices identify helpful methods for judging problematic conduct. Incompetent nursing practice is measured by nursing standards; unethical practice is determined in light of the Code for Nurses; and illegal practice is identified in terms of violation of the law.

The *Canadian Nurses' Association* has a Code of Ethics that conveys the same message as the ANA's code: "The nurse, as a member of the health care team, is obliged to take steps to ensure that the patient receives competent and ethical care."

When to blow the whistle

A health professional who makes a mistake usually wants to ensure that it won't happen again. Correcting an error usually involves admitting the mistake, expressing honest regret, and completing an *incident report.* At times, though, you may encounter a health professional who makes repeated mistakes, attempts to cover them up or minimize them, and engages in suspect or misleading behaviors. To uphold the ethical standards of your profession, you need to blow the whistle. (See *Is whistle blowing warranted?* pages 334 and 335.)

Implications of whistle blowing

Many nurses view the decision to blow the whistle as a moral choice often made at great cost to one's professional life . In fact, some nurses have had their reputations tarnished, lost their jobs, or been named in *libel* suits after reporting professional misconduct. Fortunately, such bitter retaliation is not the norm. Keep in mind, however, that the higher the professional standing of the health professional who commits misconduct, the greater the risk you face when blowing the whistle. (See *Whistle blowing: A systematic approach,* page 336.)

Reporting nurse misconduct

Most institutions have channels through which you can report the misconduct of another nurse or *nurses' aide* without fear of reprisal. Often, a nurse-manager and the hospital personnel office assume joint responsibility for investigating allegations of misconduct. For you, the only drawback is animosity from the affected staff member — and possibly from her acquaintances or sympathizers. The benefits, though, include correcting an injustice, preventing future harm, and strengthening your sense of moral integrity.

Reporting medical or management misconduct

If you report the misconduct of a doctor, a nursing supervisor, or a member of the hospital administration, expect stiffer resistance and possibly more severe retaliation, especially if management has cooperated in concealing the misconduct. Be prepared for a lengthy and hard-fought battle. That's because the accused professional may attempt to discredit you — or have you fired — rather than face the allegations honestly.

If you risk significant personal losses, you may want to make a thorough self-assessment before taking any action. If these losses may extend to

Is whistle blowing warranted?

How do you know whether or not to blow the whistle on a colleague? The decision may require careful deliberation and judgment. Review the two case studies below. Do you think that each nurse's decision to blow the whistle is justified?

Habitually late colleague

An hour after her shift began, Sylvia Myers, RN, cannot locate her co-worker Mary Calvo, RN. She checks Mary's time card; it shows that she punched in on time. A few minutes later, Sylvia sees Mary with her coat and gloves on, getting off the elevator.

Sylvia approaches Mary and asks where she's been. Mary impatiently tells her to mind her own business and adds, "You've no idea how hard it is to raise three kids and have to work."

Upset and confused, Sylvia decides that she'd better find out what's going on. After some investigation, she realizes that Allison Henkel, RN, a mutual friend, has been punching Mary in. Allison tells her that Mary arrives up to an hour late two or three times a week. She goes on to say, "Don't worry. I'll keep covering for Mary. What's important is we're helping Mary out and no one's getting hurt."

Sylvia is faced with an ethical dilemma: Should she report Mary's lateness and Allison's coverup? Or should she remain quiet; after all, Mary's lateness hasn't affected patient care thus far, and blowing the whistle might undermine her friendship with Allison.

After careful consideration, Sylvia decides that there is no getting around the fact that Mary is jeopardizing her patients' well-being. Allison shares partial responsibility. Although sympathetic to Mary's child-care problems, Sylvia recognizes

her overriding obligation to ensure the health and safety of patients.

Sylvia decides that her first step is to talk directly to Mary about the situation. If Mary's behavior persists, Sylvia will explain that she is ethically obligated to report Mary to the nurse-manager. Before taking any action, Sylvia is careful to document specific instances of Mary's lateness.

Questioning medical protocol

Rachel Kirkwood, RN, is the nurse-manager of a small oncology unit that develops treatment protocols for the National Cancer Institute. She has worked for several years on the unit, finds her position rewarding, and enjoys a good relationship with the medical staff. However, the latest protocol of the chief oncologist troubles her. None of the patients are improving with the experimental therapy. Rachel knows from her own extensive clinical experience that patients with the same condition fare much better with conventional therapy.

Rachel decides to share her concerns with the oncologist. He responds curtly, saying only that his research brings a large grant for the unit. He makes it clear that he doesn't want to discuss the matter with her any further.

Rachel is faced with a choice: Should she defer to the oncologist's knowledge and trust his sense of professional responsibility? Or should she pursue her concerns?

Rachel realizes that at this point, her options are limited: She is in no position to make charges against the chief oncologist. But she can still take steps to correct the situation. She decides to discuss

Is whistle blowing warranted? continued

the matter confidentially with another oncologist and see what insight he can provide. In addition, she begins keeping accurate records of each patient's treatment and its results. If the evidence she gathers indicates that the patients are suffering harm and the chief oncologist continues to ignore her, Rachel is ready to blow the whistle.

Rachel is committed to preparing her-

self for the long haul. She gathers numerous articles on whistle blowing and arranges to meet with a lawyer experienced in representing whistle blowers. Aware that her actions may jeopardize her job, she has begun to search for alternative employment. And she also realizes that she must emotionally prepare to deal with the wrath of co-workers, especially those who disagree with her conclusions.

your dependents, consider the situation carefully. You may have moral grounds for not blowing the whistle if your dependents could be harmed emotionally, financially, or even physically.

Working through channels

Whistle blowing can be pursued in one of two ways: by going public or by proceeding through the hospital's chain of command. You should make every effort to correct the situation internally before going public. If you work successfully through the chain of command, you'll be able to accomplish your goals with a minimum of exposure. Ethically, you owe management an opportunity to change the situation before going public. For your own legal protection, you should maintain a record of your efforts to work through channels before considering more drastic measures.

If you fail to get satisfaction from the hospital's chain of command, contact the appropriate regulatory agencies. Contact the media only as a last resort.

Providing adequate documentation

Document your disclosure carefully. Write a clear, objective summary of the relevant facts. Explain why the information is significant and what needs

to be done. Avoid focusing on personalities. Personal accusations detract from the disclosure and may invite a lawsuit for libel or *slander.* Have other professionals verify the information if possible. This will lend objectivity to the information and may shield you from retaliation.

Surviving the setbacks

Prepare yourself for possible retaliation. Management may find it more convenient to attack the whistle blower than to address the problem. Colleagues may start giving you the cold shoulder or may overtly harass you. Rumors that you're dishonest or incompetent may spread through the hospital. To protect yourself and to maintain pressure on management, meticulously document everything, including continued incidents of incompetence or negligence. Consider photocopying all the incident reports you file. Be especially vigilant in your practice, and document your nursing actions carefully. Your employer may try to distract attention from the disclosure by portraying you as a troublemaker; to counter this tactic, maintain diplomatic relations with as many colleagues as possible.

If you anticipate that whistle blowing will cause severe personal hard-

Whistle blowing: A systematic approach

Like other nursing actions, whistle blowing can be carried out successfully if it's planned, systematic, and purposeful.

Gathering facts

Begin by gathering all the facts. Then put in writing the misconduct you want to report. Be sure to include the incident's date and time, the person or people involved, and the source of your information. Above all, avoid accusations and personal opinions.

Stating the problem

Clearly state the problem and identify causative factors. Was incompetence or negligence involved? Were supplies adequate? Did equipment malfunction? Was institutional policy at fault?

When answering these questions, try to eliminate your personal biases. If possible, review the problem with a trusted colleague.

Determining your objective

State your objective in confronting the problem. For example, you may want to eliminate threats to patient safety; eliminate illegal, immoral, or illegitimate practices; uphold professional ethical standards; or put into effect needed changes in institutional policy.

Confronting the problem

Confront the person who committed the misconduct in a constructive, nonthreatening way. Express your concerns and ask for an explanation of the incident. Seek reassurance that the problem will be addressed.

Deciding whether to blow the whistle

After a reasonable duration, determine if the problem has been corrected. If it hasn't, identify the pros and cons of whistle blowing. The pros include correction of a harmful or potentially harmful situation, retained moral integrity, and an enhanced sense of moral accountability. The cons include alienation, stress, and possible loss of reputation, professional standing, and job. Once you weigh the pros and cons, talk over the issue of whistle blowing with a lawyer or other knowledgeable person before you proceed.

Next, realistically appraise your situation. Will you be able to cope if you blow the whistle? Are you secure professionally and financially? Do you have the support of your family, colleagues, and administration? How much help can you count on?

Now make your decision based on your analysis of the severity of the incident, the consequences of whistle blowing, and your resources. If you elect to blow the whistle, carefully devise a strategy that follows institutional channels. If you're fearful of losing your job as a result of your actions, consider taking a position in another institution before you blow the whistle. If you fail to get satisfaction through institutional channels, consider consulting professional organizations, regulatory agencies, and, as a last resort, the press. Be sure to document each step you take.

ship, consider mapping out a self-protection strategy. Find a new employment position before you blow the whistle, and retain a lawyer who will provide you with competent legal advice throughout your ordeal. Seek out friends and colleagues who have the moral integrity to stand behind you.

Substance abuse among nurses

An estimated 7% of the 1.9 million nurses in the United States are addicted to alcohol or drugs. In one state study, researchers found that more than 90% of disciplinary hearings for nurses in the state were related to alcohol and drug abuse. These statistics aren't surprising in light of the high stress levels in nursing today. Nurses can experience feelings of frustration and powerlessness when trying to act as patient advocates. Frequent floating to unfamiliar units, unrealistic workloads, and long or double shifts may bring on fatigue and loneliness. Many nurses today must shoulder tremendous family and financial obligations while trying to meet professional demands. And, of course, nurses are not immune to the harsh social realities of modern life. Combined with the availability of **controlled substances,** such stressors all too often lead a nurse to substance abuse.

Past attitudes toward substance abuse

In the past, nurses who were caught abusing drugs or alcohol were punished. The prevailing ethic held that a nurse who abused drugs violated the public trust and the **standards** of her profession and deserved to be subject to strong disciplinary action.

Nursing administrators were expected to report suspected substance abusers to their state nursing board. The board would then investigate the allegation and, if it found the nurse guilty, would impose punishment, such as revocation of her license.

In practice, though, many administrators didn't report substance abuse, but chose instead to fire the offending nurse. In addition, colleagues of suspected substance abusers commonly didn't report their suspicions because they knew the nurse's job would be in jeopardy. Aware of the harsh treatment that awaited them, nurses who abused drugs or alcohol switched jobs frequently rather than endure the repercussions that would follow an admission of abuse.

Ethical perspectives

From an ethical viewpoint, this punitive approach to substance abuse left much to be desired. Administrators who simply fired a substance abuser abnegated their ethical responsibility to help nurses in need and to prevent qualified nurses from dropping out of their profession. Colleagues who didn't report substance abuse because they didn't want to see a co-worker punished abandoned the best interests of both the addicted nurse and her patients. The substance abuser often switched jobs rather than ask for help. She had little motivation to change, knowing that she was unlikely to receive understanding or rehabilitation.

A more enlightened view

Fortunately, society is learning to view substance abuse as a treatable disorder; today the emphasis is on rehabilitating chemically dependent nurses. Within the nursing profession, there is a greater understanding of the importance of peer support for the nurse struggling with addiction. Nurse practice acts may include provisions that encourage chemically dependent nurses to complete a treatment program. Many hospitals now have policies for dealing with substance abuse among employees, from initial reporting through rehabilitation and returning to work. In addition, treatment programs have become commonplace, and associations for recovering nurses are available to provide needed support.

When you suspect substance abuse

Because of the high rate of chemical dependence among nurses, chances are you will encounter this problem sometime in the course of your career. Like many nurses, you may experience confusion, guilt, anger, and remorse if faced with the responsibility of confronting and reporting a nurse-addict. Numerous potential ethical conflicts may arise from this situation:

• You may resent the increased work load, risk to patients, and stress created by the nurse's drug or alcohol problem.
• You may feel torn between your obligation to protect hospital patients and your loyalty to a fellow nurse.
• You may feel that you contributed to the addiction by not acting sooner.
• If you aren't entirely certain that your suspicions are correct, you may fear the damage you could do to an innocent nurse's reputation and career.
• You may have difficulty accepting the addict's self-destructive behavior as part of her addiction.
• You may feel that you're betraying a friendship.

Though the decision to report a coworker is never an easy one, you have an ethical obligation to intervene if you suspect a colleague is abusing drugs or alcohol. Intervening enables you to fulfill your moral obligation to your colleague: By reporting the abuse, you compel her to take the first step toward regaining control over her life and undergoing rehabilitation. You also fulfill your obligation to patients by protecting them from a nurse whose judgment and care do not meet professional standards.

Recognizing substance abuse

Be aware that allegations of substance abuse are serious and potentially damaging. To make an accurate assessment, you need to be familiar with the signs of substance abuse.

Signs of drug or alcohol abuse may include:
• rapid mood swings, usually from irritability or depression to elation
• frequent absences, lateness, and use of private quarters, such as bathrooms
• frequent volunteering to administer medications
• excessive errors or problems with controlled substances, such as reports of broken vials or spilled drugs
• illogical or sloppy charting
• inability to meet deadlines or minimum job requirements
• avoidance of new and challenging assignments
• increased errors in treatment, particularly in dosage computation
• poor personal hygiene and appearance
• inability to concentrate or remember details
• alcohol on the breath
• slurred speech, unsteady gait, flushed face, or red eyes
• discrepancies in narcotics supplies detected at the end of the nurse's shift
• narcotics signed out to patients only on the nurse's shift
• patient complaints of no relief from narcotics supposedly administered when the nurse is on duty

• preference for working alone or on the night shift, when supervision is minimal
• social withdrawal
• memory loss
• alcohol-induced complications, including jaundice, bruises (from falls), and delirium.

Reporting substance abuse

If you detect signs of substance abuse, your first step is to document them. Include the time, date, and place of the incident, a description of what happened, and the names of any witnesses. Be sure to leave out personal opinions and judgments. For example, "At around 9 p.m. on November 15, 1991, Mrs. Fox in room 501 told me that my injections of morphine were much better than those the other nurse gives. I asked what she meant. She told me that June Barrett's injections never seemed to take away her pain, but that mine always did. Two nights later, at 10:15 p.m., I went to the restroom. When I opened the door, I saw June Barrett injecting some solution into her thigh using a hospital syringe. She told me to get out. I did. We didn't talk about it afterward."

Never confront or accuse the suspected nurse on your own. Once you've documented the incident, discuss it with your nurse-manager. She'll need to gather additional information by examining patient charts, medication records (especially for narcotics), and reports from patients and other nurses. Once the manager completes this review, she'll try to determine if the evidence corroborates your incident report.

Confronting the substance abuser

If the nurse-manager concludes that substance abuse is likely, she'll need to confront the nurse with the facts and explain the options. Hopefully, these options will include treatment and per-

haps eventual reinstatement in her position. (See *Steps to help an impaired colleague,* page 340.) If you're asked to be present for this confrontation, keep in mind that you best fulfill your moral obligation to the substance abuser by being honest, compassionate, and nonjudgmental and by expressing your willingness to help. Expect that she will feel threatened and may attempt to deny her condition, even if the facts are fully substantiated.

In most substance abuse cases, if the nurse is willing to enter a treatment program and successfully completes it, no disciplinary action will be taken against her. If the nurse refuses to undergo treatment, she may be reported to the state board of nursing, suspended, or dismissed.

The road back

In most instances, the recovering nurse is able to return to work. She may be placed under a special contract that stipulates conditions for continued employment. These conditions may include:
• weekly meetings with a counselor
• a 12-step program and meetings with other recovering nurses
• random blood and urine screenings
• remaining drug-free.

The nurse-manager who is responsible for the recovering nurse should carefully document all meetings and keep a copy of all contracts.

The chemically dependent nurse's colleagues must use their professional training to try to understand her condition. Co-workers play a crucial role in the recovering nurse's ultimate success or failure. When recovering from addiction, a person's needs include:
• finding ways to improve self-esteem, including assertiveness training
• developing a stronger support system
• developing stress management and coping techniques

Steps to help an impaired colleague

Colleagues can take steps to put a stop to a nurse-addict's self-destructive behavior. By using an effective, nonpunitive, group-oriented approach, they can break the cycle of addiction. In this approach, group members confront the nurse-addict, help her to acknowledge her condition, and motivate her to seek rehabilitation before she harms a patient or herself.

Intervention team

The team includes 2 to 10 carefully selected persons who are personal or professional associates of the nurse-addict. If possible, the team also includes a colleague who has successfully entered rehabilitation and a nurse who possesses experience in treating drug and alcohol addiction.

Team members must share a nonjudgmental attitude. Each must accept that the nurse's self-destructive behavior represents an aspect of her illness and doesn't indicate that she's morally deficient. What's more, each should avoid expressing judgments about her.

Confronting the colleague

Team members document all evidence of the nurse's chemical dependence, including the date, time, and place of relevant incidents. They should be careful not to include any judgmental remarks in their documentation.

The team leader reviews all important documentation, including patient charts, nurses' notes, doctor's orders, medication administration and narcotic records, and the impaired nurse's personnel file.

Team members meet with the impaired nurse in a private room away from the nurses' station. The group leader explains why the team has gathered. Participants present their evidence, always prefacing their testimony with positive remarks.

The impaired nurse is given a chance to respond.

The team leader makes clear the options available to the impaired nurse. The impaired nurse is given an opportunity to voluntarily enter a treatment program; otherwise, she may lose her job and be reported to the state board of nursing.

Arrangements are made for the team leader to monitor how the nurse is progressing in therapy.

Events of the meeting are documented.

To ease the tension stirred up by the confrontation, the team leader may arrange for follow-up discussions.

• learning to come to terms with past traumatic experiences, such as physical or sexual abuse.

Welcoming a recovering nurse back to the work setting and offering support during the critical transition period is as important as detecting and reporting signs of abuse. From an ethical point of view, working with a colleague who is a substance abuser can be frustrating and uncomfortable, but helping a nurse recognize her problem and begin the process of recovery is an act of significant moral courage and humanity.

Selected references

Brandt, M. "Confidentiality Today: Where Do You Stand?" *Journal of AHIMA* 64(12):59-64, December 1993.

Campbell, M.L., et al. "Health Care Ethics Forum '94: Perspectives on Withholding and Withdrawal of Life-Support," *ACCN Clinical Issues* 5(3): 353-59, August 1994.

Davino, M. "Advice of Counsel: When the Nurse with an Addiction Is Your Boss," *RN* 58(8):55, August 1995.

Downey, R. "Autonomy or Accountability?" *Nursing Times* 90(27):31-32, July 6-12, 1994.

Edwards, B.S. "When the Family Can't Let Go," *American Journal of Nursing* 94(1):52-56, January 1994.

Hall, S.A. "Difficult Decisions: Respecting a Patient's Right to Refuse Treatment," *Journal of Emergency Medical Services* 19(5):11-13, May 1994.

Hardingham, L.B. "Ethics in the Workplace: Power, Authority and the Nurse," *AARN Newsletter* 50(3):19, March 1994.

Milholland, D.K. "Privacy and Confidentiality of Patient Information: Challenges for Nursing," *Journal of Nursing Administration* 24(2):19-24, February 1994.

Montoya, I.D., et al. "Fostering a Drug-Free Workplace," *Health Care Supervisor* 14(1):1-13, September 1995.

Salladay, S.A. "Doctor's Negligence: Exposing the Truth," *Nursing94* 24(10):26, October 1994.

Shelor, J. "Confidant or Informer?" *AIDS Patient Care* 7(6):301, December 1993.

Nursing in a changing health care marketplace

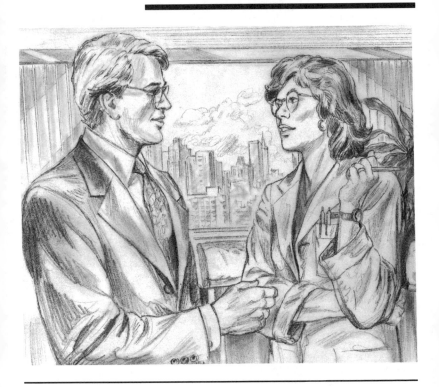

The health care industry is undergoing a rapid transformation that will profoundly affect nursing practice. Not only will these changes impact each nurse's ability to deliver quality patient care, but they will also determine the type and number of nursing job opportunities.

Nurses need to think about how they can shape future changes in the health care delivery system and how their careers can advance in uncertain times. One thing is clear—a changing health care environment will present challenges as well as opportunities for nurses. Preparation is the key to survival.

Current state of the U.S. health care marketplace

Managed care organizations and other similar entities now wield the balance of power in the delivery of health care in the United States. The implications are many, and they may not be fully understood for years to come.

During the early 1990s, it became clear that health care costs could not continue rising at their then current rate. If costs kept rising, the system would bankrupt America. President Clinton made health care reform a centerpiece of his 1992 presidential campaign. Although the Clinton administration's attempts at reform were unsuccessful, dramatic changes took place in the health care arena during the first half of the 1990s.

The marketplace responds

Traditionally, third-party payers (including insurance companies and the federal government through the Medicare and Medicaid programs) covered most expenses incurred by a patient as a result of his doctor's orders. This type of health insurance coverage, where the insurer reimburses covered individuals for the cost of their health care, is called indemnity or fee-for-service coverage.

As health care costs spun out of control in the late 1980s, third-party payers began to audit expenditures. One of the earliest forms of price control took place when third-party payers set forth what they deemed to be the "usual, customary, and reasonable charge" for a specific procedure. They then reimbursed the patient based on the usual, customary, and reasonable charge. Any charge in excess of that charge had to be absorbed by the patient.

Concern over escalating reimbursement costs eventually led to the development of managed care organizations (MCOs). MCOs are responsible for both the financing and delivery of a broad range of comprehensive health care services for an enrolled population — for a fixed fee. Most MCOs provide health care services to their covered members through affiliated providers. This differs substantially from traditional fee-for-service insurers.

By the end of 1994, more than 50 million Americans were enrolled in health maintenance organizations (HMOs), one type of MCO. From 1992 to 1994 alone, 9 million people joined HMOs. Additionally, 65% of workers insured by large and medium-sized companies were enrolled in some form of managed care — an increase from 47% only 3 years earlier. The trend away from traditional fee-for-service coverage continues at a rapid pace. (See *Trends in insurance coverage,* page 344.)

Emerging organizations

Major types of MCOs include HMOs and preferred provider organizations. Other important organizations to emerge in the new health care marketplace include disease-management companies and health care networks.

HMOs

The most well-known managed care arrangement is the HMO. Current HMO models include the *staff model,* the *group practice model,* the *network model,* and the *individual practice association* (IPA).

Kaiser Permanente is a classic example of a staff model HMO, where doctors who serve the HMO enrollees are employed by the HMO. Staff model HMOs are currently having difficulty maintaining their profitability because they are unable to reduce the compensation to doctors rapidly enough to keep up with the declining payments being made to doctors in group practice, network, or IPA model HMOs.

Group practice, network, and IPA model HMOs are in a much better competitive position in the marketplace than staff model HMOs. Each of these models requires that the HMO contract with doctors, either individually or on

Trends in insurance coverage

The U.S. marketplace for insurance coverage is undergoing radical change, with decreasing numbers of people being covered by traditional fee-for-service insurance and increasing numbers enrolled in health maintenance organizations (HMOs).

	1995	1996	1997	1998	1999
Total U.S. population	263,434,000	266,068,000	268,729,000	271,416,000	274,130,000
HMOs	61,398,000	68,766,000	75,643,000	83,207,000	91,528,000
Preferred provider organizations	62,000,000	62,000,000	60,760,000	59,545,000	58,354,000
Fee-for-service only	23,674,000	20,908,000	19,794,000	17,893,000	15,140,000
Medicare or Medicaid (not covered by managed care)	62,637,000	60,132,000	57,727,000	55,418,000	53,201,000
Military and Veterans Administration	15,000,000	15,150,000	15,302,000	15,455,000	15,610,000
Uninsured	38,725,000	39,112,000	39,503,000	39,898,000	40,297,000

Source: Incenter Strategies, Inc., *Report on Managed Care,* December 1994.

a group or network basis, for the services needed to cover people enrolled in the HMO. The HMOs currently have the upper hand as doctors struggle to respond in a competitive marketplace.

PPOs

Somewhere between the traditional fee-for-service plans and the HMO is the *preferred provider organization* (PPO). In a PPO, an employer or health care insurance carrier contracts with a group of preferred or selected participating providers. These providers typically agree to accept the PPO's reimbursement structure and payment levels. In return, the PPO limits the size of its participating provider groups and provides incentives for its covered individuals to use the participating providers instead of other providers. While PPOs are in use in a variety of forms, they usually function as a transitory way of shifting enrollees out of traditional fee-for-service programs and into HMOs.

Disease-management companies

Disease-management companies manage all aspects of treating a specific disease. Major pharmaceutical companies (including Merck, Eli Lilly, SmithKline Beecham, and others), major providers of health care (including

Johns Hopkins, the Mayo Clinic, and Memorial Sloan-Kettering), third-party payers, and others have joined forces or have gone into disease management on their own.

In a typical disease-management arrangement, an MCO, employer, or insurance company contracts with a disease-management company for coverage of its enrollees when they are diagnosed with a specific disease such as cancer. Disease-management programs rely heavily on clinical pathways or treatment guidelines designed to provide the best possible care in the most streamlined environment. Disease-management companies usually guarantee that payment won't exceed a maximum amount. At best, the arrangement has the potential advantage of providing high-quality care at the lowest possible cost.

Health care networks

Conceptually, health care networks are similar to disease-management companies. A typical health care network includes a major hub hospital, several smaller community-based hospitals, a long-term facility with subacute services and, perhaps, a rehabilitation center, home health care agency, and physician services.

In smoothly functioning health care networks, patients benefit from the reduction or elimination of fragmented delivery of care. Such networks can provide a continuum of care from one stage of illness to the next. Duplication of services is limited, and both preventive and outpatient care are encouraged.

However, powerful health care networks may eliminate competition from alternative health care providers, creating substantial controversy. And patient referrals may be ethically questionable when there is cross-ownership of different components of the health care network.

Effects of marketplace changes

For the first time in this century, increases in health care expenditures are shrinking, and the health care marketplace is undergoing a radical change of control and direction.

Increased oversight of doctors

Until now, doctors controlled the flow of health care expenditures based on what they felt was appropriate medical care. However, with the advent of managed care, doctors have had to contend with oversight from third-party payers, other health care professionals, and the government.

Greater role for primary care providers

To the extent that doctors still have an essential role in controlling the expenditure of health care dollars, it is the primary care doctor, not the specialist, who is in control.

Most HMO models will not cover any costs incurred by a patient who sees a specialist unless he is referred to that specialist by a primary care doctor who acts as a "gatekeeper." Additionally, diagnostic tests and surgery are strictly limited within certain prescribed situations.

Increased reliance on practice guidelines

Disease-management companies and health care networks increasingly rely on practice guidelines, such as clinical pathways. Although guidelines can help reduce costs and streamline care for efficiency's sake, they may stir up controversy when providers of health care disagree on the guidelines and how they should be implemented.

Questionable effects on patient care

Thirty years ago, a woman having a baby might stay in the hospital with that baby for up to a week. Today, it's not unusual for that stay to be limited to 24 hours. While advances in medical care are partially responsible for speeding up the recovery process, concerns about health care costs are also an important factor.

Continuing competition for health care dollars will force health care costs down over the near term. However, at some point, the quality of care will be compromised. Then, the pendulum may swing back as the public demands more comprehensive care.

Significantly, changes in the health care marketplace could provide additional ammunition for medical malpractice and liability lawsuits. If MCOs continue to limit the medical care being provided to their enrollees, an enrollee may claim that he was injured as a result of receiving insufficient care.

Emphasis on prevention

The growth of MCOs has been accompanied by increased emphasis on preventive medicine. But MCOs are in a quandary about preventive health care. The average time an enrollee spends in an MCO currently is 18 months to 2 years. Why should an MCO spend significant dollars promoting preventive measures if it will not be the beneficiary of the enrollees' good health?

Changing hospital environment

Hospitals are no longer the dominant providers of health care. Today, the emphasis is on providing care in less expensive ambulatory settings, including outpatient clinics and surgery centers, as well as in the patient's home.

Patients are hospitalized only for the most acute phase of their illness and then are transferred to a less intensive level of care, such as a subacute or skilled nursing unit in a long-term care facility. Hospitalized patients are typically sicker than outpatients and require more intensive services.

The length of stay for hospitalized patients has decreased sharply over the past 10 years, causing a significant decline in hospital census. The combination of fewer patient days and the deep discounts demanded by third-party payers has caused hospital reimbursement to decline as well.

As a result, hospitals are trying to do more with less. Operating budgets are being slashed, resulting in fewer dollars available for nurses' salaries. With fewer patients and improved technology, hospital executives reason that fewer nurses are needed for patient care. These executives, however, may overlook the fact that inpatients are usually very sick and that the technology used to care for them is more complex.

In an effort to contain costs, hospital executives are restructuring the delivery of patient care. In many instances, they have hired consultants to review hospital operations and to determine more cost-effective ways of delivering patient care and increasing patient (customer) satisfaction.

Restructuring seeks to achieve the following goals:
• elimination of "non-value-added" services and functions
• consolidation of management services through a reduction in the layers of management
• changes in the nursing skill mix and the cross-training of many different levels and types of personnel.

If successfully implemented, restructuring is intended to result in the breakdown of disciplinary boundaries, in improved patient care, and in significant cost reductions.

Increased implementation of cost-cutting strategies

Health care providers have adopted new strategies in their quest to overhaul patient care. These include continuous quality improvement and case management. At the core of these strategies is the desire to reduce failures in health care delivery, to minimize unnecessary variations in patient care practices, and to enhance collaboration among members of the health care team—all of which aim to produce more cost-effective, higher quality patient care.

How changes in health care will affect nursing

With dramatic changes in health care delivery in full swing, the nursing profession cannot stand still. But how will nursing change? Several important trends are apparent.

Cross-training of personnel

A major part of the work redesign process in hospitals is the cross-training of personnel to work in other specialties. For example, nurses are skilled in phlebotomy, electrocardiography, and other tasks that once were performed by technicians whose positions have been eliminated. Frequently, dietary, housekeeping, and other support personnel are cross-trained to increase flexibility and decrease costs.

Administrators hope that cross-training will lead to more effective and efficient utilization of personnel. Staff responsibilities will be broadened and increased, resulting in greater continuity of care. Cross-training practices vary from institution to institution and are governed, in large part, by state licensure requirements.

Less specialization

The need for a more flexible staff is prompting many nurses to learn new skills and become less specialized. Critical care nurses, who previously were not expected to work outside the critical care unit, are being asked to work on the general nursing units. Because the patients in hospitals are only the most seriously ill, staff nurses on general medical-surgical units must learn skills traditionally performed only by critical care nurses.

Increased use of unlicensed assistive personnel

Another major component of redesign efforts is the development of new, more cost-effective models for the delivery of nursing care. This usually includes changing the nursing skill mix and decreasing labor costs by replacing more highly paid registered nurses (RNs) with ancillary staff, often called nurse extenders or unlicensed assistive personnel (UAP).

The use of UAP will change nursing roles. For example, nurses will supervise unlicensed personnel and manage larger patient loads. These are significant changes, especially for nurses who are accustomed to working with a primary nursing model that includes an all-RN staff.

The UAP debate

Use of UAP is controversial. Opponents claim that UAP usage will lower the quality of patient care and cause poor patient outcomes. They contend that care will be fragmented, that nurses will be required to simply "manage" the care provided by the UAP, and that this may threaten patient safety and a nurse's license. Opponents argue that the workplace is being "deskilled" at a time when patients are sicker than ever before and need higher, not lower, levels of care and competence.

Proponents argue that UAP usage is a sensible way to deliver patient care less expensively. They feel that the nursing role should be expanded and enhanced and that delegating non-professional tasks to trained UAP who are closely supervised by RNs does not automatically lower the quality of care.

Like it or not, the use of UAP has become a major factor in the health care delivery system. Cost cutting and budgetary restraints are ultimately the deciding factors.

The role of nurses in shaping health care today

To protect their own interests and the interests of their patients, nurses must become involved in the changes taking place in health care delivery.

Nurses understand patient care and know how best to redesign the delivery of care while keeping the patient as the primary focus. As key players in the work redesign process, nurses can develop and implement models of nursing care that are cost-effective and that provide quality patient care.

The advantages of flexibility

The uncertainties of new work arrangements require that nurses be flexible and willing to try new ideas. What has worked in the past isn't necessarily best for the future. (See *Strategies to deal with change.*)

For example, within the scope of licensure, nurses must be willing to manage and guide UAP who have been taught to perform nonprofessional tasks that were traditionally nursing functions. Nurses are the only ones who can determine which functions can be performed by unlicensed, multiskilled workers and which functions truly require the education, knowledge, and skill of an RN. Furthermore, nurses must ensure, through the use of continuous quality improvement, that delegating tasks to UAP will not lower the quality of care.

Nurses can take control of the patient care redesign process, rather than view themselves as victims of change. Without nursing input, redesigning patient care becomes a short-term approach to cost cutting and runs the risk of becoming a long-term disaster.

The challenge of more care in less time

Any new strategy that promises to improve patient care while cutting costs will significantly change nursing practice. Nurses will be required to follow predetermined clinical pathways and guidelines and to change their practice accordingly. Nurses will have to take a proactive role in managing a patient's length of stay. They will be required to provide more care in less time and to manage their patients throughout the continuum of care, not merely through one episode of illness. Managing a patient will require that nurses interact and communicate effectively with personnel from rehabilitation centers, long-term care facilities, and home health care agencies.

These strategies will bring new members to the patient care team. Once made up solely of doctors, nurses, and physical and respiratory therapists, the patient care team may now include nondirect caregivers. For example, the role of case manager has been created in many institutions and MCOs. This person, often a nurse, works with the care team and the MCO to manage the use of resources and keep the patient on the appropriate care path. Patient care nurses will have to work with case managers and other nondirect caregivers, who will have a major voice in the management of patient care.

Strategies to deal with change

The best advice is to change the only thing you can control—your attitude.

Be flexible

● Be willing to try new ideas and roles: Open your mind and expand your horizons.

● Keep your skills and expertise updated and broaden your experience.

● Study the new situation, figure out how the game has changed, and adapt to the new rules.

● Don't try to control your situation. Generally, it's not controllable. Accept what cannot be changed, and learn ways to deal effectively with changes.

● Develop a tolerance for ambiguity and uncertainty. It is the norm in health care today and will only increase in the future.

● Accept change and move on; don't act like a victim and wallow in self-pity.

Take charge

● Instead of spending time and energy fighting change, spend your time planning how you'll succeed within the changing environment.

● Put yourself in charge of managing the pressure of change. Your own decisions determine your stress level.

● Don't look for short-term comfort. Don't spend your time and energy looking for a low-stress organization. Organizations that will survive are the very ones that are going through the painful change process.

● Proactively change your job function—add new activities and eliminate those that don't contribute to the organization's current goals. Be seen as part of the solution, not part of the problem.

● Move quickly—adapt to the changes quickly, and perform your job more quickly. Speed is a competitive advantage.

Reduce stress

● Don't be afraid of the future. Instead of worrying about the bad things that might happen, proactively create your own future.

● Choose your battles—pick battles big enough to matter, small enough to win.

● Don't let the stress of change drive a wedge between you and your work. Continue to be committed to your career and profession.

● Take personal responsibility for stress reduction, and use stress-reduction techniques on a regular basis.

Your duty as a patient advocate

As the health care delivery system evolves into a more cost-effective system, you may confront ethical conflicts brought on by difficult choices between managing costs and providing care. You will be asked to do more with less. There will be times when you feel that staffing levels are inadequate for providing safe and effective patient care. This is an extremely difficult situation for a nurse.

Use creativity and ingenuity to address and resolve each situation on an individual basis. In a health care system that increasingly stresses the "bottom line," the nurse should act as an advocate for the patient, who must always remain the primary focus in any decision about health care access, quality, and cost. Your role as a patient advocate requires you to protect the patient from institutional policies that infringe upon his rights.

Advancing your career despite downsizing

Cost cutting frequently results in a reduced staff, an increased workload, and the consolidation or elimination of services. Many nurses feel threatened by this process. This feeling is understandable because some nurses will face radical changes in their work environment and responsibilities. (Job insecurity was something that nurses rarely faced in the past.) Part of the problem for many nurses is their own inability to deal effectively with change. They are fearful and often feel powerless.

Because change is inevitable in health care, nurses need to learn new and more effective ways of coping with it. Nurses will be empowered by accepting the need for change as a matter of personal and organizational survival.

Where the jobs are

While nurses have never before faced such significant job insecurity, they've also never had such an opportunity to assume expanded roles. Nurses today are looking at pay rates and positions that didn't exist a decade ago. (See *New opportunities in nursing.*)

Within and outside the hospital

Nurses traditionally were employed in hospitals, caring for acutely ill patients. Now, with the hospital industry shrinking, the key to a successful hospital-based nursing practice is a combination of flexibility and excellent clinical skills. Even as the hospital sector is downsizing, other sectors of the health care delivery system are growing and providing greater job opportunities with increased job security. Nursing care is being provided in a variety of settings throughout the health care continuum, from hospitals to long-term care, subacute care, rehabilitation services, ambulatory care, and home health care. (See *Career management: How to achieve success,* pages 352 and 353.)

Outpatient services and long-term care

Outpatient services — particularly primary and preventive care — continue to grow, as do nursing jobs in these areas. Nurses find opportunities in surgical centers, clinics, home care services, community health, and similar settings. Certain levels of patient care that were once provided exclusively in hospitals, such as I.V. therapy and ventilator care, are now being provided in a variety of other settings, including subacute care, skilled care, and home care.

The concept of long-term care has expanded beyond the traditional custodial care provided in a nursing home to include subacute care, skilled care, rehabilitation services, and more. Patients in long-term care settings now include those with multiple acute problems. In some advanced subacute settings, the only patients who cannot be accepted are those who are hemodynamically unstable and require one-on-one nursing care and the immediate and ongoing intervention of a doctor.

Generally, fewer patient care professionals are present in the subacute, skilled, and home care settings. Nurses who choose to practice in these settings are given greater autonomy and must learn to function more independently.

Managed care

The opportunities for the professional nurse in managed care are expanding. Until recently, the focus of MCOs has been on nonclinical issues, such as network development and contracting. However, these organizations are starting to manage patients' care with

New opportunities in nursing

People with a nursing background are ideally suited to many new professional opportunities in health care.

Clinical executive: Where RN meets MBA

A new class of health care executives is emerging. They are individuals with a clinical background – primarily doctors and nurses – who have obtained a master's degree in business administration (MBA), public health, or health services administration. These clinicians are prepared to take leadership roles and can effectively manage health care professionals because they understand both patient care and administration issues.

Information systems specialists

Health care information technology continues to be a dominant force in the strategic management and daily operations of health care systems. Job opportunities are opening up for nurses as information systems specialists. In this position, nurses can help ensure that the design and application of information systems support patient-centered care and the clinical decision-making process. Nursing's influence on the functioning and development of information systems is vital in reshaping the health care industry.

Advanced practice nursing

Advanced practice is another exciting avenue of opportunity. Advanced practice nurses (APNs) include nurse practitioners (NPs), certified nurse-midwives (CNMs), clinical nurse specialists (CNSs), and certified registered nurse-anesthetists (CRNAs). Briefly, their duties include the following:

● NPs obtain medical histories, perform physical examinations, order and interpret diagnostic studies, and diagnose and treat chronic or stable acute health problems. They promote health maintenance and disease prevention through education of patients and their families.

● CNMs deliver babies and provide care before and after birth, focusing on healthy women with normal pregnancies. They work in a variety of settings, from the patient's home to birthing centers and hospitals. They may work either as partners with doctors or as independent practitioners with doctor affiliates. They refer patients with complex conditions and those who require surgery to doctors.

● CNSs care for patients with specific illnesses, such as heart disease or cancer. They are employed primarily in hospitals and provide education and clinical expertise for staff nurses.

● CRNAs deliver all types of anesthesia to patients in a variety of settings.

In the past 15 years, the scope of practice for APNs has broadened considerably. State legislators and the general public are becoming aware of the competence of APNs and the advantages they offer with regard to cutting costs. APNs continue to gain increased regulatory support for their expanded nursing role.

The strengthening role of APNs is still controversial. Some doctors feel threatened by APNs and continue to object to their growing independence. These doctors feel that APNs do not have appropriate training or expertise and, therefore, will have a negative impact on the quality of patient care. But results of initial studies suggest that APNs can match the quality of care provided by doctors. An analysis conducted for the American Nurses' Association shows that APNs score as high as, or higher than, doctors on the key measures of patient care.

Career management: How to achieve success

Because of the uncertainty in the health care marketplace, it is unrealistic and unwise to plan your career around the continuity of one organization and one role. Career management means knowing yourself and the market, then continually renewing your skills.

In a profession experiencing a dramatic metamorphosis, you can remain marketable and competitive by enhancing and fine-tuning your skills. Get as much experience and education as possible, and consider seeking national specialty certification. Today's employers are looking for experienced nurses who can work in various environments and specialties.

Look for ways to apply your skills and expertise in different roles or in alternative settings. For example, a clinical nurse specialist in a hospital may be vulnerable to downsizing; however, her skills can be transferred to a case management role with a managed care organization.

Strategies to help manage your profession

Keep informed: Stay abreast of changes and trends in health care. Assess how these changes might affect your practice. Here are some tips:
- Network with peers.
- Read professional journals.
- Attend national nursing conferences.
- Become active in your professional organization.
- Join committees that are planning your organization's future direction.
- Assess your organization's response to today's environment.
- Look beyond your organization at the big picture.

- Assess other health care organizations' ability to adapt to change
- Get involved in government, and let state and national legislators know the nursing perspective on health care.

Career milestones

All nurses, from their first position through retirement, experience tremendous personal growth and awareness. Career changes and promotions have always been part of the career span. More recently, layoffs have become an increasingly common phenomenon.

Finding your first position

When determining where to practice, consider entering the system at the hospital level so you can develop the clinical skills you'll need to practice in more autonomous settings. However, keep in mind that the number of new nursing graduates far exceeds the number of positions hospitals have to offer to inexperienced nurses. Finding that first job may require some extra effort.

Human resource professionals and nurse recruiters offer these tips for finding your first job:
- Know yourself—understand your strengths and weaknesses and your values and interests.
- Assess what you have to offer a prospective employer. Before finishing nursing school, consider seeking health care experience as a paramedic, surgical technician, or volunteer. Many new graduates are finding jobs at the hospitals where they worked as nursing assistants when they were students.
- Work at making a good impression. Present yourself as a professional.
- Prepare a professional résumé.

Career management: How to achieve success continued

Receiving a layoff notice

No matter how it's presented, a layoff always comes as a shock. No one can make you feel better, but there are guidelines you can follow to ensure that you'll receive the best possible severance package:

• Don't get angry, panic, or lash out. Don't do anything that could reduce your negotiating power. Keep a clear mind so that you can effectively negotiate your severance arrangement.

• Don't take the layoff personally – many competent and longtime employees are being laid off as more hospitals restructure and downsize.

• Get all the information about the layoff in writing, if possible.

• Determine the status of your benefits, including sick and vacation time, retirement pensions, and health insurance.

Negotiating severance

Severance packages are often negotiable. Administrators feel badly about the situation, and they also understand that if an employee is treated unfairly, she can file a grievance. Therefore, negotiate hard for a severance package that includes payment of at least 1 week's salary per year of service, outplacement services or job counseling, sick-time pay, and positive letters of reference.

Getting back to work

Once you have negotiated your severance arrangement and have left your place of employment, your goal is to find another job. Your first task will be to identify your professional strengths and areas for growth. Do a self-assessment of your life, the type of job you're looking for, and your short- and long-term career goals.

Once you have an idea of the type of position you're looking for, update your résumé. A number of good books can guide you through the process. Next, compile a list of references. Be sure to ask permission from individuals prior to giving their names as references. Keep the people on your reference list informed about your job-search progress.

Networking with colleagues is extremely important in today's job market. Let your friends and colleagues know you're looking for a job and the type of position you're pursuing.

The interview process can be tough. You can never be too good at it. Read books and articles on interviewing techniques.

Take steps to manage stress during your job search. Eat right, get plenty of rest, exercise regularly, and seek the support of family and friends.

Nurses who have successfully moved from one job to another and into new practice settings identify ongoing professional skills and training as a key survival strategy. Wise nurses are finding that continuing their nursing education bridges the gap between their basic nursing skills and the demands of new roles and changing responsibilities.

---

the goal of keeping their customers healthy.

Many MCOs are moving toward providing care within a capitated model. Under *capitation*, financial incentives encourage health care providers to keep people healthy. The essence of capitation is risk management – the organization uses a proactive strategy to identify high-risk patients, puts them under case management, and aggressively promotes healthful behavior.

Russell C. Coile, health care futurist, said, "The future of American health care is to provide more health with less care."

This change in the focus of patient care is good news for nurses, who are ideally suited to promote healthful behavior. The foundation of nursing practice is based on treating the whole person, not just an illness, and is focused on promoting wellness rather than treating disease. This holistic view of the patient is the premise of nursing. Florence Nightingale said in *Notes on Nursing* that "nature alone cures, and what nursing has to do is to put the patient in the best condition for nature to act upon him." The new health care environment will finally allow nurses to practice in the manner in which they are educated.

Within MCOs, many new job opportunities are available. Nurses may provide direct patient care or act as gatekeepers or case managers — assessing and evaluating patients by telephone to determine the proper intervention, then helping them reach the appropriate sector of the health care system.

Nurses can also function within an MCO in utilization management, quality improvement, marketing, information systems, and general management and administration.

In the managed care setting, nurses have a chance to use their creativity, take the initiative, and expand their scope of practice. Within managed care, professional nurses can provide the expertise consumers need to cope with today's health system.

Conclusion

The major challenge facing the health care industry is to find better ways to deliver quality patient care for less money. Nurses have an opportunity to dramatically influence health care.

They should embrace this opportunity and take part in shaping the new era. Their participation will be invaluable to the development of a new health care delivery system and to the profession of nursing.

Selected references

Adams, B. "Primary Care," *CQ Researcher* 7(101):217, March 17, 1995.

Andreola, N.M. "What Nursing Has Known All Along," *Nursing Spectrum D.C.* 5(16):12-13, August 7, 1995.

Buck, J.A., and Kamlet, M.S. "Problems with Expanding Medicaid for the Uninsured," *Journal of Health Politics, Policy & Law* 18(1):1-25, Spring 1993.

Coile, R. "Transformation of American Healthcare in the Post-Reform Era," *Healthcare Executive* 9(4):8-12, July-August 1994.

Curry, K. "What Networks Mean to You," *Nursing95* 25(1):49, January 1995.

Curtin, L. "Job Security: Is Nothing Sacred Anymore?" *Nursing Management* 26(7): 7-9, July 1995.

Curtin, L. *Nursing into the 21st Century.* Springhouse, Pa.: Springhouse Corp., 1996.

Doyle, E. "Advanced Practice Nurses and Managed Care," *Missouri Nurse* 64(4):6-7, July-August 1995.

Eckholm, E. "While Congress Remains Silent, Health Care Transforms Itself," *New York Times,* December 19, 1995.

Fisher, C. "Is This the Hour of Managed Care?" *Provider* 21(6):44-46, 48-50, 53 + , June 1995.

Guanowsky, G.A. "Law for the Nurse Manager. Liability in Managed Care for the Health Care Provider," *Nursing Management* 26(10):24-25, October 1995.

Hale, C. "Research Issues in Case Management," *Nursing Standard* 9(44):29-32, July 26-August 1, 1995.

Hastings, K.E. "Health Care Reform: We Need It, But Do We Have the National Will to Shape Our Future?" *Nurse Practitioner: American Journal of Primary Health Care* 20(1):52-54, 56-57, January 1995.

Hurley, M.L. "Where Will You Work Tomorrow?" *RN* 57(8):31-35, August 1994.

Jacobs, L.R. "Health Reform Impasse: The Politics of American Ambivalence Toward Government," *Journal of Health Politics, Policy & Law* 18(3, pt. 2):629-55, Fall 1993.

Jenkins, M., and Torrisi, D.L. "Marketing and Management: Nurse Practitioners, Community Nursing Centers, and Contracting for Managed Care," *Journal of the American Academy of Nurse Practitioners* 7(3):119-24, March 1995

Ketter, J. "ANA: Protecting Nurses and Patient Care in the Face of Restructuring," *The American Nurse* 26(5):1, 14, May 1994.

Longman, R. "SmithKline's Data Challenge," *In Vivo, the Business and Medicine Report* 13(1):41, January 1995.

Mason, D., and Leavitt, J. "The Revolution in Health Care: What's Your Readiness Quotient?" *American Journal of Nursing* 95(6):50, June 1995.

McLaughlin, F., et al. "Changes Related to Care Delivery Patterns," *Journal of Nursing Administration* 25(5):35-46, May 1995.

Moore, J.D. "Despite Attempts at Peace, AMA-ANA Turf War Rages On," *Modern Healthcare* 25(31):14, July 31, 1995.

Pritchett, P., et al. *A Survival Guide to the Stress of Organizational Change.* Dallas: Pritchett & Assoc., Inc., 1995.

Salmon, J.W. "A Perspective on the Corporate Transformation of Health Care," *International Journal of Health Services* 25(1):11-42, 1995.

Turner, S.O. "Laid Off? Now What?" *Nursing95* 25(5):97-98, May 1995.

Turner, S.O. "Reality Check: It's Time for Nurses to Face the Future," *Hospitals & Health Networks* 69(16):20-22, August 20, 1995.

Glossary

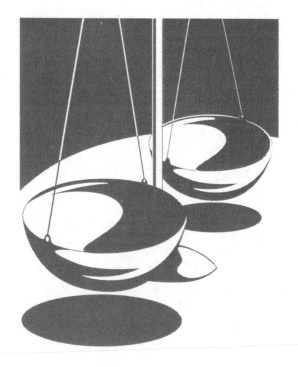

Glossary

abandonment • The unilateral ending of a professional relationship with a patient, without adequate notice and while the need for medical or nursing care still exists.

abuse of process • A civil action in which it is alleged that the legal process has been used in an improper manner. For example, an abuse of process action might be brought by a health care practitioner attempting to countersue a patient or by a psychiatric patient attempting to demonstrate wrongful confinement.

ad hoc committee • A committee commissioned for a specific purpose.

adjudicated incompetent • Declared incompetent by exercise of judicial authority. Note that a patient who has been adjudicated incompetent may still have the mental capacity to make an informed decision about his medical care. Compare ***incompetence, mental incompetence.***

administrative law • Law established by legislators, but enforced by an administrative agency on the authority of legislators.

administrative review • Investigation conducted by the state board of nursing when a nurse is accused of professional misconduct. The board first reviews the complaint and then may hold a formal hearing at which evidence is presented and witnesses examined and cross-examined. Court proceedings – and possibly legal penalties – may result from the board's findings.

administrator • Overseer of the general effectiveness and efficiency of an agency, who is concerned with organization, planning, development, growth, change, operations, budgets and evaluation.

admissible evidence • Authentic, relevant, reliable information presented during a trial, which may be used to reach a decision.

adult • *1.* One who is fully developed and matured and who has attained the intellectual capacity and the emotional and psychological stability characteristic of a mature person. *2.* A person who has reached full legal age (in most states, age 18 or 21).

advance directive • Document used as a guideline for life-sustaining medical care of a patient with advanced disease or disability who is no longer able to indicate his own wishes.

advance directive system • System implemented by health care institutions (including hospitals, nursing homes, and hospices) to ensure that every patient, at admission, is informed of his right to execute a living will or durable power of attorney for health care decisions.

advanced practice nurse • Individual whose education and certification meet criteria established by a state board of nursing. This individual is usually currently licensed as a registered nurse and has passed a postbasic certificate program in a clinical nursing specialty with national certification or has obtained a master's degree in a clinical nursing specialty.

adverse reaction • A harmful, unintended reaction to a drug administered at normal dosage.

affidavit • A written statement sworn to before a notary public or an officer of the court.

affirmative defense • A denial of guilt or wrongdoing based on new evidence rather than on simple denial of a charge. For example, a nurse who pleads immunity under Good Samaritan law is making an affirmative defense. The defendant bears the burden of proof in an affirmative defense.

age of majority • 18 or 21 years, depending on the state or Canadian provincial laws.

agency • A relationship between two parties in which the first party authorizes the second to act as agent on behalf of the first.

agent • A party authorized to act on behalf of another and to give the other an account of such actions.

AHA • See **American Hospital Association.**

Alcoholics Anonymous (AA) • An international nonprofit organization, founded in 1935, consisting of abstinent alcoholics whose purpose is to help alcoholics stop drinking and maintain sobriety through group support, shared experiences, and faith in a power greater than themselves.

alcoholism • The extreme dependence on excessive amounts of alcohol, associated with a cumulative pattern of deviant behaviors. Alcoholism is a chronic illness with a slow, insidious onset, which may occur at any age. The etiology is unknown, but cultural and psychosocial factors are suspect, and families of alcoholics have a higher incidence of alcoholism.

AMA • Against medical advice; a patient's decision to leave a health care facility against his doctor's advice. See also **American Medical Association.**

amendment • An alteration to an existing law or complaint.

American Hospital Association (AHA) • Founded in 1898, the AHA is an association of 45,000 individuals and health care institutions, including hospitals, health care systems, and preacute and postacute health care delivery organizations. The AHA is dedicated to promoting the welfare of the public through its leadership and assistance to its members in the provision of better health services for all people.

American Medical Association (AMA) • A professional association including practitioners in all recognized medical specialties as well as general primary care physicians. The AMA is governed by a Board of Trustees and House of Delegates. Trustees and delegates represent various state and local medical associations as well as such government agencies as the Public Health Service and medical departments of the Army, Navy, and Air Force.

American Nurses' Association (ANA) • The national professional association of registered nurses in the United States. It was founded in 1896 to improve standards of health and the availability of health care given in order to foster high standards for nursing, to promote the professional development of nurses, and to advance the economic and general welfare of nurses. The ANA is made up of 53 constituent associations from 50 states, the District of Columbia, Guam, and the U.S. Virgin Islands, representing more than 900 district associations. Members may join one or more of the five Divisions on Nursing Practice: Community Health, Gerontological, Maternal and Child Health, Medical-Surgical, and Psychiatric and Mental Health Nursing. These divisions are coordinated by the Congress for Nursing Practice. The Congress evaluates changes in the scope of practice, monitors scientific and educational developments, encourages research, and develops statements that describe ANA policies regarding legislation that affects nursing practice. Other commissions within the Association include the Commission on Nursing Education, the Commission on Nursing Services, the Commission on Nursing Research, and the Economic and General Welfare Commission.

American Red Cross • A nationwide organization that seeks to reduce human suffering through various health, safety, and disaster relief programs in affiliation with the International Committee of the Red Cross. The Committee and all Red Cross organizations evolved from the Geneva Convention of 1864, following the example and urging of

Swiss humanitarian Jean-Henri Dunant, who aided wounded French and Austrian soldiers at the Battle of Solferino in 1859. The American Red Cross (one of more than 120 national Red Cross organizations) has more than 130 million members in about 3,100 chapters throughout the United States. Volunteers constitute the entire staffs of about 1,700 chapters. Other chapters maintain small paid staffs and some professionals but depend largely on volunteers.

anencephaly • The congenital absence of most or all of the cerebral hemispheres. Many anencephalic infants are stillborn, but others have a functional brain stem and live for a short time after birth. The use of organs from an anencephalic infant for transplantation is controversial.

answer • The response of a defendant to the claims of a plaintiff. The answer contains a denial of the plaintiff's allegations and may also contain an affirmative defense or a counterclaim. It is the principal pleading on the part of the defense and is prepared in writing, usually by the defense attorney, and submitted to the court.

appellate court • A court of law that has the power to review the decision of a lower court. An appellate court does not make a new determination of the facts of the case; instead, it reviews the way in which the law was applied in the case.

appellee • The party in an appeal who won the case in a lower court. The appellee argues that the decision of the lower court should not be modified by the appellate court.

arbitration • The settlement of a dispute by an impartial person chosen by the disputing parties.

arbitrator • An impartial person appointed to resolve a dispute between parties. The arbitrator listens to the evidence as presented by the parties in an informal hearing and attempts to arrive at a resolution acceptable to both parties.

assault • An attempt or threat by a person to physically injure another person.

associate degree in nursing • An academic degree after satisfactory completion of a 2-year course of study, usually at a community or junior college. The recipient is eligible to take the national licensing examination to become a registered nurse. An associate degree in nursing is not available in Canada. Compare *bachelor of science in nursing.*

attending physician • The doctor who is responsible for a particular, usually private, patient. In a university setting, an attending physician usually also has teaching responsibilities and holds a faculty appointment. Also called attending (informal), *physician of record.*

attorney of record • The attorney whose name appears on the legal records for a specific case, as the agent of a specific client.

audit • A methodical examination; to examine with intent to verify. Nursing audits examine standards of nursing care.

authorization cards • Cards employees sign to authorize a union election.

autonomy • The principle of self-determination. The right to make decisions about one's own health care.

autopsy • A postmortem examination of a body to determine the cause of death.

B

bachelor of science in nursing (BSN) • An academic degree awarded upon satisfactory completion of a 4-year course of study in an institution of higher learning. The recipient is eligible to take the national licensing examination to become a registered nurse. A BSN degree is prerequisite to advancement in most systems and institutions that employ nurses. Compare *associate degree in nursing.*

bad faith • Willful, fraudulent wrongdoing that usually renders a contract null and void and that could expose an insured party to a breach of contract lawsuit.

bargaining agent • A person or group selected by members of a bargaining unit to represent them in negotiations.

bargaining unit • A group of employees who participate in collective bargaining as representatives of all employees.

BASIC • *abbr* Beginners' All-purpose Symbolic Instruction Code, a programming language widely used on personal computers and small business systems.

battered woman syndrome (BWS) • Repeated episodes of physical assault on a woman by the man with whom she lives, commonly resulting in serious physical and psychological damage to the woman. Such violence tends to follow a predictable pattern. The first phase is characterized by the man acting increasingly irritable, edgy, and tense. Verbal abuse, insults, and criticism increase, and shoves or slaps begin. The second phase is the time of the acute, violent activity. As the tension mounts, the woman becomes unable to placate the man, and she may argue or defend herself. The man uses this as the justification for his anger and assaults her, usually saying that he is "teaching her a lesson." The third stage is characterized by apology and remorse on the part of the man, with promises of change. The calm continues until tension builds again. The battered woman syndrome occurs at all socioeconomic levels, and one half to three quarters of female assault victims are the victims of an attack by a lover or husband. It is estimated that between 1 and 2 million women a year are beaten by their husbands.

battery • The unauthorized touching of a person by another person. For example, a health care professional who treats a patient beyond what the patient has consented to has committed battery.

beneficence • The promotion of good and prevention of harm.

benefits • Nonsalary forms of compensation an employer provides for employees – for example, medical and dental insurance.

binding arbitration • Process of settling disputes in which all parties agree to be bound by the determination of an arbitrator.

block charting • A method of charting in which procedures carried out during a block of time are detailed in paragraph form.

board of health • An administrative body acting on a municipal, county, state, provincial, or national level. The functions, powers, and responsibilities of boards of health vary with the locale. Each board is generally concerned with the recognition of the health needs of the people and the coordination of projects and resources to meet and identify those needs. Among the tasks of most boards of health are prevention of disease, health education, and implementation of laws pertaining to health.

borrowed servant doctrine • A legal doctrine that courts may apply in cases in which an employer "lends" his employee's services to another employer who, under this doctrine, becomes solely liable for the employee's wrongful conduct. Also called *ostensible agent doctrine.* Compare *dual agency doctrine.*

brain death • Final cessation of activity in the central nervous system, especially as indicated by a flat electroencephalogram for a predetermined length of time. The cessation of all measurable function or activity in every area of the brain, including the brain stem. Compare *death.*

breach of confidentiality • A type of invasion of privacy in which a person's trust and confidence are violated by public revelation of confidential or privileged communications without the person's consent. Breach of confidentiality usually involves a doctor's revelation of communications with a patient, but it can also extend to nurses who share privileged communication or information.

breach of contract • Failure to perform all or part of a contracted duty without justification.

breach of duty • The neglect or failure to fulfill in a proper manner the duties of an office, job, or position.

British Medical Association (BMA) • A national professional organization of doctors in the United Kingdom.

BSN • See **bachelor of science in nursing.**

C

calculus morality • An attempt to quantify or weigh the social harm and benefits of a given action in order to make an ethical decision.

Canadian Association of University Schools of Nursing (CAUSN) • A national Canadian organization of nursing schools affiliated with institutions of higher learning.

Canadian Nurses' Association (CNA) • This official national organization is a federation of 11 provincial and territorial professional nurses' associations. It represents more than 110,000 members and is the national voice of the profession in Canada.

capitation • A per-member, monthly payment to a health care provider that covers contracted services and is paid in advance of delivery. In essence, a provider agrees to provide specified services to enrollees for this fixed payment for a specified term, regardless of how many times the member uses the service.

captain of the ship doctrine • A legal doctrine that considers a surgeon responsible for the actions of his assistants when those assistants are under the surgeon's supervision. Similar to the **borrowed servant doctrine.**

care maps • A charting format that shows the relationships of sets of interventions to sets of intermediate outcomes along a time line.

case management • The process by which a designated health care professional, usually a nurse, manages all health-related matters of a patient. Case managers coordinate and ensure continuity of care. They develop a plan to efficiently utilize health care resources and achieve the optimum patient outcome in the most cost-effective manner. They also match the appropriate intensity of services to the patient's needs.

causa mortis • Latin phrase meaning "in anticipation of approaching death." The state of mind of a person approaching death.

Centers for Disease Control and Prevention (CDC) • An agency of the United States government that provides facilities and services for the investigation, identification, prevention, and control of disease.

central processing unit (CPU) • In data processing: the group of physical components of a computer system containing the logical, arithmetical, and control circuits for the system. Also called hardware.

certification • A statement of recognition that a nurse is specially qualified, based on predetermined standards, to provide nursing care in a particular area of nursing practice.

chain of custody • Evidentiary rule requiring that each individual having custody of a piece of evidence be identified and that the transfer of evidence from one custodian to another be documented so that all evidence is accounted for. Also called chain of evidence.

challenge • An objection by a party (or his lawyer) to the inclusion of a particular prospective juror as a member of the jury that is to hear the party's cause or trial, with the result that the prospective juror is disqualified.

challenge for cause • A challenge based upon a particular reason (such as bias) specified by law or procedure as a reason that a party (or his lawyer) may use to disqualify a prospective juror.

charting by exception • A shorthand method for documenting normal findings that's based on clearly defined standards of practice and predetermined criteria for nursing assessments and interventions.

child abuse • The physical, sexual, or emotional mistreatment of a child. It may be overt or covert and often results in permanent physical or psychological injury, mental impairment or, sometimes, death. Child abuse results from complex factors involving both parents and child and is compounded by various stressful environmental circumstances, such as poor socioeconomic conditions, inadequate physical and emotional support within the family, and any major life change or crisis, especially those crises arising from marital strife. Also called battered child syndrome in children under age 3. Compare *child neglect.*

child neglect • The failure by parents or guardians to provide for the basic needs of a child by physical or emotional deprivation that interferes with normal growth and development or that places the child in jeopardy. Compare *child abuse.*

child welfare • Any service sponsored by the community or special organizations that provides for the physical, social, or psychological care of children in need.

chronic care • A pattern of medical and nursing care that focuses on long-term care of people with chronic diseases or conditions, either at home or in a medical facility. It includes care specific to the problem and measures to encourage self-care, promote health, and prevent loss of function.

circumstantial evidence • Testimony based on inference or hearsay rather than actual personal knowledge or observation of the facts in question.

civil defense laws • That body of statutory law that is invoked when the jurisdiction is under attack – for example, during a war.

civil penalty • Fines or money damages imposed as punishment for a certain activity.

civil rights violation • A wrongful act against another person that violates a civil rights statute. The most common civil rights violations in the health care setting involve an administration's decisions about hiring or terminating employees; disputes over due process (such as committing a patient to a mental health facility without following the proper procedure) and an institution's provision of care based on sex, race, or creed.

claims-made policy • A professional liability insurance policy that covers the insured only for a claim of malpractice made while the policy is in effect.

claims review agency • An agency that investigates claims for payment made to an insurance company. The claims review agency determines whether the claim is legitimate, assesses how severe the loss is, and determines the amount the insurance company is required to pay.

clinical nurse specialist (CNS) • A registered nurse who holds a master of science degree in nursing (MSN) and who has acquired advanced knowledge and clinical skills in a specific area of nursing and health care.

clinical pathways • A clinical tool used by case managers to achieve better quality and cost outcomes by outlining and sequencing the usual and desired care for particular groups of patients. Clinical pathways incorporate care requirements from preadmission through postdischarge.

clinical practice guidelines • A decision-making tool to help practitioners determine how diseases or disorders can most effectively and appropriately be prevented, diagnosed, treated, and clinically managed. These guidelines include advice and information from recognized clinical experts.

closed shop • See *union shop.*

CNA • See *Canadian Nurses Association.*

CNM • *abbr* certified nurse-midwife. See *midwife.*

CNS • See *clinical nurse specialist.*

code • *1.* A published body of statutes, such as a civil code. *2.* A collection of standards and rules of behavior, such as a dress code. *3.* A symbolic means of representing information for communication or transfer, such as a genetic code. *4.* *Informal.* A discreet signal used to summon a special team to resuscitate a patient without alarming patients or visitors. See also *no-code order.*

codes • A system of assigned terms designed by a medical institution for quick and accurate communication during emergencies or for patient identification.

collaborative decision making • The process of resolving dilemmas in consultation with other health care professionals to arrive at an objective decision.

collective bargaining • A legal process in which representatives of organized employees negotiate with employers about such matters as wages, hours, and conditions.

collectively bargained contract • Contract negotiated by a labor organization or union. Also called a collective contract.

Commission on Graduates of Foreign Nursing Schools *(CGFN)* • An organization established in 1977 to ensure safe nursing care for the American public and to protect graduates of foreign nursing schools from employment exploitation.

commitment • *1.* The placement or confinement of an individual in a specialized hospital or other institutional facility. *2.* The legal procedure of admitting a mentally ill person to an institution for psychiatric treatment. The process varies from state to state but usually involves judicial or court action based on medical evidence certifying that the person is mentally ill. *3.* A pledge or contract to fulfill some obligation or agreement, used especially in some forms of psychotherapy or marriage counseling.

common law • Law derived from previous court decisions as opposed to law based on legislative enactment (statutes). Also called case law. In the absence of statutory law regarding a subject, the judge-made rules of common law are the law on that subject.

comparative negligence • Determination of liability in which damages may be apportioned among multiple defendants. The extent of liability depends on each defendant's relative contribution to the harm done, as determined by the jury.

compensation • *1.* All forms of payment from an employer to an employee, including salary and benefits. *2.* Anything given as an equivalent, or to make amends for a loss, damage, unemployment, etc.

complaint • *1.* In a civil case, a pleading by a plaintiff made under oath to initiate a suit. It is a statement of the formal charge and the cause for action against the defendant. In a criminal case, a serious felony prosecution requires an indictment with evidence presented by a state's attorney. *2. Informal.* Any ailment, problem, or symptom identified by the patient, member of the patient's family, or other knowledgeable person. The chief complaint is usually the reason the patient has sought health care.

computerized medical record system • A system that stores medical records in the memory bank of a computer.

confidentiality • A professional responsibility to keep all privileged information private. In some instances, confidentiality is mandated by state or federal statutes and case law.

consent form • A document, prepared for a patient's signature, that discloses his proposed treatment in general terms.

consequential damages • See **special damages.**

consumer • A person who buys goods or services for his own needs and not for resale or to use in the production of other goods or services for resale.

continuity of care • A pattern of health care that is centrally focused on the patient and coordinated among various members of the health care team. It begins with the patient's entrance into the health care system and continues until discharge.

continuum of care • The full range of health care services, from health promotion and disease prevention through delivery of primary care, acute care, home health care, and long-term care.

contract defense • An answer to an allegation that a breach of contract has occurred. Compare **impossibility defense.**

contract duties • Duties defined in a contract, such as an employment contract.

contract violations • Actions that break mutually accepted contract provisions, such as those of an employment contract.

controlled substance • Any substance that is strictly regulated or outlawed because of its potential for abuse or addiction. Controlled substances include cannabis, depressants, hallucinogens, narcotics, and stimulants. Compare **prescription drug.**

convalescent home • See **extended care facility.**

cooperation strategy • A plan for bringing about change in which the person who initiates change influences others to adapt to the change, using open communication and interpersonal skills.

coronary care unit (CCU) • A specially equipped hospital area designed for the treatment of patients with sudden, life-threatening cardiac conditions. Such units contain resuscitation and monitoring equipment and are staffed by personnel specially trained and skilled in recognizing and immediately responding to cardiac emergencies with cardiopulmonary resuscitation techniques, the administration of antiarrhythmic drugs, and other appropriate therapeutic measures.

coroner • A public official who investigates the causes and circumstances of a death occurring within a specific legal jurisdiction or territory, especially a death that may have resulted from unnatural causes. Also called medical examiner.

corporate liability • The legal responsibility of a corporation and its officers. A corporation's liability is normally limited to its assets; the shareholders are thus protected against personal liability for the corporation.

counterclaim • A claim made by a defendant establishing a cause for action in his favor against the plaintiff. The purpose of a counterclaim is to oppose or detract from the plaintiff's claim or complaint.

countersignature • A signature obtained from another health care professional to verify that information is correct and is within the verifier's personal knowledge.

critical care unit • A hospital unit in which patients requiring close monitoring and critical care are housed for as long as needed. A critical care unit contains highly technical and sophisticated monitoring devices and equipment, and the staff in the unit is educated to give critical care as needed by the patients.

critical paths • See **clinical pathways.**

CRNA • *abbr* certified registered nurse anesthetist. See **nurse anesthetist.**

cross-examination • The questioning of a witness by the attorney for the opposing party.

CRT • *abbr* Cathode-ray tube, or the display screen on a computer terminal or heart monitor, similar to a television screen.

custodial care • Services and care of an unskilled nature provided on a long-term basis, usually for convalescent and chronically ill individuals. Custodial care may include providing board and personal assistance.

damages • An amount of money a court orders a defendant to pay the plaintiff, when the case is decided in favor of the plaintiff.

DEA • See **Drug Enforcement Administration.**

death • *1.* The final and irreversible cessation of life as indicated by the absence of heartbeat or respiration. *2.* The total absence of meaningful activity in the brain and the central nervous, cardiovascular, and respiratory systems, as observed and declared by a doctor. See also **brain death.**

declared emergency • The situation when a government official formally identifies a state of emergency.

decree of educational equivalency • An official decision stating that a person's experience is of equal value to an academic degree.

default judgment • A judgment rendered against a defendant because of the defendant's failure to appear in court or to answer the plaintiff's claim within the proper time.

defendant • The party that is named in a plaintiff's complaint and against whom the plaintiff's allegations are made. The defendant must respond to the allegations. See also **answer.**

defense independent medical examination (IME) • In malpractice litigation, a medical examination of the injured party by a doctor selected by the defendant's attorney or insurance company.

delinquency • *1.* Negligence or failure to fulfill a duty or obligation. *2.* An offense, fault, misdemeanor, or misdeed; a tendency to commit such acts.

delinquent • *1.* Characterized by neglect of duty or violation of law. *2.* Behavior characterized by persistent antisocial, illegal, violent, or criminal acts; a juvenile delinquent.

deontology • An ethical theory based on moral obligation or commitment to others.

dependent nursing function • A function the nurse performs, with another health care professional's written order, on the basis of that professional's judgment, and for which that professional is accountable.

deposition • A sworn pretrial testimony given by a witness in response to oral or written questions and cross-examination. The deposition is transcribed and may be used for further pretrial investigation. It may also be presented at the trial if the witness cannot be present or changes his testimony. Compare *discovery device, interrogatories.*

diagnosis-related group (DRG) • A system that classifies patients by age, medical diagnosis, and surgical procedure to predict the use of hospital resources and length of stay and to set predetermined Medicare reimbursement rates.

direct access • The right of a health care provider and a patient to interact on a professional basis without interference.

direct contract model HMO • A health maintenance organization that contracts directly with individual doctors to provide services to its members.

directed verdict • A verdict given by a jury at the direction of the trial judge.

direct examination • The first examination of a witness called to the stand by the attorney for the party the witness is representing.

direct patient care • Care of a patient provided in person by a member of the staff. Direct patient care may involve any aspect of the health care of a patient, including treatments, counseling, self-care, patient education, and administration of medication.

disclosure laws • Legislation requiring that potentially confidential information be reported — for example, laws that mandate nurses report suspected child abuse or neglect.

discovery device • A pretrial procedure that allows the plaintiff's and defendant's attorneys to examine relevant materials and question all parties to the case. Compare *deposition, interrogatories, defense independent medical examination.*

discovery rule • Rule stating that the statute of limitations begins to run when a patient discovers the injury. This may take place many years after the injury occurred and af-

ter the applicable statute of limitations has formally run out.

discretionary powers • The freedom of a public officer to choose courses of action within the limits of his authority.

disease management • An effort to provide cost-effective care for a chronic condition by emphasizing treatment protocols and changes in personal habits. It is a comprehensive approach to lowering costs and improving patient outcomes, applied on a disease-by-disease basis.

dismiss • To discharge or dispose of an action, suit, or motion trial.

dispense • To take a drug from the pharmacy and give or sell it to another person.

distributive justice • The principle that advocates equal allocation of benefits and burdens to all members of society.

Doctor of Medicine (MD) • See *physician.*

Doctor of Osteopathy (DO) • See *physician.*

documentation • The preparing or assembling of written records.

drug abuse • The use of a drug for a non-therapeutic effect, especially one for which it was not prescribed or intended. Some of the most commonly abused substances are amphetamines, barbiturates, tranquilizers, and cocaine. Drug abuse may lead to organ damage, addiction, and disturbed patterns of behavior. Some illicit drugs, such as lysergic acid diethylamide, phencyclidine hydrochloride, and heroin, have no recognized therapeutic effect. Use of these drugs can incur criminal penalties in addition to the potential for physical, social, and psychological harm. See also *drug addiction.*

drug addiction • A condition characterized by an overwhelming desire to continue taking a drug to which one has become habituated through repeated consumption because it produces a particular effect, usually an alteration of mental activity, attitude, or outlook. Addiction is usually accompanied by a compulsion to obtain the drug, a tendency to increase the dose, a psychological or physical dependence, and detrimental consequences for the individual and society. Common addictive drugs are barbiturates, cocaine, crack, and morphine and other narcotics, especially heroin, which has slightly greater euphorigenic properties than other opium derivatives. See also *alcoholism, drug abuse.*

Drug Enforcement Administration (DEA) • An agency of the federal government empowered to enforce regulations regarding the import or export of narcotic drugs and certain other substances or the traffic of these substances across state lines.

dual agency doctrine • A legal doctrine that states that both the agency and the "borrowing" party may be held liable for the actions of the agent. Under this doctrine, a nurse from a nurses' registry may be held to be the agent of both the registry and the hospital. Compare *borrowed servant doctrine.*

due process • The specific procedures or steps one must follow to ensure a fair resolution of a conflict.

due process rights • Personal rights based on the principle that the government may not deprive an individual of life, liberty, or property unless certain rules and procedures required by law are followed.

durable power of attorney • An instrument authorizing another person to act as one's agent or attorney, an "attorney-in-fact," if the principal person becomes incompetent. This power is revoked when the principal person dies. Compare *power of attorney.*

duty • A legal obligation owed by one party to another. Duty may be established by statute or other legal process, as by contract or oath supported by statute, or it may be voluntarily undertaken. Every person has a duty to avoid causing harm or injury to others by negligence.

duty-to-rescue laws • Legislation requiring certain people – those who perform rescues as part of their jobs – to rescue people in need. These people include fire fighters, police officers, and emergency medical technicians. Only a few states apply duty-to-rescue laws to nurses.

egoism • An ethical theory that considers self-interest the goal of all human actions.

emancipated minor • A minor who's legally considered free from the custody, care, and control of his parents before the age of majority. Emancipated minors lose the right to parental support but may gain certain other rights, such as the right to consent to their own medical care and the right to enter into binding contracts.

Emergency Medical Service (EMS) • A network of services coordinated to provide aid and medical assistance from primary response to definitive care, involving personnel trained in the rescue, stabilization, transportation, and advanced treatment of trauma or medical emergency patients. Linked by a communications system that operates on both a local and regional level, EMS is usually initiated by a citizen calling an emergency number. Stages include the first medical response; involvement of ambulance personnel, medium and heavy rescue equipment, and paramedic units, if necessary; and continued care in the hospital with emergency department nurses and doctors, specialists, and critical care nurses and doctors.

emergency nursing • Nursing care provided to prevent imminent severe damage or death or to avert serious injury. Activities that exemplify emergency nursing care include basic life support, cardiopulmonary resuscitation, control of hemorrhage, and burn care.

endorsement • The act of giving approval, support, or sanction. A policy whereby the state board of nursing will accept an out-of-state license to practice nursing.

ethical diagnosis • The determination that a moral dilemma exists, followed by classification of the dilemma by type.

ethics • An area of philosophy that examines values, actions, and choices to determine right and wrong. The study of standards of conduct and moral judgments.

euthanasia • Deliberately bringing about the death of a person who's suffering from an incurable disease or condition, either actively (for example, by administering a lethal drug) or passively (for example, by withholding treatment).

evaluation • Determining the extent to which nursing care has achieved its goals.

exclusionary rule • A constitutional rule of law that states that otherwise admissible evidence may not be used in a criminal trial if it was obtained as a result of an illegal search and seizure.

exclusive provider organization (EPO) • Managed care organization similar to a preferred provider organization (PPO) in which health services are purchased from a select group of providers. Unlike a PPO, an EPO will reimburse beneficiaries only for health care services obtained from participating providers. Compare **preferred provider organization.**

executing a contract • Carrying out all the terms of a contract.

exemplary damages • See **punitive damages.**

expert witness • A person who has special knowledge of a subject about which a court requests testimony. Special knowledge may be acquired by experience, education, observation, or study and is not possessed by the average person. An expert witness gives expert testimony or expert evidence. This evidence usually serves to educate the court and the jury about the subject under consideration.

express contract • A verbal or written agreement between two or more people to do, or not do, something.

extended care facility • An institution devoted to providing medical, nursing, or custodial care for an individual over a prolonged period of time, as during the course of a chronic disease or during the rehabilitation phase after an acute illness. Kinds of extended care facilities are intermediate care facilities and skilled nursing facilities. Also called **convalescent home, nursing home.**

extraordinary life-support measures • Resuscitative efforts and therapies that maintain or prolong a patient's life, usually at great expense and suffering.

false imprisonment • The act of confining or restraining a person without his consent for no clinical or legal reason.

family nurse practitioner (FNP) • A nurse practitioner possessing skills necessary for the detection and management of acute self-limiting conditions and the management of chronic stable conditions. An FNP provides primary, ambulatory care for families, in collaboration with primary care physicians.

FDA • See **Food and Drug Administration.**

federal tort claims act • A federal law that regulates how and under what circumstances the United States government can be sued. Sections of the law include the statute of limitations for filing suits, the procedure for filing suits, and causes of action that may be alleged against the government.

fee for service • *1.* A charge made for a professional activity, as for a physical examination. *2.* A system for the payment of professional services in which the practitioner is paid for the particular service rendered, rather than receiving a salary for providing professional services as needed during scheduled hours of work or time on call.

felony • Any serious criminal offense (the U.S. legal system lacks a more specific definition). A felony is considered more serious than a misdemeanor and carries with it a greater penalty, usually a fine or imprisonment for a year or more. Examples of felonies include murder, manslaughter, assault, kidnapping, and controlled substance violations.

fidelity • Faithfulness to agreements that one has accepted.

fiduciary • A person having a duty, created by his undertaking, to act primarily for the benefit of another in matters connected with that undertaking.

fiduciary relationship • A legal relationship of trust and confidence that exists whenever one person relies on another – for example, a doctor-patient relationship.

first aid • The immediate care given to an injured or ill person. It includes self-help and home care measures.

flexible staffing patterns • Work schedules that vary – for example, 10- and 12-hour shifts, shorter workweeks, and special weekend schedules.

flextime, flexitime • A system of staffing that allows flexible work schedules. A person working 7 hours daily might choose to work from 7 to 3, 9 to 5, or other hours. Use of the system tends to improve morale and decrease turnover.

floating • The temporary assignment of a nurse who normally works on one unit to work on another unit, usually to fill a staff shortage.

FNP • See *family nurse practitioner.*

Food and Drug Administration (FDA) • The federal agency responsible for the enforcement of federal regulations regarding the manufacture and distribution of food, drugs, and cosmetics.

forensic medicine • A branch of medicine that deals with the legal aspects of health care. The application of medical knowledge to questions of law affecting life or property.

fraud • Intentional deception resulting in damage to another, whether to his person, rights, property, or reputation. Fraud usually consists of a misrepresentation, concealment, or nondisclosure of a material fact, or at least misleading conduct, devices, or contrivance.

#

garnishment • The court's seizure of a defendant's wages or property to pay fines or damages awarded to a plaintiff.

gatekeeper • Usually a doctor or a nurse who screens people seeking medical care and eliminates costly and sometimes unnecessary medical interventions or referrals to specialists for diagnosis and management.

general damages • Compensation for losses that are directly referrable to a legal wrong but that are abstract in nature, such as pain and suffering or a worsening change in lifestyle. Compare *punitive damages, special damages.*

gerontologic nursing • Nursing care that provides for the physical, intellectual, and emotional needs of elderly people. As defined by the American Nurse's Association, gerontologic nursing is the care and treatment of an older adult holistically, not just as a diseased or sick person. Nurses may choose gerontologic nursing as an area of clinical specialty.

good faith • Total absence of intention to seek unfair advantage or to defraud another party; an intention to fulfill one's obligations.

Good Samaritan acts • State or provincial laws that provide civil immunity from negligence lawsuits for individuals who stop and render care in an emergency.

grace period • In general, any period specified in a contract during which payment is permitted, without penalty, beyond the due date of the debt.

grandfather clause • A provision permitting persons who were engaged in an activity before passage of a law affecting that activity to receive a license without having to meet the new requirements.

grievance • A complaint about working conditions or contract violations brought by an employee or union against an employer.

grievance procedure • Steps agreed upon by employees and their employer to settle disputes in an orderly fashion. A labor contract may outline grievance procedures.

gross negligence • The flagrant and inexcusable failure to perform a legal duty in reckless disregard of the consequences.

ground rules • Rules governing a particular situation that describe legitimate behavior.

group model HMO • A health maintenance organization that contracts with a multi-specialty group of doctors to provide all doctor services to its members. The doctors are employed by the group practice, not the HMO, and may treat outside patients.

guardian ad litem • A person appointed by the court to safeguard a minor's or another incompetent person's legal interests during certain kinds of litigation.

health care consumer • Any actual or potential recipient of health care, as a patient in a hospital, a client in a community mental health center, or a member of a prepaid health maintenance organization.

health care industry • The complex of preventive, remedial, and therapeutic services provided by hospitals and other institutions, nurses, doctors, dentists, government agencies, voluntary agencies, noninstitutional care facilities, pharmaceutical and medical equipment manufacturers, and health insurance companies.

health care professional • Any person who has completed a course of study in a field of health care, such as a nurse. The person is usually licensed by a governmental agency, such as a board of nursing, and becomes registered or licensed in that health care field. In some instances, the person is certified by a state regulatory body, such as with a certified nurses' aide.

health maintenance organization (HMO) • An organization that provides basic and supplemental health maintenance and treatment services to voluntary enrollees who prepay a fixed periodic fee that is set without regard to the amount or kind of services received. Individuals and families who belong to an HMO are cared for by member doctors with limited referral to outside specialists.

health provider • Any individual who provides health services to health care consumers.

homestead laws • Laws protecting any property designated as a homestead – any house, outbuildings, and surrounding land owned and used as a dwelling by the head of a family – from seizure and sale by creditors.

hospice • A system of family-centered care designed to assist the chronically ill person to be comfortable and to maintain a satisfactory life-style through the terminal phases of dying. Hospice care is multidisciplinary and includes home visits, professional medical help available on call, teaching and emotional support of the family, and physical care of the client. Some hospice programs provide care in a center as well as in the home.

hospital information system (HIS) • A computer-based information system with multi-access units to collect, organize, store, and make available data for problem solving and decision making.

hospital quality assurance program • A program developed by a hospital committee that monitors the quality of the hospital's diagnostic, therapeutic, prognostic, and other health care activities.

human investigations committee • A committee established in a hospital, school, or university to review applications for research involving human subjects in order to protect the rights of the people to be studied. Also called **human subjects investigation committee.**

human subjects investigation committee • See **human investigations committee.**

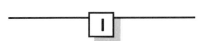

ICCU • *abbr* intensive coronary-care unit.

ICU • See **intensive care unit.**

illegal abortion • Induced termination of a pregnancy under circumstances, or at a ges-

tational time, prohibited by law. Many illegal abortions are performed under medically unsafe conditions. Also called criminal abortion. Compare **legal abortion, therapeutic abortion.**

immunity from liability • Exemption of a person or institution, by law, from a legally imposed penalty.

immunity from suit • Exemption of a person or institution, by law, from being sued.

implementation • *1.* A deliberate action performed to achieve a goal, such as carrying out a plan in caring for a patient. *2.* In the nursing process: a category of nursing behavior in which the actions necessary for accomplishing the health care plan are initiated and completed.

implied conditions • Elements of a contract that are not stated, but are assumed to be part of the contract.

implied consent • A patient's presumed agreement to a medical procedure or test, usually in a life-threatening emergency when the patient cannot grant an informed consent.

implied contract • A contract manifested by conduct rather than words. Also called a quasi-contract, an implied contract is based on an obligation created by law for reasons of justice and fairness.

implied-in-law contract • Obligations imposed upon a person by the law, without his agreement and against his will or design, because the circumstances between the parties are such as to render it just that the one should have a right, and the other a corresponding liability, similar to those that would arise from a contract between them.

impossibility defense • A contract defense that says circumstances rendered the violation of a contract (such as not showing up for work) impossible to avoid. Compare **contract defense.**

incident • An event that is inconsistent with ordinary routine, regardless of whether injury occurs.

incident report • Formal written report that informs hospital administration (and the hospital's insurance company) about an incident and serves as a contemporary, factual statement of it in the event of a lawsuit.

incompetence • The inability or lack of legal qualification or fitness to discharge the required duty. Compare **adjudicated incompent, mental incompetence.**

indemnification • Repayment or compensation for a loss. A person who has compensated another for injury, loss, or damage caused by a third party may file a suit seeking indemnification from the third party.

independent contractor • A self-employed person who renders services to clients and independently determines how the work will be done.

independent practice • The practice of certain aspects of professional nursing that are encompassed by applicable licensure and law and require little or no direct supervision or direction from others. Nurses in independent practice may have an office in which they see patients and charge fees for services. State practice acts may define aspects of nursing practice that are independent as well as those to be done only under supervision of another individual, usually a doctor.

independent practice association (IPA) model HMO • A health maintenance organization that contracts with an association of doctors to provide doctor services to its members. The doctors maintain their independent practices.

independent practitioner organization (IPO) • A hybrid form with characteristics of both IPAs and medical associations, they're often organized by community doctors to provide a mechanism for evaluating and negotiating participation in HMOs.

individual contract • A contract negotiated with an employer by an individual employee.

informed consent • Permission obtained from a patient to perform a specific test or procedure after the patient has been fully informed about the test or procedure.

injunction • A court order restraining a person from committing a specific act or requiring the individual to do something.

in loco parentis • Latin phrase meaning "in the place of the parent." The assumption by a person or institution of the parental obligations of caring for a child without adoption.

inpatient • **1.** A patient who has been admitted to a hospital or other health care facility for at least an overnight stay. **2.** Pertaining to the treatment of such a patient or to a health care facility to which a patient may be admitted for 24-hour care.

institutional licensure • The process by which a state government regulates institutions that provide health care services.

insurance adjuster • One who determines the amount of an insurance claim and then makes an agreement with the insured as to a settlement.

intensive care • Constant, complex, detailed health care as provided in various acute, life-threatening conditions. Special training is necessary to provide intensive care. Also called critical care.

intensive care unit (ICU) • A hospital unit in which patients requiring close monitoring and intensive care are housed for as long as needed. An ICU contains highly technical and sophisticated monitoring devices and equipment, and the staff in the unit is educated to give critical care as needed by the patients.

intentional tort • A willful act that violates another person's rights or property.

intermediate care • A level of medical care for certain chronically ill or disabled individuals in which room and board are provided but skilled nursing care is not.

International Council of Nurses (ICN) • The oldest international health organization, the ICN is a federation of nurses' associations from 93 nations and was one of the first health organizations to develop strict policies of nondiscrimination based on nationality, race, creed, color, politics, sex, or social status. The objectives of the ICN include promoting national associations of nurses, improving standards of nursing and the competence of nurses, improving the status of nurses within their countries, and establishing an authoritative international voice for nurses.

International Red Cross Society • An international philanthropic organization, based in Geneva, concerned primarily with the humane treatment and welfare of the victims of war and calamity and with the neutrality of hospitals and medical personnel in times of war. See also ***American Red Cross.***

interrogatories • A series of written questions submitted to a witness or other person having information of interest to the court. The answers are transcribed and are sworn to under oath. Compare ***deposition, discovery device.***

intervention • **1.** Any act performed to prevent harm from occurring to a patient or to improve the mental, emotional, or physical function of a patient. A physiologic process may be monitored or enhanced, or a pathologic process may be arrested or controlled. **2.** The fourth step of the nursing process. This step includes nursing actions taken to meet patient needs as determined by nursing assessment and diagnosis.

invalid contract • Any contract concerning illegal or impossible actions; no legal obligation exists.

JCAHO • See ***Joint Commission on Accreditation of Healthcare Organizations.***

job description • A written statement describing responsibilities of a specific job and the qualifications an applicant for that job should have.

Joint Commission on Accreditation of Healthcare Organizations (JCAHO) • A private, nongovernmental agency that establishes guidelines for the operation of hospitals and other health care facilities, conducts accreditation programs and surveys, and encourages the attainment of high standards of institutional medical care. Members include representatives from the American Medical Association, American College of Physicians, and American College of Surgeons.

joint practice • **1.** The (usually private) practice of a doctor and a nurse practitioner who work as a team, sharing responsibility for a group of patients. **2.** In inpatient nursing, the practice of making joint decisions about patient care by committees of the doctors and nurses working on a division.

joint statement • A statement, opinion, or recommendation issued jointly by two or more organizations or committees.

judicial bypass statutes • Statutes that allow a minor to avoid a strict parental notification or consent requirement for obtaining an abortion by going before a judge.

just cause • A lawful, rightful, proper reason to act; a defendant establishes a cause for action in his favor.

L

law • *1.* In a field of study: a rule, standard, or principle that states a fact or a relationship between factors, as Dalton's law regarding partial pressures of gas or Koch's law regarding the specificity of a pathogen. *2. a.* A rule, principle, or regulation established and promulgated by a government to protect or to restrict the people affected. *b.* The field of study concerned with such laws. *c.* The collected body of the laws of a people, derived from custom and from legislation.

lay jury • A jury made up of people who are not from a particular profession. For example, a lay jury in a medical malpractice trial would not contain any doctors, nurses, or other members of medical professions.

legal abortion • Induced termination of pregnancy by a doctor before the fetus has developed sufficiently to live outside the uterus. The procedure is performed under medically safe conditions prescribed by law. Compare **illegal abortion, therapeutic abortion.**

legal death • See **death.**

legal guardian • An officer or agent of the court who is appointed to protect the interests of minors or incompetent persons and to provide for their welfare, education, and support.

liability • Legal responsibility for failure to act and so causing harm to another person, or for actions that fail to meet standards of care, so causing another person harm.

liable • Legally bound or obligated to make good any loss or damage; responsible.

liaison nurse • A nurse who acts as an agent between a patient, the hospital, and the patient's family, and who speaks for the entire health care team.

libel • A tort consisting of a false, malicious, unprivileged publication aiming to defame a living person or to damage the memory of one dead. Compare **slander.**

licensed practical nurse (LPN) • A person trained in basic nursing techniques and direct patient care who practices under the supervision of a registered nurse or other health care provider. An LPN must complete a course of training that usually lasts 1 or 2 years, pass the NCLEX-PN examination, and meet the requirements set forth by the board of nursing for licensure in her state. In Canada an LPN is called a nursing assistant. Also called **licensed vocational nurse** (U.S.).

licensed vocational nurse (LVN) • See **licensed practical nurse.**

licensure • The granting of permission by a competent authority (usually a governmental agency) to an organization or person to engage in a practice or activity that would otherwise be illegal. Kinds of licensure include the issuing of licenses for general hospitals or nursing homes; for health care professionals, such as doctors; and for the production or distribution of biologic products. Licensure is usually granted on the basis of education and examination rather than performance. It is usually permanent, but a periodic fee, demonstration of competence, or continuing education may be required. Licensure may be revoked by the granting agency for incompetence, criminal acts, or other reasons stipulated in the rules governing the specific area of licensure.

lie detector • An electronic device or instrument used to detect lying or anxiety in regard to specific questions. A commonly used lie detector is the polygraph recorder, which senses and records pulse, respiratory rate, blood pressure, and perspiration. Some experts hold that certain patterns indicate the presence of anxiety, guilt, or fear, emotions that are likely to occur when the subject is lying.

litigant • A party to a lawsuit. See also *defendant, plaintiff.*

litigate • To carry on a suit or to contest a suit.

living will • A witnessed document indicating a patient's desire to be allowed to die a natural death, rather than be kept alive by heroic, life-sustaining measures. The will applies to decisions that will be made after a terminally ill patient is incompetent and has no reasonable possibility of recovery. Compare *testamentary will.*

living will laws • Laws that help to guarantee that a patient's documented wishes regarding terminal illness procedures will be carried out. Living will laws may set forth testator and witness requirements for executing a living will and medical requirements for terminating treatment. Living will laws may also address other issues, such as authorization of a proxy for health care decisions, immunity from liability for following a living will's directives, and the withholding or withdrawal of tube feedings. Also called *natural death laws.*

locality rule • Allowance made, when considering evidence in a trial, for the type of community in which the defendant practices his profession, and the standards of that community.

LPN • See *licensed practical nurse.*

LVN • *abbr* *licensed vocational nurse.* See *licensed practical nurse.*

M

---

malfeasance • Performance of an unlawful, wrongful act. Compare *misfeasance, nonfeasance.*

malice aforethought • The intent to commit an unlawful act. For example, murder is defined as the unlawful killing of another person with malice aforethought.

malicious prosecution • A situation in which a person is forced to be a defendant in a legal action when no foundation for the action exists. A person can prove malicious prosecution only if he was found innocent in the original trial, the court action against him was initiated without sufficient and probable cause, the court action was conducted with malice, and he suffered harm to his reputation, person, or property as a result of the case.

malpractice • A professional person's wrongful conduct, improper discharge of professional duties, or failure to meet standards of care, which results in harm to another person.

malpractice insurance • An insurance policy in which an insurer agrees to provide monetary compensation coverage to a professional who is liable for acts of professional negligence.

managed care organizations (MCOs) • Organizations reponsible for the financing and delivery of health care services to covered individuals for a fixed fee. Most MCOs provide services by means of contracts with selected providers.

mandatory bargaining issues • Issues such as wages and working conditions that an employer must address during collective bargaining.

mandatory licensure • The legal requirement that a person earning compensation in a licensed profession must obtain a license to use the title of the profession and to practice its skills and services.

master's degree program in nursing • A postbaccalaureate program in a school of nursing, based in a university setting, that grants the degree Master of Science in Nursing (MSN) to successful candidates. Nurses with this degree usually work in leadership roles in clinical nursing, as consultants in various settings, and in faculty positions in certain schools of nursing. Some programs also prepare the nurse to function as a nurse practitioner in a specific specialty.

MD • *abbr* **Doctor of Medicine.** See *physician.*

Medicaid • A program that subsidizes medical care for low-income women and children, some men, and people with certain disabilities. Although passed by Congress in 1965, Medicaid is a state-level program, with each state defining income levels and other standards of eligibility and the federal government subsidizing a portion of the expenses.

medical directive/physician's directive • A comprehensive advance care document that covers preferred treatment goals and specific scenarios of patient incompetence. It also includes the option to designate a proxy decision maker or power of attorney for the event of incompetence, the option to record a personal statement, and a place to designate wishes for organ donation.

medical record • A written, legal record of every aspect of the patient's care. A record of a person's illnesses and their treatment.

medical release form • The form an institution asks a patient to sign when he refuses a medical treatment. The form protects both the institution and the health care professional from liability if the patient's condition worsens because of his refusal.

Medicare • Federally funded national health insurance authorized by the Social Security Act for persons age 65 or older.

medicolegal • Of or pertaining to both medicine and law. Medicolegal considerations are a significant part of the process of making many patient care decisions and in setting policies regarding the treatment of mentally incompetent people and minors, the perfor-

mance of sterilization or therapeutic abortion, and the care of terminally ill patients. Medicolegal considerations, decisions, definitions, and policies provide the framework for informed consent, professional liability, and many other aspects of health care practice.

mental competence • The ability to understand information and to act reasonably. A mentally competent person is capable of understanding explanations and is able to comprehend the results of his decisions.

mental incompetence • The inability to understand the nature and effect of the action a person is engaged in. A mentally incompetent person is incapable of understanding explanations and is unable to comprehend the results of his decisions. Compare *adjudicated incompetent, incompetence.*

mental status examination • A diagnostic procedure for determining the mental status of a person. The trained interviewer poses certain questions in a carefully standardized manner and evaluates the verbal responses and behavioral reactions.

midwife • *1.* In traditional use: a person who assists women in childbirth. *2.* According to the International Confederation of Midwives, the World Health Organization, and the Federation of International Gynecologists and Obstetricians, "a person who, having been regularly admitted to a midwifery educational program fully recognized in the country in which it is located, has successfully completed the prescribed course of studies in midwifery and has acquired the requisite qualifications to be registered and/or legally licensed to practice midwifery." Among the responsibilities of the midwife are supervision of pregnancy, labor, delivery, and puerperium. The midwife conducts the delivery independently, cares for the newborn, procures medical assistance when necessary, executes emergency measures as required, and may practice in a hospital, clinic, maternity home, or in a woman's home. *3.* A lay-midwife. *4.* A nurse-midwife or certified nurse-midwife *(CNM)*.

minor • A person not of legal age; beneath the age of majority. Minors may not be able to consent to their own medical treatment unless they are legally emancipated. However, in many jurisdictions, parental consent is no longer necessary for certain types of medical and psychiatric treatment.

misdemeanor • An offense that is considered less serious than a felony and carries with it a lesser penalty, usually a fine or imprisonment for less than 1 year. Examples of misdemeanors include criminally negligent involuntary manslaughter (the unintentional killing of another person through failure to act when one has a duty to act), failure to report certain injuries or illnesses, failure to provide emergency services (if the hospital's failure is willful and causes injury to a patient), fraudulent business activities, and violation of professional practice acts or health and safety acts. Note that a crime that is usually classified as a misdemeanor may be considered a felony if the evidence shows sufficient criminal intent and significant harm to an individual or society.

misfeasance • An improper performance of a lawful act, especially in a way that might cause damage or injury. Compare *malfeasance, nonfeasance.*

misrepresentation • The statutory crime of giving false or misleading information, usually with the intent to deceive or be unfair.

moral dilemma • An ethical problem caused by conflicts of rights, responsibilities, and values.

moral relativism • An ethical theory that holds that there are no ethical absolutes, that whatever an individual feels is right is right for him at that moment.

moral turpitude • Vileness or dishonesty of a high degree. A crime of moral turpitude

demonstrates depravity in the private and social duties a person owes to others, contrary to what is accepted and customary.

MSN • *abbr* **Master of Science in Nursing.** See **master's degree program in nursing.**

National Council of Licensure Examination (NCLEX) • An examination, administered separately by licensing authorities of each state, that measures competence to practice as a licensed RN, LPN, or LVN. The test is commonly referred to as the "state boards." All 50 states (and some Canadian provinces) require candidates for RN licensure to take the NCLEX-RN test. Candidates for LPN or LVN licensure must take the NCLEX-PN test. The NCLEX-RN consists of approximately 375 multiple-choice items, which appear as case situations. Most of the test questions require the examinee to apply nursing knowledge to patient care situations.

National League for Nursing (NLN) • An organization concerned with the improvement of nursing education, nursing service, and the delivery of health care in the United States. Its members include nurses and other health care professionals, nursing educational institutions, agencies, departments of nursing in hospitals and other health care facilities, home and community health services, and community members interested in health. Among its many activities are accreditation of nursing programs at all levels, provision of preadmission and achievement tests for nursing students, and compilation of statistical data on nursing manpower and on trends in health care delivery.

natural death laws • See *living will laws.*

negligence • Failure to act as an ordinary prudent person would under similar circumstances. Conduct that falls below the standard established by law for the protection of others under the same circumstances.

negligent nondisclosure • The failure to completely inform a patient about his treatment.

negotiation • A meeting at which an employer and employees confer, discuss, and bargain to reach an agreement.

network model HMO • A health maintenance organization that contracts with more than one group practice to provide doctor services to its members.

next of kin • One or more persons in the nearest degree of relationship to another person.

NLN • See **National League for Nursing.**

no-code order • An order, written in the patient record and signed by a doctor, instructing staff not to attempt to resuscitate a patient if he suffers cardiac or respiratory failure.

nonfeasance • A failure to perform a task, duty, or undertaking that one has agreed to perform or that one has a legal duty to perform. Compare **malfeasance, misfeasance.**

nonmaleficence • An ethical principle based on the obligation to do no harm.

nurse • **1.** A person educated and licensed in the practice of nursing. The nurse acts to promote, maintain, or restore the health of the patient. The American Nurses' Association defines nursing as the "diagnosis and treatment of human responses to actual and potential health problems." The nurse may be a generalist or a specialist and, as a professional, is ethically and legally accountable for the nursing activities performed and for the actions of others to whom the nurse has delegated responsibility. **2.** To provide nursing care. **3.** To breast-feed an infant. See also **nursing, registered nurse.**

nurse anesthetist • A registered nurse qualified by advanced training in an accredited program in the specialty of nurse anesthetist to manage the anesthetic care of the patient in certain surgical situations.

nurse clinician • A nurse who is prepared to identify and diagnose problems of patients by using the expanded knowledge and skills gained by advanced study in a specific area of nursing practice. The specialist may function independently within standing orders or protocols and collaborates with associates to implement a plan of care that is focused on the patient.

nurse-midwife • See **midwife.**

nurse practice act • A law enacted by a state's legislature outlining the legal scope of nursing practice within that state.

nurse practitioner • A nurse who, by advanced training and clinical experience in a branch of nursing (as in a master's degree program in nursing or a certification program), has acquired expert knowledge in a specialized branch of practice.

nurses' notes • A means of documenting the care the nurse provides and the patient's response to that care; a legal document that can be submitted as admissible evidence in a court of law.

nurses' registry • An employment agency or listing service for nurses who wish to work in a specific area of nursing, usually for a short period of time or on a per diem basis.

nursing • **1.** The professional practice of a nurse. **2.** The process of acting as a nurse, of providing care that encourages and promotes the health of the person being served. **3.** According to the American Nurses' Association, the "diagnosis and treatment of human responses to actual and potential health problems." **4.** Breast-feeding an infant. See also **nurse.**

nursing administrator • A nurse who's responsible for overseeing the efficient management of nursing services.

nursing assessment • The first step of the nursing process, which involves the systematic collection of information about the patient from multiple sources, including the history, physical examination, and laboratory findings. This information is analyzed and the nurse formulates inferences or impressions about the patient's needs or problems.

nursing audit • A thorough investigation designed to identify, examine, or verify the performance of certain specified aspects of nursing care using established criteria. A concurrent nursing audit is performed during ongoing nursing care. A retrospective nursing audit is performed after discharge from the care facility, using the patient's record. In many instances, a nursing audit and a medical audit are performed collaboratively, resulting in a joint audit.

nursing care plan • A plan that is based on a nursing assessment and a nursing diagnosis, devised by a nurse. It has four essential components: the identification of the nursing care problems and a statement of the nursing approach to solve those problems; the statement of the expected benefit to the patient; the statement of the specific actions taken by the nurse that reflect the nursing approach and the achievement of the goals specified; and the evaluation of the patient's response to nursing care and the readjustment of that care as required. See also ***nursing assessment, nursing diagnosis.***

nursing diagnosis • Descriptive interpretations of collected and categorized information indicating the problems or needs of a patient that nursing care can affect. According to the North American Nursing Diagnosis Association, "a clinical judgment about individual, community, or family responses to actual or potential health problems or to life processes. Nursing diagnoses provide the basis of selection of nursing interventions for which the nurse is accountable."

nursing home • See ***extended care facility.***

nursing liability • A nurse's legal responsibility for harm caused to a patient by an inappropriate nursing action or by a failure to perform a required nursing action.

nursing process • An organizational framework for nursing practice, encompassing all the major steps a nurse takes when caring for a patient. These steps are assessment, diagnosis, planning, implementation, and evaluation.

nursing skills • The cognitive, affective, and psychomotor abilities a nurse uses in delivering nursing care.

nursing specialty • A nurse's particular professional field of practice, such as surgical, pediatric, obstetric, or psychiatric nursing. Compare ***subspecialty.***

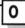

obligationism • An ethical theory that attempts to resolve ethical dilemmas by balancing distributive justice with beneficence.

occurrence policy • Professional liability insurance policy that protects against an error of omission occurring during a policy period, regardless of when the claim is made.

ombudsman • A person who investigates complaints, reports findings, and helps to achieve equitable settlements.

open shop • A place of employment where employees may choose whether or not to join a union.

oral contract • Any contract that is not in writing or that is not signed by the parties involved.

ordinary negligence • The inadvertent omission of the care that a reasonably prudent nurse would ordinarily provide under similar circumstances.

original position • The underlying principle of the social contract theory, which states that people in a society determine the principles of justice by which all members are bound to live.

ostensible agent doctrine • See *borrowed servant doctrine.*

outcomes management • A process of systematically tracking a patient's clinical treatment and responses. This system encourages caregivers to follow a set of guidelines (practice guidelines or critical pathways) that research has shown to be the "one best way" to treat a medical condition.

parens patriae • A doctrine that appoints the state as legal guardian of a child or an incompetent adult when a person hasn't been appointed as guardian.

Parents Anonymous (PA) • An international organization, founded in 1970, dedicated to the prevention and treatment of child abuse.

paternalism • The belief that health care professionals know what is best for the patient and that the patient need not question the nature of the care provided.

patient • *1.* A health care recipient who is ill or hospitalized. *2.* A client in a health care service.

patient advocate • A person (often a nurse) who seeks to protect a patient's rights from infringement by institutional policies.

patient anti-dumping laws • Amendments to the Social Security Act intended to prevent hospitals from turning away patients who are uninsured or unable to pay. They require that

hospitals participating in Medicare provide medical screening and stabilizing treatment for any patient who has an emergency condition or is in labor and provide guidelines and require documentation for transfers to other facilities or for hospital discharge.

patient classification systems • Ways of grouping patients so that the size of the staff needed to care for them can be estimated accurately.

patient overload/staffing shortage • The situation that occurs when the number of patients exceeds an institution's medical, nursing, and support staff resources to care for them properly.

patient record • A collection of documents that provides a record of each time a person visited or sought treatment and received care or a referral for care from a health care facility. This confidential record is usually held by the facility, and the information in it is released only to the person or with the person's written permission, except in certain situations, such as when release is required by law. It contains the initial assessment, health history, laboratory reports, and notes by nurses, doctors, and consultants, as well as order sheets, medication sheets, admission records, discharge summaries, and other pertinent data. A problem-oriented medical record also contains a master problem list. The patient record is usually a collection of papers held in a folder, but increasingly, hospitals are computerizing the records after every discharge, making the past record available on visual display terminals. Also called chart (informal).

patient's bill of rights • Documents that define a person's rights while receiving health care. Bills of rights for patients are designed to protect such basic rights as human dignity, privacy, confidentiality, informed consent, and refusal of treatment. The American Hospital Association, the National League for Nursing, the American Civil Liberties Union, and other organizations, as well as many health care institutions, have prepared patient's bills of rights. Concepts expressed in these documents may be incorporated into law. Although bills of rights issued by health care institutions and professional organizations don't have the force of law, nurses should regard them as professionally binding.

pediatric nurse practitioner (PNP) • A nurse practitioner who, by advanced study and clinical practice, has gained expert knowledge in the nursing care of infants and children.

peremptory challenge • A right given to attorneys at trial to dismiss a prospective juror for no particular reason; the number of times an attorney can invoke this right is usually limited.

permissive licensure • A form of licensure that regulates the use of professional titles rather than professional actions.

persistent vegetative state • A state of severe mental impairment in which only involuntary bodily functions are sustained.

physician • *1.* A health professional who has earned a degree of Doctor of Medicine (MD) after completion of an approved course of study at an approved medical school and satisfactory completion of National Board Examinations. *2.* A health professional who has earned a degree of Doctor of Osteopathy (DO) by satisfactorily completing a course of education in an approved college of osteopathy.

physician of record • See *attending physician.*

physician's assistant (PA) • A person trained in certain aspects of the practice of medicine to provide assistance to a doctor. A physician's assistant is trained by doctors and practices under the direction and supervision and within the legal license of a doctor. Training programs vary in length from a few months to 2 years. Health care experi-

ence or academic preparation may be a prerequisite to admission to some programs. Most physician's assistants are prepared for the practice of primary care, but some practice subspecialties, including surgical assisting, dialysis, or radiology. National certification is available to qualified graduates of approved training programs. The national organization is the American Association of Physician's Assistants (AAPA). Also called *physician's associate.*

physician's associate • See *physician's assistant.*

plaintiff • A person who files a civil lawsuit initiating a legal action. In criminal actions, the prosecution is the plaintiff, acting in behalf of the people of the jurisdiction.

PNP • See *pediatric nurse practitioner.*

policy • A definite course or method of action selected from among alternatives and in the light of given conditions to guide, and usually determine, present and future decisions. Compare *rule.*

policy defense • Rationale for denying coverage given by professional liability insurance carriers when a client submits a claim. Reasons for denial may include failure to pay a premium on time or failure to renew the policy.

power of attorney • An instrument authorizing another person to act as one's agent or attorney, an "attorney-in-fact." Power of attorney continues to operate only with the continued consent of the person who granted it. If the grantor of the power should become incompetent, the power of attorney is automatically revoked. It is also revoked when the principal person dies. Compare *durable power of attorney.*

practicing medicine without a license • Practicing activities defined under state or provincial law in the medical practice act without medical supervision, direction, or control.

practicing pharmacy without a license • Practicing activities defined under state or provincial law in the pharmacy practice act without pharmacist supervision, direction, or control. These laws give pharmacists the sole legal authority to prepare, compound, preserve, and dispense drugs.

practitioner • A person qualified to practice in a special professional field, such as a nurse practitioner.

preferred provider organization (PPO) • Managed care organization in which an employer or insurance carrier purchases health care services from a select group of health care providers. These providers agree to accept the PPOs reimbursement structure and payment levels.

prescription drug • Any drug restricted from regular commercial purchase and sale. Compare **_controlled substance._**

presumed consent • The legal principle based on the belief that a rational and prudent person would consent in the same situation, if able to. Applies primarily to emergency care of unconscious patients but may be expanded to cadaver organ donors.

privacy • One's private life or personal affairs. The right to privacy refers to the right to be let alone and to be free from unwanted publicity.

privileged communication • A conversation in which the speaker intends the information given to remain private (between himself and the listener).

privilege doctrine • A doctrine that protects the privacy of persons within a fiduciary relationship, such as a husband and wife, a doctor and patient, or a nurse and patient. During legal proceedings, a court cannot force either party to reveal communications

between them unless the party who would benefit from the protection agrees.

probate • The act of proving that a purported will was signed and executed in accordance with the law, and of determining its validity. Combined result of all procedures necessary to establish the validity of a will.

probation period • A period of time during which an individual is observed and evaluated to ascertain fitness for a particular job or duty.

problem-oriented medical record • A record-keeping system in which all members of the health care team combine their information in a special format that goes by the acronym SOAP. Each note combines Subjective data, Objective data, Assessment data, and Plans. Also, the patient's active and inactive problems are documented on a master problem list. See also **_SOAP._**

problem patient • A patient who displays inadequate coping abilities, which lead to inappropriate behaviors that his nurses find irritating and frustrating.

pro-choice • The philosophy that a woman has the right to choose either to continue or to terminate her pregnancy.

professional corporation (PC) • A corporation formed according to the law of a particular state for the purpose of delivering a professional service.

professional liability • A legal concept describing the obligation of a professional person to pay a patient or client for damages caused by the professional's act of omission, commission, or negligence, after a court determines that the professional was negligent. Professional liability better describes the responsibility of all professionals to their clients than does the concept of malpractice, but the idea of professional liability is central to malpractice.

professional liability insurance • A type of liability insurance that protects professional persons against malpractice claims made against them.

professional licensure • A legal method to control the quality of a profession by establishing a minimum level of competence for the professional to be licensed.

professional organization • An organization created to deal with issues of concern to its members, who share a professional status.

professional RN • Defined by the ANA as a nurse who has graduated from a baccalaureate or higher degree program. Professional RNs develop policies, procedures, and protocols, and set standards for practice. Compare *technical RN.*

pro-life • The philosophy that the unborn fetus has the right to develop to term and to be born.

proprietary hospital • A hospital operated as a profit-making organization. Many are owned and operated by doctors primarily for their own patients, but they also accept patients from other doctors. Others are owned by investor groups or large corporations.

protocol • A code providing and prescribing strict adherence to guidelines for and authorization of particular practice activities.

Provincial Territorial Nurses' Association (PTNA) • An association of nurses organized at the provincial or territorial level. The Canadian Nurses' Association is a federation of the 11 PTNAs.

proviso • A condition or stipulation. Its general function is to except something from the basic provision, to qualify or restrain its general scope, or to prevent misinterpretation.

proximate cause • A legal concept of cause and effect, which says a sequence of natural

and continuous events produces an injury that wouldn't have otherwise occurred.

proxy • The recipient of a grant of authority to act or speak for another.

psychiatric nurse practitioner • A nurse practitioner who, by advanced study and clinical practice, has gained expert knowledge in the care and prevention of mental disorders.

public health service • Any organization dedicated to protecting and improving the health of the entire community or public through applying preventive medicine and sanitary and social sciences. Compare *United States Public Health Service.*

punitive damages • Also called *exemplary damages,* punitive damages are compensation in excess of actual damages that are a form of punishment to the wrongdoer and reparation to the injured. These damages are awarded only in rare instances of malicious and willful misconduct. Compare *general damages, special damages.*

qualified privilege • A conditional right or immunity granted to the defendant because of the circumstances of a legal case.

quality of life • A legal and ethical standard that is determined by relative suffering or pain, not by the degree of disability.

quasi-intentional tort • A voluntary act that directly causes injury or distress without intent to injure or cause distress.

RCP • See *Royal College of Physicians.*

RCPSC • See *Royal College of Physicians and Surgeons of Canada.*

RCS • See *Royal College of Surgeons.*

reasonable patient standard • The amount of information that a reasonable patient needs to know about a test or procedure before granting informed consent.

reasonably prudent nurse • The standard a court uses to judge a nurse in a negligence suit. The court considers whether another nurse would have acted similarly to the defendant under similar circumstances.

rebuttable presumption • A presumption that may be overcome or disputed by contrary evidence.

Red Cross • *1.* See *International Red Cross Society.* *2.* See *American Red Cross.*

redefinition • A rewriting of the fundamental provision of a nurse practice act. This changes the basic premise of the entire act without amending or repealing it.

registered nurse (RN) • *1. In the United States:* A professional nurse who has completed a course of study at an approved school of nursing, passed the NCLEX-RN, and met the requirements for licensure set forth by the board of nursing in her state. A registered nurse may use the initials RN following her signature. RNs are licensed to practice by individual states. *2. In Canada:* A professional nurse who has completed a course of study at an approved school of nursing and who has taken and passed an examination administered by the Canadian Nurses' Association Testing Service. See also *nurse, nursing.*

registered nursing assistant • *Canada.* A person trained in basic nursing techniques and direct patient care who practices under the supervision of a registered nurse.

registry • *1.* An office or agency in which lists of nurses and records pertaining to nurses seeking employment are maintained.

2. In epidemiology: a listing service for incidence data pertaining to the occurrence of specific diseases or disorders, as a tumor registry.

remand • To send back. An appellate court may send a case back to the lower court that considered the case, ordering that further action be taken there.

res ipsa loquitur • Latin phrase meaning "the thing speaks for itself." A legal doctrine that applies when the defendant was solely and exclusively in control at the time the plaintiff's injury occurred, so that the injury would not have occurred if the defendant had exercised due care. In addition, the injured party cannot have contributed to his own injury. When a court applies this doctrine to a case, the defendant bears the burden of proving that he was not negligent.

respondeat superior • Latin phrase meaning "let the master answer." A legal doctrine that makes an employer indirectly liable for the consequences of his employee's wrongful conduct while the employee is acting within the scope of his employment.

restraint of trade • Illegal restraints interfering with free competition in commercial transactions, which tend to restrict production, affect prices, or otherwise control the market to the detriment of consumers of goods and services.

resuscitative life-support measures • Actions taken to reverse an immediate, life-threatening situation (for example, cardiopulmonary resuscitation).

review committee • A group of individuals delegated to inspect and report on the quality of health care in a given institution.

right-of-conscience laws • Based on freedom of thought or of religion, such laws allow a health care provider to refuse to care for a patient when an objection to the care or non-care exists.

right-to-access laws • Laws that grant a patient the right to see his medical records.

right-to-die laws • Laws that uphold a patient's right to choose death by refusing extraordinary treatment. Also referred to as **natural death laws** or **living will laws.**

right to notice • **1.** A due process right requiring that the accused receive timely notice of both the pending charges and the hearing date. **2.** An employee's right to receive sufficient notification or warning before termination. This allows the employee time to protest or appeal the termination, and to seek employment elsewhere.

risk management • The identification, analysis, evaluation, and elimination or reduction, to the extent possible, of risks to hospital patients, visitors, or employees. Risk management programs are involved with both loss prevention and loss control, and handle all incidents, claims, and other insurance- and litigation-related tasks.

risk manager • A person who identifies and treats exposures to potential accidental losses. Almost always, a risk manager deals with situations in which the only possible outcome is a loss or no change in the status quo. Examples of the responsibilities of a risk manager include purchasing and managing insurance policies, inviting engineering professionals to examine the structural integrity of a building, or examining hospital policies and procedures to eliminate unnecessary risks.

RN • See **registered nurse.**

Royal College of Physicians (RCP) • A professional organization of physicians in the United Kingdom.

Royal College of Physicians and Surgeons of Canada (RCPSC) • A national Canadian organization that recognizes and confers membership on certain qualified physicians and surgeons.

Royal College of Surgeons (RCS) • A professional organization of surgeons in the United Kingdom.

rule • A guide for conduct that describes the actions that should or should not be taken in specific situations. Compare **policy.**

school nurse practitioner (SNP) • A registered nurse qualified by postgraduate study to act as a nurse practitioner in a school.

scope of practice • In nursing, the professional nursing activities defined under state or provincial law in each state's (or Canadian province's) nurse practice act.

self-determination • An individual's right to decide, without interference from others, how and where to live. Informed consent is based on the ethical principle of self-determination.

service of process • The delivery of a writ, summons, or complaint to a defendant. The original of the document is shown; a copy is served. Service of process gives reasonable notice to allow the person to appear, testify, and be heard in court. See also **summons.**

settlement • An agreement made between parties to a suit before a judgment is rendered by a court.

shared governance • A means of involving staff nurses in all nursing-related decisions through participation in a formal nursing staff organization that establishes standards of practice, quality, education, management, research, and professionalism. The organizational structure consists of a nurse-executive board and various councils and their committees.

signature code • A code of letters or numbers that are entered into a computer to identify the user.

skilled nursing facility (SNF) • An institution or part of an institution that meets criteria for accreditation established by the sections of the Social Security Act that determine the basis for Medicaid and Medicare reimbursement for skilled nursing care, including rehabilitation and various medical and nursing procedures.

slander • Spoken words that may damage another's reputation. Compare *libel.*

slippery slope principle • An ethical principle based on the belief that once an ethical or legal barrier has been lowered, desensitization to the ethical or legal principle occurs.

slow-code order • An illegal verbal or implicit order from a doctor instructing staff to delay resuscitation so that CPR, once begun, is unlikely to succeed.

SNF • See *skilled nursing facility.*

SOAP • An acronym for the format used in problem-oriented record keeping; it represents: *S*ubjective data, *O*bjective data, *A*ssessment data, and *P*lans.

socialized medicine • A system for the delivery of health care in which the expense of care is borne by the government.

source-oriented records • A record-keeping system in which each professional group within the health care team keeps separate information on the patient.

sovereign immunity doctrine • A privilege granted to the elected government and its appointed agents – government employees – giving them immunity from lawsuits.

special damages • Compensation for indirect loss or injury, such as present and future medical expenses, past and future loss of earnings, or decreased earning capacity. Also called *consequential damages.* Compare *general damages, punitive damages.*

specialization • Concentration in a specific branch of nursing, or in a particular clinical area, through focused work experience or formal education, or both.

specialty standard • The standard of care that applies to a given nursing specialty.

staff • *1.* The people who work toward a common goal and are employed or supervised by someone of higher rank, such as the nurses in a hospital. *2.* A designation by which a staff nurse is distinguished from a head nurse or other nurse. *3.* In nursing education: the nonprofessional employees of the institution, such as librarians, technicians, secretaries, and clerks. *4.* In nursing service administration: the units of the organization that provide service to the "line," or administratively defined hierarchy, as the personnel office is "staff" to the director of nursing and the nursing service administration.

staffing pattern • In hospital or nursing administration: the number and kinds of staff assigned to the particular units and departments of a hospital. Staffing patterns vary with the unit, department, and shift.

staff model HMO • A health maintenance organization in which the doctors who serve the HMO are its salaried employees.

standard • *1.* A criterion that serves as a basis for comparison for evaluating similar phenomena or substances, as a standard for the practice of a profession. *2.* A pharmaceutical preparation or a chemical substance of known quantity, ingredients, and strength that is used to determine the constituents or the strength of another preparation. *3.* Of known value, strength, quality, or ingredients.

standard death certificate • A form for a death certificate commonly used throughout the United States. It is the preferred form of the U.S. Census Bureau.

standards of care • Criteria that serve as a basis of comparison when evaluating the quality of nursing practice. In a malpractice lawsuit, a measure by which the defendant's alleged wrongful conduct is compared – acts performed or omitted that an ordinary, reasonably prudent nurse, in the defendant's position, would have done or not done.

standing orders • A written document containing rules, policies, procedures, regulations, and orders for the conduct of patient care in various stipulated clinical situations.

state of emergency • A widespread need for immediate action to counter a threat to the community.

statute • An act of the federal or state legislature that becomes the law governing the conduct within its scope. Statutes are enacted to prescribe conduct, define crimes, create inferior government bodies, appropriate public monies and, in general, promote the public welfare.

statutes of limitations • Laws that set forth the length of time within which a person may file specific types of lawsuits.

statutory law • A law passed by a federal or state legislature. The nurse practice acts of the 50 states and the District of Columbia are examples of statutory law.

statutory rape • Sexual intercourse with a female below the age of consent (age of consent varies from state to state).

steward • A union representative.

subacute care • Designed for patients who don't need acute-care hospitalization but need more hours of nursing care per day than the typical nursing home resident.

subpoena • A writ issued under authority of a court to compel the appearance of a witness at a judicial proceeding; disobedience may be punishable as contempt of court.

subspecialty • A subordinate field of specialization. For example, dialysis nursing might be considered a subspecialty of renal care. Compare *nursing specialty.*

substantive laws • Laws that define and regulate a person's rights.

substitute consent • Permission obtained from a parent or legal guardian of a patient who is a minor or who has been declared incompetent by the court.

substitute judgment • A legal term indicating the court's substitution of its own judgment for that of a person the court considers unable to make an informed decision, such as an incompetent adult.

sudden emergency exception • Defense used by hospitals in liability cases involving understaffing when staffing shortages could not have been anticipated, as opposed to chronic understaffing.

summary judgment • A judgment requested by any party to a civil action to end the action when it is believed that there is no genuine issue or material fact in dispute.

summons • A document issued by a clerk of the court upon the filing of a complaint. A sheriff, marshal, or other appointed person serves the summons, notifying a person that an action has been begun against him. See also *service of process.*

support group • People whom a person confides in and draws on for support, either as individuals or in a group setting. Organized self-help and support groups have gained popularity because they provide people with needed support outside of their existing social network. Support groups may promote changes in behavior (Co-dependents Anonymous or Alcoholics Anonymous, for example), provide support for families (Al-Anon), or focus on a specific illness (Alzheimer's Association) or lifestyle (Parents without Partners). Referral to a support group may be included in a patient's nursing care plan.

surrogate motherhood • A practice in which a woman gives birth after carrying the fertilized ovum of another woman or, more commonly, after being artificially inseminated with sperm from the biological father; in the latter case, the infant is then legally adopted by the wife of the biological father.

technical RN • Defined by the ANA as a nurse who has graduated from an associate degree program. Technical RNs follow policies, procedures, and protocols developed by professional RNs. Compare *professional RN.*

teleology • An ethical theory that determines right or good based on an action's consequences.

temporary practice permit • Permission granted by a state board of nursing to an out-of-state nurse enabling her to legally practice nursing until she can obtain a license from that state.

terminate • In contract law: to fulfill all contractual obligations or to absolve oneself of the obligation to fulfill them.

termination process • The procedure an employer follows to fire an employee.

testamentary • Any document, such as a will, which doesn't take effect until after the death of the person who wrote it.

testamentary will • A will whose provisions take effect after death. Compare *living will.*

testator • One who makes and executes a testament or will.

therapeutic abortion • Induced termination of pregnancy to preserve the health, safety, or life of the woman. Compare *illegal abortion, legal abortion.*

therapeutic privilege • A legal doctrine that permits a doctor to withhold information from the patient if he can prove that disclosing it would adversely affect the patient's health.

third-party reimbursement • Reimbursement for services rendered to a person in which an entity other than the giver or receiver of the service is responsible for the payment. Third-party reimbursement for the cost of a subscriber's health care is commonly paid by insurance plans.

time charting • A method of charting in which the care administered to a patient at a particular time is detailed at regular time intervals – for example, every half hour.

tort • A civil wrong outside of a contractual relationship.

total quality management (TQM) • A system of management that seeks to ensure organizational efficiency, effectiveness, and quality through organizational teamwork and excellence. In a TQM system, employees are given more authority over their work and greater autonomy in decision making; the focus is on results rather than daily activities. Employees are trained to make decisions that improve both the quality of the work and the productivity of workers. Strategic planning is based on a long-term commitment to productivity and quality. First introduced to business organizations in the United States in the 1970s, TQM is being used by some health care organizations today as a model for management.

traditional staffing patterns • Work schedules that follow 8-hour shifts, 7 days a week, including evening and night shifts.

trial de novo • A proceeding in which both issues of law and issues of fact are reconsidered as if the original trial had never taken place. New testimony may be introduced or the matter may be determined a second time on the basis of the evidence already produced.

trial process • A systematic method of legal decision making that begins with the initiation of a complaint and ends with a final judgment.

true emergency • A situation in which a patient faces death or serious bodily injury unless immediate medical or nursing care is rendered.

unfair labor practices • Actions taken by an employer that are prohibited by state and federal labor laws. This term commonly refers to tactics used by an employer to discourage employees from participating in union activities. For example, under the National Labor Relations Act, unfair labor practices include interfering with, restraining, or coercing employees who exercise their right to organize.

Uniform Anatomical Gift Act • A law, in all 50 states, that allows anyone over age 18 to sign a donor card, donating some or all of his organs after death.

unintentional tort • A wrongful (though unintended) act against another person or another person's property.

union shop • A place of employment in which employees must join a union.

United States Public Health Service (USPHS) • An agency of the federal government responsible for the control of the arrival from abroad of any people, goods, or substances that may affect the health of U.S. citizens. The agency sets standards for the domestic handling and processing of food and the manufacture of serums, vaccines, cosmetics, and drugs. It supports and performs research, aids localities in times of disaster and epidemics, and provides medical care for certain groups of Americans.

utilization management • Evaluation of the necessity, appropriateness, and efficiency of medical services, procedures, and facilities. This includes review of admissions, services ordered and provided, length of stay, and discharge practices on a concurrent and retrospective basis.

value conflict • Incompatibilities or inconsistencies in beliefs, ideals, or concepts experienced by an individual who is faced with opposing choices of action. Value conflicts can arise when professional demands violate one's personal beliefs – for example, when a nurse must decide whether to follow a doctor's order to administer an unusually high dose of a narcotic drug.

values • Strongly held personal and professional beliefs about worth and importance. The social principles, goals, or standards held by an individual or society.

verbal order • A spoken order given directly and in person by a doctor to a nurse.

verdict • A formal decision rendered by a jury in a trial.

voluntary bargaining issues • Issues such as noneconomic fringe benefits that an employer or union may or may not address during collective bargaining.

witness • *1.* One who gives evidence in a case before a court and who attests or swears to facts or gives testimony under oath. *2.* To observe the execution of an act, such as the signing of a document, or to sign one's name to authenticate the observation.

workers' compensation • Compensation to an employee for an injury or occupational disease suffered in connection with his employment, paid under a government-supervised insurance system contributed to by employers.

writ of habeas corpus • Literally means "you have the body"; a process whereby an individual detained or imprisoned asks the court to rule on the validity of the detainment or imprisonment. If the person is granted the writ, he must be released immediately.

wrongful death statute • A statute existing in all states that provides that the death of a person can give rise to a cause of legal action brought by the person's beneficiaries in a civil suit against the person whose willful or negligent acts caused the death. Prior to the existence of these statutes, a suit could be brought only if the injured person survived.

wrongful life action • A civil suit usually brought against a doctor or health care facility on the basis of negligence that resulted in the wrongful birth or life of an infant. The parents of the unwanted child seek to obtain payment from the defendant for the medical expenses of pregnancy and delivery, for pain and suffering, and for the education and upbringing of the child. Wrongful life actions have been brought and won in several situations, including unsuccessful tubal ligations and vasectomies. Failure to diagnose pregnancy in time for abortion and incorrect medical advice leading to the birth of a defective child have also led to malpractice suits for a wrongful life.

wrongful treatment • A medical or nursing intervention that violates a patient's right to self-determination or the family's wishes.

Appendices

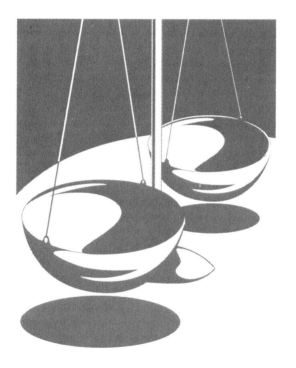

Types of law

Constitutional, administrative, and criminal law deal with the individual's relationship to the federal government and the state. Contract law, tort law, and protective reporting laws deal with relationships between people.

Constitutional law

Constitutional law deals with the individual's rights and responsibilities under the federal and state constitutions, as the U.S. and state courts interpret them. The patient's right to self-determination in refusing treatment, as well as the right to life, liberty, and religious freedom, are all founded in constitutional law.

Administrative law

Administrative law concerns administrative agencies, boards, and commissions legislated by Congress or the state legislatures. For nurses, the most important administrative agency is the state or provincial board of nursing created under the provisions of each state's nurse practice act.

Criminal law

Criminal law concerns state and federal criminal statutes, which define criminal actions such as murder, manslaughter, criminal negligence, theft, and illegal possession of drugs. Nurses risk violating criminal laws when they become involved in such actions as removing life-support systems, carrying out no-code orders, administering high doses of pain-killing medication to terminally ill patients, or failing to nourish or medicate deformed newborns, and when they perform obviously criminal acts such as stealing medications or narcotics. Nurses also may be involved in criminal court proceedings as witnesses, if they care for victims of rape, shootings, and other violent crimes.

Contract law

Contract law involves agreements between two or more parties to do something, for some type of remuneration—a "bargained-for exchange." In essence, a contract is a promissory agreement between two or more persons that creates, modifies, or destroys a legal relationship. In many situations, an oral agreement is also legally binding.

Tort law

Tort law concerns the reparation of civil wrongs or injuries. A tort is a breach of a legal duty that exists by virtue of society's expectations regarding interpersonal conduct (as opposed to a legal duty that exists by virtue of a contractual relationship). More generally, you may define a tort as "any action or omission that harms somebody." Common causes of tort litigation include professional malpractice, negligence, assault and battery, invasion of privacy, false imprisonment, and defamation.

Protective reporting laws

Protective reporting laws are enacted to protect the individual's health and well being. Examples of protective reporting laws include laws requiring nurses to report child abuse or elder abuse and the federal Privacy Act of 1974, which protects a person's legal right to obtain and correct information held by the government. Protective reporting laws may be considered criminal law, depending on how the state has classified them.

The chart at right provides examples of constitutional, administrative, and criminal laws and contract, tort, and protective reporting laws.

Types of law continued

CONSTITUTIONAL LAW	ADMINISTRATIVE LAW	CRIMINAL LAW OR CODE
Federal		
• U.S. Constitution • Civil Rights Act	• Food, Drug, and Cosmetic Act • Social Security Act (Medicare/Medicaid) • National Labor Relations Act	• Comprehensive Drug Abuse Prevention and Control Act (Controlled Substance Acts) • Kidnapping laws
State		
• State constitution	• Nurse practice act • Medical practice act • Pharmacy act • Workers' compensation laws • State labor relations act • Employment security act	• Criminal codes that define murder, manslaughter, criminal negligence, rape, fraud, illegal possession of drugs (and other controlled substances), theft, assault, battery

CONTRACT LAWS	TORT LAWS OR CLAIMS	PROTECTIVE REPORTING LAWS
Federal		
• Laws that govern business or employment relationships with the federal government	• Federal Torts Claims Act (allow tort claims against the federal government)	• Child Abuse Prevention and Treatment Act of 1984 • Privacy Act of 1974 (protects the legal right of a U.S. citizen or permanent resident alien to obtain and correct information about him held by the government or governmental agencies)
State		
• Laws that govern entering into business or employment contracts • Uniform commercial code (a state statute that governs sales, banking documents, and credit transactions)	• State and local government tort claims acts (allow tort claims against the state or local government) • Malpractice statutes (establish professional liability) • Other tort claims, such as negligence, assault, battery, false imprisonment, invasion of privacy, libel	• Age of consent statutes for obtaining medical treatment • Privileged communications statute • Abortion statute • Good Samaritan act • Child abuse and neglect statute • Elderly abuse statute • Domestic violence statute • Involuntary hospitalization statute • Advance directives legislation (laws dealing with living wills and durable powers of attorney for health care)

Understanding the judicial process

The judicial process in the United States is based on court jurisdiction and consists of state and federal court systems. *Court jurisdiction* refers to a court's authority to hear a case and determine judicial action in a given place at a given time. Jurisdiction is determined by several factors, including type of case (for example, a tort action or a criminal case) and location of the transgression or dispute.

Appeal is a legal process whereby a party dissatisfied with the decision of a lower court can seek a more favorable decision from a higher court. Either the

Probate Courts
Hear lawsuits involving wills and inheritances

Local Courts
Specific courts hear lawsuits according to the types of charges, such as small claims, traffic, and housing.

Criminal Courts
Hear criminal lawsuits

Lower Trial Courts
Hear civil and criminal lawsuits, and may hear appeals from probate, criminal, and family or juvenile courts

Intermediate Court of Appeals
Hears appeals from lower courts (23 states have an intermediate court of appeals)

Family/ Juvenile Courts
Hear lawsuits involving delinquent or neglected children

plaintiff or the defendant can appeal an unfavorable decision from a lower court to a higher court.

Courts in the federal and state systems

The diagram below depicts selected courts within the federal and state judicial systems. The arrows indicate pathways for appeal. Note that this diagram does not include the complete federal court structure and that not all states follow the model depicted here.

State Supreme Court
Hears appeals from lower state courts. Makes final decisions except when lawsuits involve constitutional rights.

Supreme Court of the United States
Consists of a chief justice and eight associate justices appointed by the President with advice and consent of the U.S. Senate. Hears lawsuits between states, appeals from the U.S. Court of Appeals, and appeals from state supreme courts if cases involve federal law or constitutional rights.

U.S. Court of Customs and Patent Appeals
Hears appeals from the U.S. Customs Court

U.S. Court of Appeals
Hears appeals from U.S. district courts and the U.S. Tax Court

U.S. Court of Claims
Hears lawsuits against the federal government that involve a constitutional right, federal laws or regulations, or government contracts

U.S. Customs Court
Hears lawsuits involving the U.S. Patent and Trademark Office and other federal agencies

U.S. Tax Court
Hears lawsuits involving tax disputes

U.S. District Courts
Hear federal, criminal, and civil lawsuits

How to interpret legal citations

You may obtain information on a specific court case or law (statute or regulation) from your county courthouse law library or local law school library. If you're looking for an overview or summary of a court case or law, look up the citation in a standard legal reference, such as a legal encyclopedia *(Corpus Juris Secundum)* or a legal text *(Restatements of Law)*.

If you have a full citation, you can locate the complete text of a court case. A full citation includes the name of the court case and a series of identifying numbers and letters. If you're missing some or all of the identifying information, you can look up the case name in the index of a legal reference.

In the court case citation index of this handbook, most of the court cases on the state level will have two complete series of identifying numbers. The first series is the *official citation,* indicating where the case can be found in that state's set of court case decisions. The second series is the *unofficial citation,* indicating where the case can be found in a commercially published set of court case decisions

grouped by region. Keep in mind that an "unofficial" legal reference does not have any less authority than an "official" legal reference.

Each citation includes an abbreviation for the legal reference that contains the law or case. For example, "U.S.L.W." stands for *United States Law Week.* To find out what the abbreviations used in the *Nurse's Handbook of Law and Ethics* stand for, see the list of legal reference abbreviations at right. For more information on legal citations, see *A Uniform System of Citation* (The Harvard Law Review Association, 15th ed., 1991).

The number that precedes the abbreviation indicates either a volume number or title classification within the legal reference. A title classification is a body of laws or cases on a particular subject, such as malpractice. A title can be one book or many books, depending on the amount of cases that bear on the titles.

Two sets of numbers follow the abbreviation. The first set indicates the page where you'll find the case. The second set, in parentheses, indicates the year of the decision.

Court case

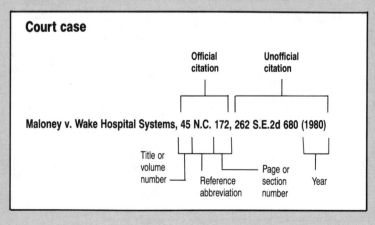

How to interpret legal citations continued

TYPE OF LAW/CASE	LEGAL REFERENCE	ABBREVIATION
Federal court decisions	*United States Law Week* (unofficial reporter containing recently issued Supreme Court decisions)	U.S.L.W.
	United States Reports (official reporter containing Supreme Court decisions)	U.S.
	Supreme Court Reporter (unofficial reporter containing Supreme Court decisions)	S. Ct.
	Lawyers Edition, United States Supreme Court (unofficial reporter containing Supreme Court decisions)	L. Ed.
	Federal Reporter (contains court of appeals decisions)	F., F.2d
	Federal Supplement (contains Federal District Court of Appeals decisions)	F. Supp.
State court decisions	About two thirds of the states publish state court decisions in official state sets. The *Uniform System of Citation* lists all state reporters and instructs how to cite them.	Standard state abbreviations
	All states are included in the commercially published National Reporter System, which groups state court decisions by region:	
	North Eastern Reporter	N.E., N.E.2d
	Atlantic Reporter	A., A.2d
	South Eastern Reporter	S.E., S.E.2d
	Southern Reporter	So., So. 2d
	North Western Reporter	N.W., N.W.2d
	South Western Reporter	S.W., S.W.2d
	Pacific Reporter	P., P.2d
Miscellaneous abbreviations	New York Supreme Court, appellate division	A.D.
	New York Miscellaneous Reports	Misc. 2d
	West's New York Supplement	N.Y.S.2d
	Dominion Law Reports (Canada)	D.L.R.
	Western Weekly Reports (Canada)	W.W.R.
	Ontario Reports	O.R.
	Ontario Law Reports	O.L.R.
	Labour Arbitration Cases (Canada)	L.A.C.
	Canadian Cases on the Law of Torts	CCLT
	Reports of Family Law (Canada)	RFL
	National Labor Relations Board	N.L.R.B.
		(continued)

How to interpret legal citations continued

TYPE OF LAW/CASE	LEGAL REFERENCE	ABBREVIATION
Federal statutes	*United States Law Week* (contains chronologic list of recently enacted statutes)	U.S.L.W.
	United States Statutes at Large (contains chronologic lists of all statutes enacted during a single legislative session)	STAT. or STAT. AT L.
	United States Code (contains all statutes arranged by title)	U.S.C.
State statutes	All states publish state statutes in official state sets	Standard state abbreviations
Federal regulations	*Code of Federal Regulations* (contains federal regulations arranged by title)	C.F.R.
	The Federal Register (contains updates to the C.F.R.)	F.R.
State regulations	All states publish state regulations in official state sets	Standard state abbreviations

Indexes

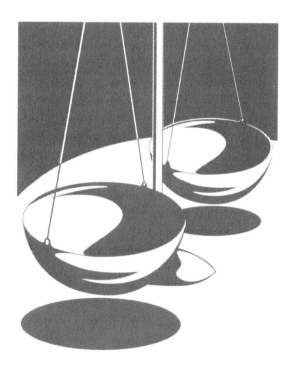

Court Case Citation Index

Italicized numbers refer to book pages.

Collins v. Davis, 254 N.Y.S. 2d 666, 44 Misc. 2d 622 (1964), *pp. 83, 145*

Collins v. Westlake Community Hospital, 57 Ill. 2d 388, 312 N.E. 2d 614 (1974), *p. 238*

Colorado State Board of Nurse Examiners v. Hohu, 129 Colo. 195, 268 P. 2d 401 (1954), *p. 37*

Commissioner of Correction v. Myers, 379 Mass. 255, 399 N.E. 2d 452 (1979), *p. 154*

Commonwealth v. Gordon, 431 Pa. 512, 246 A. 2d 325 (1968), *p. 151*

Commonwealth v. Porn, 196 Mass. 326, 82 N.E. 31 (1907), *p. 39*

Commonwealth v. Storella, 6 Mass. App. 310, 375 N.E. 2d 348 (1978), *p. 151*

Cooper v. National Motor Bearing Co., 136 Cal. App. 2d 229, 288 P. 2d 581 (1955), *pp. 40, 51*

Crowe v. Provost, 52 Tenn. App. 397, 374 S.W. 2d 645 (1963), *p. 206*

Cruzan v. Director, Mo. Dept. of Health, 110 S. Ct. 2841, 111 L. Ed. 2d 224 (1990), *pp. 62, 76, 155*

D. v. D., 108 N.J. Super. 149, 260 A. 2d 255 (1969), *p. 89*

Darling v. Charleston Community Memorial Hospital, 33 Ill. 2d 326, 211 N.E. 2d 253 (1965), *pp. 107, 121*

Dembie, 21 RFL 46 (1963), *p. 88*

Derrick v. Portland Eye, Ear, Nose and Throat Hospital, 105 Ore. 90, 209 P. 344 (1922), *p. 123*

Dessauer v. Memorial General Hospital, 96 N.M. 92, 628 P. 2d 337 (N.M. Ct. App. 1981), *p. 124*

Doe v. Roe, 400 N.Y.S. 2d 668, 93 Misc. 2d 201 (Sup. Ct. 1977), *p. 90*

In re Doe Children, 402 N.Y.S. 2d 958, 93 Misc. 2d 479 (1978), *p. 89*

Dowey v. Rothwell, [1974] 5 W.W.R. 311 (Alberta), *p. 51*

Eastern Maine Medical Center v. NLRB, 658 F. 2d 1 (1st. Cir. 1981), *p. 269*

Edith Anderson Nursing Homes, Inc. v. Bettie Walker, 232 Md. 442, 194 A. 2d 85 (1963), *p. 46*

Eisenstadt v. Baird, 405 U.S. 438, 92 S. Ct. 1029 (1972), *p. 85*

Emory University v. Shadburn, 47 Ga. App. 643, 171 S.E. 192 (Ct. App. 1933), *p. 46*

Estelle v. Gamble, 429 U.S. 97, 97 S. Ct. 285 (1976), *p. 154*

Feeney v. Young, 181 N.Y.S. 481, 191 A.D. 501 (1920), *p. 89*

Q

In re Quinlan, 137 N.J. Super. 227, 348 A. 2d 801 (Ch. Div. 1975); modified, 70 N.J. 10, 355 A. 2d 647 (1976), *pp. 62, 76*

R

Ramos v. Lamm, 639 F. 2d 559 (10th Cir. 1980), *p. 154*

Richardson v. Brunelle, 119 N.H. 104, 398 A. 2d 838 (1979), *pp. 9, 33*

Rochin v. California, 342 U.S. 165, 72 S. Ct. 205 (1952), *p. 151*

Roe v. Wade, 410 U.S. 113, 93 S. Ct. 705 (1973), *p. 85, 87*

Rogers v. Kasdan, 612 S.W. 2d 133 (Ky. 1981), *p. 246*

Rohde v. Lawrence General Hospital, 34 Mass. App. Ct. 584, 614 N.E. 2d 686 (1993), *p. 147*

Rust v. Sullivan, 59 U.S.L.W. 4451 (1991), *p. 85*

S

Salgo v. Leland Stanford Jr. Univ. Board of Trustees, 154 Cal. App. 2d 560, 317 P. 2d 170 (1957), *p. 72*

In re Sampson, 328 N.Y.S. 2d 686, 278 N.E. 2d 918 (1972), *p. 83*

Sanchez v. Bay General Hospital, 116 Cal. App. 3d 776, 172 Cal. Rptr. 342 (1981), *pp. 108, 207*

Re SAS, 1 LMQ 139 (1977), *p. 88*

Schloendorff v. Society of New York Hospitals, 211 N.Y. 125, 105 N.E. 92 (1914), *p. 72*

Schmerber v. California, 384 U.S. 757, 86 S. Ct. 1826 (1966), *p. 150*

Schneckloth v. Bustamonte, 412 U.S. 218, 93 S. Ct. 2041 (1973), *p. 150*

Secretary of Public Welfare v. Institutionalized Juveniles, 442 U.S. 640, 99 S. Ct. 2523 (1979), *p. 136*

Sengstack v. Sengstack, 4 N.Y. 2d 502, 176 N.Y.S. 2d 337; 151 N.E. 2d 887 (1958), *p. 148*

Sermchief v. Gonzales, 660 S.W. 2d 683 (Mo. 1983), *pp. 42, 240*

Sheffield v. State Education Department, 174 A.O. 2d 865, 571 N.Y.S. 2d 350 (1991), *p. 15*

Simonsen v. Swenson, 104 Neb. 224, 177 N.W. 831 (1920), *p. 89*

Snelson v. Culton, 141 Me. 242, 42 A. 2d 505 (1949), *p. 33*

Stack v. Wapner, 368 A. 2d 292 244 (Pa. Super. Ct. 278, 1976), *p. 245*

Stahlin v. Hilton Hotels Corp., 484 F. 2d 580 (7th Cir. 1973), *pp. 40, 51*

T

U

V

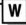

W

General Index

E

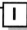

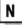

O

PQ

Past practice violation, 272
Patient advocate
  ethics and, 284, 287
  job protection for, 50
  nurse's duty as, 349-350
  right to die and, 293
Patient safety
  decreasing liability for, 122
  determining liability for, 121-122
  disease transmission and, 120
  equipment and, 120
  falls and, 119
  hospital's responsibility for, 120-121
  legal responsibility for, 118-122
  restraints and, 119
  standards of care and, 118-119
  suicide prevention and, 119-120
Patient Self-Determination Act, 62, 80
Patient rights, 60-99
  ACLU bill of, 65-66
  age of majority and, 76
  AHA's statement on, 61, 62, 63-64
  confidentiality and, 89-90
  congressional action on, 62, 64, 66
  deceased patient and, 96-99
  discharge against medical advice and, 92-96
  documents upholding, 61-70
  evolution of, 61-62, 64, 66
  in geriatric facilities, 49-50
  guidelines for upholding, 69-70
  hospice bill of, 67-68
  informed consent and, 71-76
  interpreting, 68-69
  job protection for advocate of, 50
  legal status of, 66, 68
  living will and, 79
  medical record disclosure and, 90-92
  NLN's statement on, 61, 62, 69, 70
  nurse's role in, 60
  Patient Self-Determination Act and, 62, 80
  Pennsylvania Insurance Department and, 61, 62, 64
  privacy and, 84-85, 87-89
  refusal of treatment and, 76-78, 80, 83-84
  right to die and, 78, 80
Patient teaching, 127-129
  colleague cooperation in, 128-129
  LPN's role in, 128
  patient's rejection of, 128
  patient's right to, 127-128
  standards of, 127

Pennsylvania Insurance Department, patient's
    bill of rights and, 61, 64
Perinatal ethics, 304-307
  "Baby Doe" regulations and, 306
  courts and, 306
  critically ill neonate and, 307
  ethics committee and, 306
  health care team as decision makers in, 305
  nurse's role in, 306
  parents as decision makers in, 305
  quality-of-life decision and, 305
  sanctity of life vs. quality of life and, 305
PIE charting, 242
Policy defense, insurance companies and, 223,
    226, 228
Policy violations, employer, 272
Postanesthesia care unit. *See* Special care
    units.
Power of attorney, 80. *See also* Durable power of
    attorney.
PPOs. *See* Preferred provider organizations.
Practice guidelines, 246
Practice parameters, 246
Preferred provider organizations, 344
Prisoners, detention of, 96
Privacy, right to, 84-90
  abortion and, 85, 87
  ANA Code of Ethics and, 329
  child abuse and, 89
  criminal cases and, 89-90
  ethical conflicts about, 330-331
  government requests and, 90
  lawful disclosure and, 88-89
  mandatory disclosure and, 89-90
  privilege doctrine and, 87-88
  protecting, 88
  vs. protection of public, 89
  vs. public's right to know, 90
  state law and, 87
  U.S. Constitution and, 85
Private-duty nurse, 45-47
  advantages of, 45
  financial burdens of, 46
  home care and, 45-46
  hospital care and, 46
  as independent contractor, 45-46
  legal risks of, 45-46
  tasks performed by, 45
  working with, 46-47
Privileged communication, 228
Privilege doctrine, 87-88
Problem-oriented documentation system, 241
Professional liability insurance. *See* Liability in-
    surance.

V

WXYZ